VIDEOFLUOROSCOPY

VIDEOFLUOROSCOPY: A MULTIDISCIPLINARY TEAM APPROACH

Roger D. Newman, MSc, BSc (Hons), CertMRSCLT
Highly Specialist Speech and Language Therapist,
Lancashire Teaching Hospitals NHS Trust, Preston, UK
Senior Lecturer, University of Manchester, UK
Honorary Lecturer, University of Salford, UK

Julie M. Nightingale, PhD, MSc, DCR(R)
Director of Radiography,
University of Salford,
Greater Manchester, UK

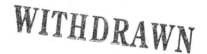

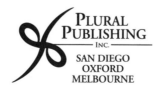

PLURAL
PUBLISHING
INC.
SAN DIEGO
OXFORD
MELBOURNE

MW

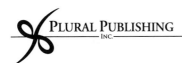

PLURAL PUBLISHING
INC.

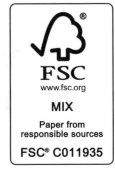
FSC
www.fsc.org
MIX
Paper from
responsible sources
FSC® C011935

5521 Ruffin Road
San Diego, CA 92123

e-mail: info@pluralpublishing.com
Web site: http://www.pluralpublishing.com

49 Bath Street
Abingdon, Oxfordshire OX14 1EA
United Kingdom

Library of Congress Cataloging-in-Publication Data

Videofluoroscopy : a multidisciplinary team approach / [edited by] Roger Newman, Julie
Nightingale.
    p. ; cm.
Includes bibliographical references and index.
ISBN-13: 978-1-59756-439-7 (alk. paper)
ISBN-10: 1-59756-439-7 (alk. paper)
I. Newman, Roger (Roger D.) II. Nightingale, Julie.
[DNLM: 1. Deglutition Disorders. 2. Fluoroscopy. 3. Video Recording. WI 250]

616.3'23 — dc23
                    2012012010

4/22/13

CONTENTS

Foreword   *vii*
Contributors   *ix*

PART I: OVERVIEW   **1**

1 Introduction to the Videofluoroscopic Swallowing Study   3
   Roger D. Newman

2 Alternative Investigations   19
   Justin Roe

3 Improving Patient Experience and Minimizing Risk   35
   Julie M. Nightingale, Tracy Lazenby-Paterson, and Hannah Crawford

4 Anatomy and Physiology of Swallowing   53
   Claire Butler and Paula Leslie

5 The Neurophysiology of Swallowing   81
   Maggie-Lee Huckabee and Sebastian H. Doeltgen

6 Biomechanical Analysis   107
   James L. Coyle

7 The Normal Aging Swallow   123
   Margaret Coffey

8 Effective Use of Imaging Technology   137
   Elizabeth Judson and Julie M. Nightingale

PART II: CLINICAL INDICATIONS   **157**

9 Stroke   159
   Stephanie K. Daniels and Joseph Murray

10 Neuromuscular Conditions   177
   Julie Regan and Margaret Walshe

11 Pediatric Videofluoroscopy   197
   Joanne Marks and Rebecca Howarth

12 Videofluoroscopy in Learning Disabilities   213
   Tracy Lazenby-Paterson and Hannah Crawford

13 Dementia   227
   Pamela A. Smith and Paula Leslie

14 Head and Neck Cancers   239
   Jo Patterson and Margaret Coffey

15 Structural Causes of High Dysphagia   263
   Roger D. Newman

16 Standardized Clinical Reporting: Writing for the Reader   281
   Martin B. Brodsky

Glossary   *297*
Index   *307*

FOREWORD

Being able to image the swallow is seen by most as a boon to dysphagia management. In the right hands, videofluoroscopy provides a potentially useful view of the interaction of barium and bulbar structures. In persons with dysphagia, that view supports hypotheses about why bolus flow is misdirected, incomplete, or too fast or slow. In turn, these hypotheses provide a portion of the support necessary for effective, efficient, humane management decisions. Like the then newly developed procedure of visual field testing that Freud worried would supplant all other forms of patient evaluation, the videofluoroscopic swallowing examination's popularity has attracted critical attention. Critics remind users that what they see are shadows; and that what they conclude from what they see is biased by the technical competence of the procedure, the examiner's training and expectations, and the swallower's compliance. And as Coyle reminds readers in Chapter 6 of this edited volume, clinicians treat the patient and not the barium. Barium is a message, sometimes not even the most important one, and it is never the messenger.

Like Coyle, this volume's other contributors recognize this reality. What they intended and what they achieve is a thoughtful and data-based guide to making barium's message maximally intelligible, coherent, and useful. As Newman says in Chapter 1, the book's purpose is to explore "the complexities of the videofluoroscopic swallowing study and offer guidance on best practice." They do so. Chapter 3 by Nightingale, Lazenby-Paterson, and Crawford is devoted to the specifics of reducing patients' risks and maximizing their comfort. Chapter 8 by Judson and Nightingale is a primer on radiation science and safety. The authors' theme is that patient, clinician, and

carer safety is paramount and that a first step is to "ascertain that the potential benefits of the procedure outweigh the potential harm." Brodsky, in Chapter 16, provides the reader with a standard reporting protocol preceded by a thoughtful argument about why standardization can be good patient care. Coffey's Chapter 7 on swallowing in normal aging is motivated by an awareness that without such information, "there is a risk of over-managing swallowing in the elderly with subsequent threats to quality of life." Seven of the book's chapters describe the special challenges and opportunities provided by special populations — stroke, written by Daniels and Murray; neuromuscular conditions such as ALS, written by Regan and Walshe; pediatrics, written by Marks and Howarth; the learning disabled, defined as those with intelligent quotients of 70 or less, written by Lazenby-Paterson and Crawford; dementia, written by Smith and Leslie; head and neck cancers, written by Patterson and Coffey; and other structural causes of dysphagia, written by Newman. These seven chapters are unfailingly thorough and emphasize the potential challenges, risks, rewards, and ethical implications of videofluoroscopy with these populations.

Edited books can be published Towers of Babel, but not this one. Several themes echo throughout. One of the most compelling for modern practitioners is that videofluoroscopy provides only a portion of what is necessary for management and is sometimes not as useful as another tool. Chapter 2 — early in the book, lest one overlook it — is a discussion of other instrumented investigations, written by Roe. All chapters highlight the importance of screening, taking a good history, and completing a careful clinical examination. And for readers responsible for establishing or improving the safety, efficiency, and pleasure of eating and drinking, all authors endorse the importance of normal and abnormal physiology to treatment planning. The bases for doing so are provided by three substantive chapters. Swallowing anatomy and physiology is described in Chapter 4 by Butler and Leslie. The neurophysiology of normal and abnormal swallowing is described by Huckabee and Doeltgen in Chapter 5. These authors also remind readers that "instrumental imaging in the absence of sound clinical understanding is incomplete and can be misleading." Coyle applies anatomy and physiology to treatment planning and execution in a chapter called "Biomechanical Analysis." Do not be threatened by the title; your patients will suffer if you are.

The authors promise an evidence-based book and they deliver. References are bountiful throughout. They know that a book about imaging needs images and they deliver. Perhaps best of all, they have not written a polemic. They mention videofluoroscopy as a gold standard, but they put those two words in quotation marks. I had the feeling as I read the book that they do not care what you believe as you begin reading. They may not even care what you believe when you finish, although I am less sure of that. On the other hand, the hard writing that makes this book easy reading makes me think they would be dispirited if their themes did not at least occasionally cause each reader to lay the book aside for a few minutes of contemplation about the rigors and rewards of clinical practice in dysphagia.

John C. Rosenbek, PhD
Professor
University of Florida

CONTRIBUTORS

Martin B. Brodsky, PhD, CCC-SLP
Assistant Professor
Department of Physical Medicine and
    Rehabilitation
Johns Hopkins University
Baltimore, Maryland
Chapter 16

**Claire Butler, BMedSci, MSc,
CertMRCSLT**
Clinical Lead Speech and Language
    Therapist
Adult Dysphagia
RCSLT Adviser in Adult Dysphagia
Chapter 4

Margaret Coffey, MA, MSc, CertMRCSLT
Research Speech and Language Therapist
Charing Cross Hospital
Imperial College Healthcare Trust
NIHR Clinical Doctoral Fellow
Imperial College
London, United Kingdom
Chapters 7 and 14

James L. Coyle, PhD, CCC-SLP, BRS-S
Assistant Professor
Communication Sciences and Disorders
University of Pittsburgh
Pittsburgh, Pennsylvania
Board Recognized Specialist, Swallowing and
    Swallowing Disorders
Chapter 6

Hannah Crawford, MSc, CertMRCSLT
Consultant Speech and Language Therapist
Tees, Esk and Wear Valleys NHS Foundation
    TMST
RCSLT Professional Advisor
Middlesbrough, United Kingdom
Chapters 3 and 12

Stephanie K. Daniels, PhD
Visiting Associate Professor
Department of Communication Sciences
    and Disorders
University of Houston
Research Speech Pathologist
Michael E. DeBakey VA Medical Center
Assistant Professor
Department of Physical Medicine and
    Rehabilitation
Baylor College of Medicine
Houston, Texas
Chapter 9

Sebastian H. Doeltgen, PhD
NHMRC Postdoctoral Research Fellow
Neuromotor Plasticity and Development
    Research Group
Robinson Institute
School of Paediatrics and Reproductive
    Health
University of Adelaide
Adelaide, Australia
Chapter 5

Rebecca Howarth, BSc, CertMRCSLT
Pathology and Therapeutics
Senior Specialist Speech and Language
    Therapist
Royal Manchester Children's Hospital
Manchester, United Kingdom
Chapter 11

Maggie-Lee Huckabee, PhD
Senior Lecturer,
Senior Researcher,
Swallowing Rehabilitation Research Laboratory
The New Zealand Brain Research Institute
Department of Communication Disorders
The University of Canterbury
Christchurch, New Zealand
Chapter 5

Elizabeth Judson, MSc, DCR(R)
Imaging Service Manager
Sunderland City Hospitals Foundation Trust
Sunderland
Tyne and Wear, United Kingdom
Chapter 8

Tracy Lazenby-Paterson, BA, BSc, MSc, CertMRCSLT
Specialist Speech and Language Therapist
Learning Disabilities Service
NHS Lothian
Edinburgh, United Kingdom
Chapters 3 and 12

Paula Leslie, PhD, FRCSLT, CCC-SLP
Associate Professor
Communication Sciences and Disorders
University of Pittsburgh
Pittsburgh, Pennsylvania
Chapters 4 and 13

Joanne Marks, BSc, CertMRCSLT
Speech Pathology and Therapy
Lead Speech and Language Therapist in
    Paediatric Dysphagia
Royal Manchester Children's Hospital
Manchester, United Kingdom
Chapter 11

Joseph Murray, PhD, CCC-SLP
Chief, Audiology/Speech Pathology Service
VA Ann Arbor Healthcare System
Ann Arbor, Michigan
Chapter 9

Roger D. Newman, MSc, BSc (Hons), CertMRCSLT
Highly Specialist Speech & Language
    Therapist
Lancashire Teaching Hospitals NHS Trust,
Preston, United Kingdom
Senior Lecturer, University of Manchester,
    United Kingdom
Honorary Lecturer, University of Salford,
    United Kingdom
Chapters 1 and 15

Julie M. Nightingale, PhD, MSc, DCR(R)
Director of Radiography,
University of Salford,
Greater Manchester
United Kingdom
Chapters 3 and 8

Jo Patterson, PhD, MSc, BSc (Hons) CertMRCSLT
Macmillan Speech & Language Therapist
Research Associate
Sunderland Royal Hospital
Newcastle University
Newcastle upon Tyne, United Kingdom
Chapter 14

Julie Regan, MSc, BSc, CertMRCSLT
Clinical Specialist Speech and Language
    Therapist (Neurology)
PhD Student, School of Clinical Medicine
Trinity College
Research Fellow, Health Research Board
Dublin, Ireland
Chapter 10

Justin Roe, MSc, CertMRCSLT
Research Speech and Language
    Therapist—Head and Neck Oncology
Head and Neck Unit
The Royal Marsden NHS Foundation Trust
London, United Kingdom
Chapter 2

Pamela A. Smith, PhD, CCC-SLP
Associate Professor of Speech Pathology
Department of Audiology and Speech
    Pathology
Bloomsburg, Pennsylvania
Chapter 13

Margaret Walshe, PhD, MSc, MRCSLT
Assistant Professor
Department of Clinical Speech and
    Language Studies
Trinity College
Dublin, Ireland
Chapter 10

Part

I

OVERVIEW

Chapter

1

INTRODUCTION TO THE VIDEOFLUOROSCOPIC SWALLOWING STUDY

Roger D. Newman

INTRODUCTION

The last decade has seen an enormous upheaval within all aspects of health care, and the videofluoroscopy service is no exception. There is an ever-increasing need for the objective examination of swallowing to create a baseline for the patient as part of their diagnosis and subsequent treatment. However, a fundamental lack of standardization exists within videofluoroscopy service provision, not only between organizations within any particular country, but also a worldwide variability of practice is evident. There are many reasons for this variability, the most profound being the very wide range of referrals for this examination: from infants to the elderly and infirm, and for clinical investigations for a multitude of different conditions resulting in swallowing difficulty. Variability of practice in such circumstances is inevitable; however, the diversity creates problems for the practitioner in identifying what is best practice. This book

explores the complexities of the videofluoroscopy swallowing study (VFSS) in an attempt to offer evidence-informed guidance to the practitioner on what is "best" practice. The editors have adopted a multidisciplinary team approach to the compilation of this text, collaborating with a renowned team of experts from across the globe to give an international perspective.

This chapter introduces the reader to the relevant context for the videofluoroscopic swallowing study, and signposts the reader to subsequent chapters for more detailed information.

Fluoroscopy is a general term used within radiology to encompass any procedure which uses real-time acquisition and display of x-ray images using an image intensification system. The "real-time" examination is displayed on a TV monitor, although this is often for the purposes of accurate positioning and centering, with static 2D image capture for archiving; see Chapter 8, Effective Use of Imaging Technology. A barium enema procedure to demonstrate the large intestine is one example of the use of conventional fluoroscopy. In contrast, videofluoroscopy refers to imaging in real time, where the dynamic images demonstrate features of physiology and function that contribute to the diagnosis. Images can be captured as "stills" or may be recorded in real time on video, DVD, or more increasingly a picture archiving and communication system (PACS). This is a recent addition to imaging technology enabling storage of, and access to, any obtained images from the majority of computer stations throughout, and beyond, the hospital.

Videofluoroscopy has been used in demonstrating subtle joint movements, and in "capturing" physiological processes such as *micturating cystography* or *defecating proctography*. However, its most widespread application has been in the demonstration of the swallowing process. The videofluoroscopic swallowing study (VFSS), sometimes known as a modified barium swallow (MBS), utilizes a contrast agent (usually a barium sulfate preparation) which is swallowed by the patient in order to examine the oropharyngeal and upper esophageal swallowing function and to identify any associated risks of aspiration (Logemann, 1983). VFSS remains the most common clinical method for instrumental assessment and investigation of swallowing (dys)function (Frowen, Cotton, & Perry, 2008), and is considered the "gold standard" of swallowing examinations by many researchers (Daniels, McAdam, Brailey, & Foundas, 1997; Robbins, Coyle, Rosenbek, Roecker, & Woods, 1999). This is further qualified by other researchers who show that no other examination comes close to it in terms of sensitivity of specificity (Martino, Pron, & Diamont, 2000 and Singh, Berry, Brockbank, Frost, Tyler, & Owens, 2009).

The Royal College of Speech and Language Therapists (RCSLT) (2006) provide the general definition of VFSS as being a dynamic fluoroscopic imaging procedure and modification of the standard barium swallow examination whereby the physiology of swallowing is graphically revealed, usually by means of providing a range of food and fluid consistencies. There is a huge variation in the etiology and presentation of swallowing disorders, many of which are described in later chapters. These disorders can occur at any age and arise from many causes, but their effect on the patient covers a spectrum of psychosocial issues that may be related solely to the oropharyngeal swallowing disorder (or *dysphagia*) and not the disorder from which it arises. Dysphagia is defined by Logemann (1998) as a disorder of swallowing food or fluid from the mouth to the stomach. Ultimately, dysphagia can be a socially debilitating or even life-threatening disorder, and the patient may be experiencing emotions such as anxiety, isolation, frustration, and depression. As a result, all professionals involved in VFSS must be aware of the potential physical and social consequences of dysphagia when commencing the VFSS.

Functional Versus Structural Interpretation

VFSS examines the *function* of the oropharyngeal swallowing mechanism, whereas a standard barium swallow studies the pharyngoesophageal *structures*, highlighting any structural abnormality. Such structural abnormalities usually fall into two categories: congenital and acquired, both of which significantly vary in prevalence. However, subtle overlaps exist between the two radiological examinations, and although both may investigate motility, standard barium swallows primarily examine both the proximal and distal esophagus, and VFSS examines any functional deficit of motility at the oral, pharyngeal, and (to a certain extent) the proximal esophageal stages. The density of x-ray contrast used typically differs depending on whether structural or functional anomalies are being investigated: barium swallows require a high density contrast with good coating of the mucosa, whereas low density contrast with minimal coating properties would be used in VFSS. However, examination of a structural anomaly that subsequently leads to a functional deficit of oropharyngeal deglutition may indeed be the aim of the VFSS. This may be the case in congenital disorders such as cleft lip/palate, or acquired disorders in adolescence and adulthood including cervical osteophytes. In instances like this, the density and type of contrast may be altered accordingly. This is discussed in Chapter 11, Pediatric Videofluoroscopy, and Chapter 15, Structural Causes of High Dysphagia.

VFSS also incorporates modifications to the volumes and consistencies of the contrast agents used to replicate the consistencies of everyday food and fluid (Newman, 2010). This then demonstrates any dysfunction of oropharyngeal deglutition, enabling appropriate treatment and therapy aims to be devised. Another major benefit of VFSS is that it provides an objective baseline to which future examinations can be compared as a measure of improvement (or deterioration) and thus enable management and treatment strategies to be formulated accordingly.

Indications for Videofluoroscopic Examination

Patient Groups

Various client groups who present with dysphagia may benefit from VFSS if an objective examination of the oropharyngeal swallowing function is required:

Stroke: A large proportion of patients who have suffered a stroke will present with some form of oropharyngeal dysphagia. See Chapter 9, Stroke.

Neurological Disorders/Diseases: Patients of any age who have a congenital or acquired neuromuscular disorder may also present with dysphagia requiring examination via VFSS. For more information about the neurology of swallowing and their impairments in children and adults, see Chapter 5, The Neurophysiology of Swallowing; Chapter 10, Neuromuscular Conditions; and Chapter 11, Pediatric Videofluoroscopy.

Pediatrics: The normal swallowing function in babies and young children is quite different to that of older children and adults, and the disorders with which babies and children present reflects this. In addition, there may be congenital abnormalities such as cerebral palsy that can significantly impede the child's feeding and swallowing. The VFSS procedure must be undertaken extremely cautiously given the child's reduced understanding of the need to examine the swallowing function in detail. See Chapter 11, Pediatric Videofluoroscopy.

Learning Disabilities: Learning disabilities often do not present as an isolated cognitive deficit, but a group of clinical presentations including dysphagia may form the complete disorder or syndrome. This again may warrant investigation via VFSS. See Chapter 12, Videofluoroscopy in Learning Disabilities.

Dementia: Patients diagnosed with any form of dementia will usually present with some level of feeding and/or swallowing disorder. Examination using VFSS may prove extremely difficult as a result of the cognitive deficit forming the main presentation of dementia and may not always be indicated, but in some cases it may be warranted to highlight any modification or risk. For more information on this, and to differentiate it from the normal elderly swallow, see Chapter 7, The Normal Aging Swallow; and Chapter 13, Dementia.

Head and Neck Cancers: Secondary to malignancies of the head and neck, the swallowing mechanism often becomes highly dysfunctional due to damage to the intricate innervation of oropharyngeal deglutition, structural damage caused by the removal of any such malignancy, or subsequent radiotherapy tissue damage. For more information on the normal anatomy, physiology, and neurology of swallowing, and the impact of head and neck cancers upon the swallowing function, see Chapter 4, Anatomy and Physiology of Swallowing; Chapter 5, The Neurophysiology of Swallowing; and Chapter 14, Head and Neck Cancers.

Structural Causes of Dysphagia: The pharyngeal space may be affected by a number of non-malignant obstructions, often related to the aging process. These include degeneration of tissue, including external impingement by cervical osteophytes, or intrinsic obstructions, both congenital and acquired (e.g., Zenker's diverticulum or postcricoid web). See Chapter 15, Structural Causes of High Dysphagia.

A shortcoming of VFSS is that not all patients are deemed suitable to undergo the examination. The pre-VFSS clinical swallowing examination (CSE), usually completed by a speech-language pathologist (SLP), assesses if the patient is safe to commence oral intake, but also ascertains if they are appropriate for a videofluoroscopic investigation of their swallowing. The clinical/bedside examination and objective instrumental examinations such as VFSS and fiberoptic endoscopic evaluation of swallowing (FEES) yield useful information for the assessment and management of patients with dysphagia (Swigert, 2007). However,

each of these has benefits and disadvantages. The SLP must establish which assessment(s) are required for particular patients and critically appraise the evidence base for each, as they hold ultimate responsibility for the well-being and safety of their patient; see Chapter 2, Alternative Investigations.

Both the RCSLT (2006) and the American Speech-Language-Hearing Association (ASHA) (2000) concur that the purpose of VFSS includes:

- Visualization and evaluation of the oropharyngeal structures and upper gastrointestinal tract.
- Assessment and evaluation of swallowing physiology, including lip and tongue function, velopharyngeal closure, base of tongue retraction; hyolaryngeal elevation; pharyngeal contraction; upper esophageal sphincter (UES) function; and airway protection mechanisms, inclusive of assessment with a range of consistencies to replicate normal food/fluids.
- Identify the risks and presence of aspiration, plus the patients' response.
- Assessment of the impact of therapeutic mechanisms over time.
- Biofeedback.
- Patient, carer, and health care professional education.
- Contribution to a diagnostic profile.

There are, however, occasions when instrumental assessment of swallowing via VFSS is contraindicated. The patient and their condition must be assessed on an individual basis. Some of the contraindications to VFSS are now discussed.

Contraindications to VFSS

A VFSS examination requires access to fluoroscopy equipment situated within an x-ray department, requiring the patient to be transported there from their current location. The patient therefore needs to be medically stable, and capable of cooperating with the procedure (Cichero & Langmore, 2006). For example, very frail patients (young and old alike) or those requiring a high level of medical support who present with dysphagia may be unable to withstand transportation away from a safe ward environment where emergency treatment is more readily available.

Videofluoroscopy enables a pathophysiological diagnosis of swallowing dysfunction to be formed, and allows a secondary therapeutic approach to be created (Terre & Mearin, 2007). However, patient cooperation plays a very large role in the capture of the images. If a patient is unable to cooperate with the procedure it is unlikely that they would benefit from a VFSS and must therefore be deemed unsuitable. This could be due to behavioral or cognitive deficits that present as a risk of injury to themselves or others; damaging equipment; an inability to maintain concentration for long enough to follow verbal or non-verbal instructions; or simply being unnecessarily exposed to an excess dose of radiation due to an increased length of examination (Wright, Boyd, & Workman, 1998).

Patient pregnancy is another contraindication for VFSS, and whereas radiation doses are reported to be minimal for videofluoroscopy (Zammit-Maempel, Chapple, & Leslie, 2007), exact radiation dose will depend (among other things) on patient size, imaging equipment, operator experience, and length of procedure (Hurwitz et al., 2006). Abdominal shielding with a lead rubber gown may be used for fetal protection, but radiographic imaging during pregnancy should only be considered in extreme cases where non-ionizing methods of imaging are inappropriate.

In addition, in an age of rising obesity rates (Cai, Lubitz, Flegal, & Pamuk, 2010), an obese patient may not be able to be positioned correctly, or indeed fit in the prescribed space limitations that fluoroscopic imaging equipment allows (Cichero & Langmore, 2006); see Chapter 8, Effective Use of Imaging Technology. Paradoxically, research suggests that the incidence of stroke is increasingly observed in obese patients (Towfighi, Zheng, & Ovbiagele, 2010) and therefore this client group may in fact be the ones who potentially require a VFSS in the long term.

If a patient is placed nil by mouth (NBM)/ nil per oris (NPO) for any reason other than oropharyngeal dysphagia, for example following gastrointestinal tract surgery for fear of anastomotic dehiscence (Osland, Yunus, Khan, & Memon, 2009), VFSS would not be appropriate. The ingestion of oral intake or contrast (of any kind) could potentially pose a significant threat to the patient by penetrating the upper or lower gastrointestinal tract wall and invading the thoracic or peritoneal cavities.

Though very rare, the patient may have had a previous adverse reaction to the x-ray contrast (Idee, Pines, Pringent, & Corot 2005), in which case the VFSS procedure could be potentially life threatening. An alternative means of investigation should therefore be identified. Prior to all VFSS procedures, the patient, carer or representative should be questioned regarding any known allergy or adverse reaction to any contrast media.

Finally, if in the clinicians' judgment the investigation would not change the clinical management of the patient, this is a definite contraindication. This principle is referred to as "Justification" under the UK Ionising Radiation (Medical Exposure) Regulations (2000), and both radiographers and radiologists are legally obliged to justify all imaging procedures that they undertake.

However, most importantly, the etiology of any dysphagia is notably diverse (Chau & Kung, 2009), but the initial disorder leading to its onset must be taken into account, often as a priority. In other words, the presenting dysphagia is often only one manifestation of a wider condition (e.g., stroke), and when presenting acutely it may be in the patient's best interests to receive further treatment to improve the wider condition prior to undertaking the dysphagia investigation (Cichero & Langmore, 2006). All of the factors mentioned above need to be taken into account when assessing patient suitability for instrumental investigation via the pre-VFSS CSE.

Patient Positioning

Usually, a standard VFSS is performed in the lateral view (Cheung, Chen, Hsin, Tsai, & Leong, 2010) and regions of visualization include the oral cavity, pharyngeal cavity, larynx, and cervical esophagus (Martin-Harris & Jones, 2008). This demonstrates bolus preparation, anterior-posterior (AP) control and bolus propulsion, timing of oropharyngeal trigger, and occurrence of laryngeal penetration and aspiration. However, the lateral plane alone does not allow for viewing laterality of deficit, for example, post-swallow residue in the pyriform sinuses. The AP projection (or viewing plane) is employed to enable decisions to be made regarding equilibrium of bolus flow, lateral pharyngeal wall contraction, and symmetry of structure and function (Martin-Harris & Jones, 2008), and, ideally, all patients should be examined in both the lateral and AP positions.

However, in the case of a bedbound patient who is only able to manage supine positioning, AP viewing may be the only possibility. Within a fluoroscopy suite equipped with a C-arm, manipulation of the x-ray tube to the side of the patient will enable lateral viewing, but in a traditional fluoroscopy room this is not possible and viewing is limited to AP positioning; see Chapter 8, Effective Use of Imaging Technology. Although this has benefits for assessment of laterality of deficit, full assessment of laryngeal penetration and aspiration is not as clear as in the lateral position, and all attempts should be made to examine in the lateral viewing plane.

Positional Modifications

Analysis of the oropharyngeal swallowing mechanism during a VFSS may identify an "unsafe" swallow, whereby the clinician detects either an overt or covert threat to the airway, or observes residual pooling of the contrast agent following the swallow. In these instances, trials of positional modifications and/or swallowing maneuvers under fluoroscopic control are indicated. Table 1–1 (Newman, 2010) outlines the potential positional modifications available to the clinician during the VFSS, and the reasons for their use. If successful, these modifications can then be explained to the patient (and/or carers) so that they can be employed when eating/drinking, thus enabling oral intake to commence to a certain degree.

In addition to positional modification, airway protection strategies designed to specifically assist the strength and safety of swallowing can (if appropriate) be attempted during VFSS. These are outlined below, but should only be used with those patients deemed appropriate by the clinician from the CSE and/or the VFSS:

Supraglottic Swallow: Gently take a breath and hold it, take the bolus into the mouth and swallow while holding the breath. Immediately after the swallow, breathe out, and cough or clear the throat and swallow again. This will prevent any residue sitting in the laryngeal inlet from being aspirated beyond the level of the vocal folds.

Super-supraglottic Swallow: This is the next step on from the supraglottic swallow whereby a deep breath is taken and held tightly, the patient is encouraged to bear down tightly or pull up on the chair or bed with great strength and swallow while

Table 1–1. *The Role of Positional Modifications to the VFSS Procedure*

Positional Modification	Disorder and Presentation
Chin tuck Chin is tucked down so the patient is "looking into their lap"	• Reduced base of tongue movement—residue in the valleculae • Delayed pharyngeal trigger—overspill of contrast into the pharynx prior to onset of the swallow • Laryngeal penetration—contrast evident in the laryngeal inlet and/or resting on the vocal folds • Aspiration—residue evident in the airway below the true vocal folds
Chin lift Chin is lifted up so the patient is looking up to a 45° angle	• Poor lip seal—anterior spillage of contrast • Reduced oral strength—poor formation and manipulation of the bolus, often resulting in anterior spillage or premature overspill • Nasal regurgitation—contrast noted to enter the nasopharynx
Head turn Patient turns the head to the affected side if the damage is unilateral (e.g., unilateral pharyngeal weakness post-stroke)	• Unilateral pharyngeal wall disorder—residue in the affected pyriform sinus • Reduced opening of the cricopharyngeal sphincter— residue in the pyriform sinuses (often bilateral)
Lean/Head tilt Patient leans, or tilts their head to the stronger side	• Oral **and** pharyngeal weakness—residue noted in the mouth and pharynx on the same side
Lie down Patient reclines beyond 45° angle.	• Reduced laryngeal elevation—residue at the entrance to the larynx • Bilateral pharyngeal weakness—equal amounts of residue evident in bilateral pyriform fossae after swallowing

Source: Newman, R. D. (2010). Videofluoroscopy. In J. M. Nightingale & R. L. Law (Eds.), *Gastrointestinal tract imaging: An evidence-based practice guide* (p. 108). Copyright © 2010 Elsevier. All rights reserved. Used with permission.

bearing down. After swallowing, a forced cough/throat clear is used to expel any residue into the oral cavity, and immediately swallowed again prior to inhaling, or if necessary, expectorated.

Mendelsohn Maneuver: Designed to voluntarily prolong laryngeal elevation (Singh & Hamdy, 2005), the patient is instructed to hold the swallow at the height of vertical movement of the larynx (Cichero, 2006) which subsequently lengthens airway clo-

sure and holds open the cricopharyngeal sphincter in an aim to allow safer passage of the bolus into the esophagus.

Effortful Swallow: This technique is simply instructing the patient to swallow very hard. In doing so, increased posterior tongue base movement is generated (Logemann, 1997) which compensates for posterior pharyngeal weakness, allowing the bolus to be propelled effectively through the pharynx and reduces the likelihood of pooling/residue.

All of the positional modifications and compensatory strategies should be used with caution, and not all are appropriate for particular patients. The clinician must therefore use expertise and clinical discretion to establish from the VFSS which techniques are most applicable and ultimately safest for the patient.

Evolution of the Examination

The enormous upheaval within all aspects of health care over the last 10 years has created pressure to perform to a high standard, but also introduced a foundation for independent learning and practitioner development, and the videofluoroscopy service is no exception. The United Kingdom's National Health Service (NHS) has been repeatedly restructured since 1991 (Sheaff, 2009), a factor which typically is demonstrated in the majority of modern health care systems worldwide. There is ever-increasing need for the objective examination of swallowing to create a baseline for the patient as part of their diagnosis and subsequent treatment. Historically, the SLP would perform the procedure and interpret the results with a radiologist (Logemann, 1997), while radiographers/radiologic technologists were involved in booking appointments, patient preparation, image storage, and patient safety (Power, Laasch, Kasthuri, Nicholson, & Hamdy, 2006). However, due to recent significant changes in health care provision all over the world, initiatives now exist for VFSS clinics to be operated solely by radiographers and SLPs. An extension of the traditional radiography responsibility now exists to incorporate a specialist fluoroscopic radiographer role that includes working alongside the SLP in the joint SLP-radiographer-led VFSS clinic. This incorporates image acquisition, protocol formation/selection, image interpretation and joint clinical reporting. The changes may have been brought about

by reduced availability of radiologists in VFSS examinations, particularly in the United Kingdom, but, as Power et al. (2006) explain in their research, specialist training in VFSS for all professionals is extremely limited, and formal training in VFSS for radiologists was negligible. In addition to this, Power et al. (2006) went on to report that it is usual for the SLP to lead the investigation, with the radiologist role in the procedure being the capturing of images and subsequent interpretation. With appropriate training this could therefore be achieved by a radiographer.

However, although valid opportunities exist for SLP-radiographer-led VFSS clinics to be created and operate extremely successfully without the presence of a radiologist, variables exist at all levels: local, national, and international. The SLP should be aware of local policy/protocol, plus governing body and state legal or regulatory issues regarding the presence of a radiologist or other physician. In the United States and other countries where health care is funded by outside agencies including private insurance companies, the need for radiologist presence will not only be dictated in third-party payer requirements (ASHA, 2004), but also by the level of radiographer training and their entitlement to contribute to an imaging report. Whoever the professionals involved in the VFSS examination are, it is vital to remember that capturing images whereby artificial radiopaque food materials are administered is "one moment in time" (Newman, 2010), and the examination requires the presence of an astute observer (who has valuable knowledge and experience) to conduct and interpret the outcome of the investigation. Bearing in mind the research by Power et al. (2006) which shows negligible formal training for radiologists, combined with lesser experience and overreliance upon the SLP, this potentially highlights (alongside an increased radiologist portfolio of duties), an enthusiasm for radiographer role advancement, and opportunities for new ways of working within VFSS clinics.

Other Professionals Involved in VFSS

As the VFSS evidence base evolves, other professions from the multidisciplinary team (MDT) whose traditional boundaries may not have included the objective examination of swallowing have become centrally involved in VFSS services. Though potentially not directly linked with the procedure itself, their input is vital to maintain a high level of ongoing patient care and intervention, and to facilitate smooth running of the service. The professionals incorporated in the wider VFSS service (and a brief explanation of their role[s]) are as follows:

Nursing Staff: Potentially required to accompany the patient to monitor their vital signs to ensure risk is minimized; assist with moving and handling for correct screening positioning; patient reassurance (particularly in pediatrics, elderly, learning disabilities, and any other client group where there is a potential for fear and anxiety to impact upon the assessment); complete oral suction if incomplete clearance is noted; and provide feedback of the results of the investigation to the ward staff and medical team in the interim period between examination completion and final reporting.

Physiotherapist: Required if the patient is known to present with a high risk of aspiration and complete immediate chest physiotherapy and deep pharyngeal suction to minimize the implications of greater amounts of contrast in the airway and lungs. If the patient has a tracheostomy in situ, deeper suction directly into the trachea may be required if significant aspiration is noted. In many cases, a physiotherapist may be the only professional in the MDT

who is trained (and deemed competent) in deep tracheal suctioning. They can also assist in specific moving and handling if the patient is known to have individual needs.

Dietician: Provide specific guidance of any individual feeding requirements that the patient may have, e.g. diabetes mellitus and gluten allergy. This will assist the decision of which contrast to use and which foodstuffs to mix them with to replicate a more viscous bolus. In addition, if the patient is to remain on a modified diet, or indeed NBM/NPO, the dietician will need to be aware of this and provide alternative nutritional recommendations and arrangements as necessary.

Ear, Nose, and Throat (ENT) Surgeon: The ENT specialists may wish to be present during the examination to obtain a "real time" appreciation of the swallowing anatomy and function, and if necessary make comparisons with clinical and endoscopic examinations that they may have undertaken themselves. This may help in guiding their decision-making for differential diagnostic purposes. For example, though more detailed radiological investigations may have been completed, e.g., CT or MRI scans, the VFSS can be included in the investigation procedure to ascertain the location, size, and importantly, the impact of a subcutaneous tumor; see Chapter 14, Head and Neck Cancers.

Plastic Surgeon/Maxillofacial Surgeon: The plastic surgeon or maxillofacial surgeon may be the professional taking the lead role in the VFSS, particularly within pediatrics presenting with cleft lip and/or palate. They may wish to see exactly the nature the disorder is having on the child's swallowing, and because of incomplete fusion of the hard palate, speech will also be significantly affected.

Professionals Involved Following VFSS Completion

Once the VFSS is complete and a more holistic view of the patient's swallowing has been obtained, referral to other specialists within the multidisciplinary team may be necessary. For example, if the patient's dysphagia is seen to have a functional nature, whereby the presentation is atypical and no neurological, structural, mechanical, or other cause can be found, referral to a psychologist or psychiatrist may be the next option. The mental health team holds a significant role in the MDT as some disorders of swallowing may be psychological in nature and require further investigation.

In addition, patients who have received a distressing diagnosis such as a progressive neuromuscular disease or head and neck cancer are ultimately bound to feel fear regarding their potential prognosis, and how it may affect their family, work, and social lives. Specialist nurse counselors and/or clinical psychologists are appropriately trained professionals from the MDT to address these emotions and provide ongoing support to these particular patients and relatives/carers.

This is where close MDT working is required. The dietician will need to remain involved to ensure that the patient continues to receive adequate nutrition; the physiotherapist will need to maintain a patent airway; the appropriate medic/surgeon may be more regularly involved; and the SLP will need to frequently review the case in clinics and wards, and undertake the VFSS with the radiographer/radiologist as appropriate.

Any change or modification in practice in the VFSS service requires close liaison between all professionals involved with different knowledge and clinical objectives, and also for them to highlight the level of skill and experience each professional can share with the rest of the team to enhance the VFSS clinic and maximize its potential for further development. This will then enable protocol formation and agreement which acts both to meet patients' needs and protect the practitioner. This highlights the need to amplify the MDT knowledge of the VFSS procedure, as agreement is fundamental to the extension of traditional roles; see Chapter 3, Improving Patient Experience and Minimizing Risk.

Legal and Ethical Considerations

Access to a VFSS service offered by the team of SLPs, radiographers, and radiologists should be based on clinical need and be available regardless of age, disability (bearing in mind the individual's suitability for the examination), ethnicity, gender, or creed (RCSLT, 2007).

Consent

In addition to an individual's suitability for, and ability to cooperate with the procedure, consent must be obtained prior to VFSS. According to the legal doctrine of informed consent, sufficient information must be provided to the individual undergoing the investigation for consent to be seen as adequate, as accepting consent based on insufficient information may constitute malpractice (Munetz & Roth, 1985). Despite this, some reports state that it is unlikely that informed consent is ever completely achieved as it requires a detailed understanding of anatomy and physiology (Stanley, Walters, & Maddern, 1998). However, the important question for the clinician is how much, and what kind of information constitutes enough for a patient to make an informed decision. Ideally, information should be as specific as possible while still being simple and easy to understand, which explains the details of the procedure and any potential complications that may arise. If a patient chooses not to undergo the VFSS, then the potential consequences of their actions must be clearly explained to them. Their wishes regarding consent should be fully documented by the clinician. A detailed section on consent can be found in Chapter 3, Improving Patient Experience and Minimizing Risk.

Risk

In some instances, the patient may not comply with the results of the VFSS and continue to take food or fluid orally against advice; these actions are known to cause adverse conditions (Low, Wyles, Wilkinson, & Sainsbury, 2001). In addition to this, nursing staff in acute and long-term care may not understand the complexity of the VFSS and the resulting feeding instructions, and as a result compliance with the feeding protocols may be as low as 50% (Colodny, 2001). In these instances, discussion of the VFSS recommendations must be in collaboration with the appropriate department or directorate, and full documentation is warranted. Patients' decisions to comply with the findings and subsequent recommendations of the VFSS may be influenced by medical or social issues, quality of life, cultural or other personal factors (Sharp & Geneson, 1996). The clinician must respect these choices, but risk management is necessary via recommendation of the safest consistency/consistencies (and/or positions) but may require close consultation with the patient's physician(s) and the clinical risk officer. For more information, see Chapter 3, Improving Patient Experience and Minimizing Risk.

Ethical Dilemmas

When considering VFSS as an investigation of the oropharyngeal swallow, the clinician must be sure *why* the examination is being completed, and the question, "What is going to be achieved?" should be asked. There are bound to be instances where a VFSS would the perfect examination of choice, but if it is not going to change a particular treatment or course of action, then it would not be beneficial to put the patient through it, and unnecessarily expose them to radiation. An example of this could be an elderly patient who is suffering from an acute chest infection, and a bedside assessment of swallowing is inconclusive as no coughing or choking is evident upon oral trials. However, if the patient is investigated via VFSS and is seen to be at significant risk of aspirating, it is likely that alternative means of nutrition and hydration will be recommended and the patient kept NBM/NPO. This undoubtedly will have a considerable psychosocial impact on the life of the individual and their family (Miller & Carding, 2008). In addition to this, as eating and drinking are highly social activities, the patient's social circle will also be affected, therefore potentially reducing their quality of life. It is in instances like this where the *full* consequences of a poor outcome on VFSS must be explained to the patient beforehand so they can make a decision as to whether or not to consent. The elderly patient may wish to continue to eat and drink orally and accept the risk of aspiration, and refuse to consent to the investigation.

There are other such disorders where an ethical dilemma may become apparent, for example in neurodegenerative conditions where the outcome may again be negative and oral feeding may be considered to be unsafe. However, as long as the clinician is sure why the examination is being completed, the decision to continue with the VFSS can then be discussed with the patient.

To Diagnose or Not?

Various reporting styles exist, ranging from narrative style with broad range headings (Murray, 2003), to very prescriptive detailed checklists as described by Logemann (1998). A long-awaited universal style of reporting is explained by Dr. Martin Brodsky in Chapter 16.

A patient presenting with dysphagia undergoing a VFSS should expect to have the salient features of the swallowing function described, with the results highlighting any risk to the airway and the factors causing such risk. However, one thing which is agreed between many speech pathology governing bodies is that medical practitioners are the only people qualified to make a medical diagnosis (Kelly, Hydes, McLaughlin, & Wallace 2007), and no diagnosis should be rendered by the SLP (ASHA, 2004). However, although independent radiographer reporting of medical images is supported by some professional bodies (College of Radiographers, 2006, 2010), it is believed that the multiprofessional combination report will provide the patients and referring clinicians with the most effective service.

Where a radiologist is present during the examination, a potential medical diagnosis seen on x-ray can be discussed with them, but they must document the findings, as it is not the role of the SLP. Where a radiologist is not present in the VFSS and a suspicious finding is highlighted, contact must be made with them immediately to discuss this. If suspicions are confirmed, the radiologist should take over the VFSS (or the reporting of it), and suggest further/alternative investigation(s) where necessary. The SLP should then simply document the outcome of the VFSS, highlighting the fact that consultation with a radiologist was necessary and that their findings and recommendations should be awaited.

Financial Implications

Being both a time consuming and costly examination, it is vital that the actual VFSS procedure runs as smoothly as possible (Newman,

2010). The cost of the procedure has many variables that will differ locally and internationally, but the main financial implications depend on the number of staff involved in the procedure, radiologist presence, type and amount of contrast medium used, length of procedure, and imaging equipment or PACS transfer technology. Additional costs include internal and external staff training to bring their competency to an acceptable level, and any foodstuffs used to mix with contrast to replicate "normal" foods taken when eating. Barium sulfate is the medium of choice due to its high level of radiopacity with few side effects, but also (and importantly) it has the advantage of being a cheap medium with which to work (Leferre et al., 2005). Its relative low cost of approximately £1 to £2 ($1.60 to $3.20) per examination, compared to between £10 to £50 ($15 to $80) per examination for an iodine-based water-soluble contrast, means that unpredictability of cost is high. The main expense is radiologist presence, and in a report written by Newcastle Acute Hospitals Trust (2009) that promotes SLP-radiographer-led VFSS clinics, the cost of *one* procedure was seen to decrease from £345 to £215 ($550 to $340), simply by eliminating radiologist presence. The implications of this over a period of one financial year are significant.

However, demands of some private insurance companies, particularly in the United States, mean that radiologist presence is frequently required, and a VFSS is often a prerequisite to create a baseline against which further levels of therapy can be calculated. The financial repercussions are therefore removed from the SLP and radiography service and dealt with at a tertiary level by the insurance company themselves.

Combining the VFSS with a follow-up swallowing rehabilitation plan can decrease the cost and time for rehabilitation of patients with dysphagia. In some cases the patient can begin safe oral intake immediately after the examination, and therapy may not be needed if consistent spontaneous recovery is anticipated (Logemann, 1997). As a result, there is a definite need for patient pathway protocols to be designed, which include VFSS costing to open up the investigation to more patients, and allow greater freedom for SLPs and radiographers to create a fully functioning, low cost, and appealing service.

Summary

Although local and worldwide variation exists in many areas of the VFSS service provision, including availability, funding, imaging equipment and contrast(s) used, VFSS remains the supreme example of instrumental swallowing assessment against which others are measured, and no other comes as close. It remains the only examination where all stages of the swallow can be examined in detail and highlight both oropharyngeal structure and bolus flow. SLPs have utilized the technique to their advantage and skills have progressed to enable baselines to be created against which future examinations can be compared. However, the need for further development continues, and, in order to maintain professional standards, there is a requirement for regular involvement in VFSS investigations, and a commitment to continuing professional development. Professional boundaries need to be maintained and respected, and any variation in service provision between departments and countries should be appreciated. The fact that VFSS continues to evolve should act as an innovation to clinicians, and also serve as a drive for new skills/techniques to be adopted and regularly audited.

Although VFSS is an excellent investigation, its limitations should be duly noted and clinicians should be aware that not all patients will be suitable candidates for such an examination. Because the patient is exposed to lim-ited amounts of radiation, attention is drawn to the fact that VFSS remains a MDT procedure and knowledge and responsibility should be shared with other members of the team.

In an increasingly demanding financial climate where health care systems continue to evolve, the VFSS service must continue to remain in the good standing that it has over the last decade. SLPs and radiographers must maintain their skills and prove their worth as the clinicians of choice to complete this objective instrumental examination of swallowing, working in close collaboration with the multidisciplinary team. Research, innovation, and training are the key to the continued success of VFSS in the ever-changing health care environment.

REFERENCES

American Speech-Language-Hearing Association. (2004). *Guidelines for speech-language pathologists performing videofluoroscopic swallowing studies* [Guidelines]. Retrieved February 16, 2011, from http://www.asha.org/policy

Cai, L., Lubitz, J., Flegal, K., & Pamuk, E. R. (2010). The predicted effects of chronic obesity in middle age on medicare costs and mortality. *Medical Care, 48*(6), 510–517.

Chau, K. H. T., & Kung, C. M. A. (2009). Patient dose during videofluoroscopy swallowing studies in a Hong Kong public hospital. *Dysphagia, 24*, 387–390.

Cheung, S. M., Chen, C. J., Hsin, Y. J., Tsai, Y. T., & Leong, C. P. (2010). Effect of neuromuscular electrical stimulation in a patient with Sjogren's syndrome with dysphagia: A real-time videofluoroscopic swallowing study. *Chang Gung Medical Journal, 33*, 338–345.

Cichero, J. (2006). Improving swallowing function: Compensation. In J. Cichero & B. Murdocj (Eds.), *Dysphagia: Foundation, theory and practice*. Chichester, UK: John Wiley & Sons.

Cichero, J., & Langmore, S. (2006). Imaging assessments. In J. Cichero & B. Murdocj (Eds.),

Dysphagia: Foundation, theory and practice. Chichester, UK: John Wiley & Sons.

College of Radiographers. (2006). *Medical image interpretation and clinical reporting by non-radiologists: The role of the radiographer.* London, UK: The COR.

College of Radiographers. (2010). *Medical image interpretation by radiographers: Definitive guidance.* London, UK: The COR.

Colodny, N. (2001). Construction and validation of the mealtime and dysphagia questionnaire: An instrument designed to assess nursing staff reasons for noncompliance with SLP dysphagia and feeding recommendations. *Dysphagia, 16,* 263–271.

Daniels, S. K., McAdam, C. P., Brailey, K., & Foundas, L. (1997). Clinical assessment of swallowing and prediction of dysphagia severity. *American Journal of Speech-Language Pathology, 6*(4), 17–23.

Frowen, J. J., Cotton, S. M., & Perry, A. R. (2008). The stability, reliability, and validity of videofluoroscopy measures for patients with head and neck cancer. *Dysphagia, 23*(4), 348–363.

Hurwitz, L. M., Yoshizumi, T., Reiman, R. E., Goodman, P. C., Paulson, E. K., Frush, D. P., . . . Barnes, L. (2006). Radiation dose to the fetus from body MDCT during early gestation. *American Journal of Roentgeneology, 186,* 871–876.

Idée, J. M., Pines, E., Pringent, P., & Corot, C. (2005) Allergy-like reactions to iodinated contrast agents: A critical analysis. *Fundamental and Clinical Pharmacology, 19*(3), 263–281.

Ionising Radiation (Medical Exposure) Regulations. (2000). London, UK: The Stationary Office.

Kelly, A. M., Hydes, K., McLaughlin, C., & Wallace, S. (2007). *Fibreoptic Endoscopic Evaluation of Swallowing (FEES): The role of speech and language therapy.* RCSLT Policy Statement.

Leferre, P., Gryspeerdt, S., Marrannes, J., Baekelandt, M., & Van Holsbeeck, B. (2005). CT colonography after fecal tagging with a reduced cathartic cleansing and a reduced volume of barium. *American Journal of Roentgenology, 184,* 1836–1842.

Logemann, J. (1983). *Evaluation and treatment of swallowing disorders.* Austin, TX: Pro-Ed.

Logemann, J. A. (1997). Role of the modified barium swallow in management of patients with dysphagia. *Otolaryngology—Head and Neck Surgery, 116*(3), 335e8.

Logemann, J. A. (1998). *Evaluation and treatment of swallowing disorders* (2nd ed.). Austin, TX: Pro-Ed.

Low, J., Wyles, C., Wilkinson, T. & Sainsbury, R. (2001). The effect of compliance on clinical outcomes for patients with dysphagia on videofluoroscopy. *Dysphagia, 16,* 123–127.

Martin-Harris, B., & Jones, B. (2008). The videofluorographic swallowing study. *Physical Medicine and Rehabilitation Clinics of North America, 19*(4), 769–785.

Martino, R., Pron, G., & Diamont, N. (2000). Screening for oropharyngeal dysphagia in stroke: Insufficient evidence for guidelines. *Dysphagia, 15*(1), 19–30.

Miller, N., & Carding, P. (2008). Dysphagia: Implications for older people. *Reviews in Clinical Gerontology, 17,* 177–190.

Murray, J. (2003, October 21). Responding to the dysphagia consult: A report-writing primer. *ASHA Leader.*

Munetz, M. R., & Roth, L. H. (1985). Informing patients about tardive dyskinesia. *Archives of General Psychiatry, 42,* 866–871.

Newcastle Acute Hospitals Trust. (2009). Speech therapist led videofluoroscopy for swallowing assessments. Retrieved March 6, 2011, from http://www.evidence.nhs.uk/qualityand productivity

Newman, R. D. (2010). Videofluoroscopy. In J. M. Nightingale & R. L. Law (Eds.), *Gastrointestinal tract imaging: An evidence-based practice guide.* New York, NY: Elsevier.

Osland, E., Yunus, R., Khan, S., & Memon, M. A. (2009). Early enteral nutrition within 24h of intestinal surgery versus later commencement of feeding: A systematic review and meta-analysis (Letter to the Editors). *Journal of Gastrointestinal Surgery, 13*(6), 1163–1165.

Power, M., Laasch, H. U., Kasthuri, R. S., Nicholson, D. A., & Hamdy, S. (2006). Videofluoroscopic assessment of dysphagia: A questionnaire survey of protocols, roles and responsibilities of radiology and speech and language therapy personnel. *Radiography, 12,* 26–30.

Robbins, J. A., Coyle, J. L. Rosenbek, J. C., Roecker, E. B. & Woods, J. L. (1999). Differentiation of normal and abnormal airway protection during swallowing using the penetration-aspiration scale. *Dysphagia, 14*(4), 228–232.

Royal College of Speech and Language Therapists. (2006). *Videofluoroscopic Evaluation of Oropharyngeal swallowing disorders (VFS) in adults: The role of speech and language therapists.* Policy Statement: RCSLT.

Sharp, H. M., & Genesen, L. B. (1996). Ethical decision-making in dysphagia management. *American Journal of Speech-Language Pathology, 5*(1), 15–22.

Sheaff, R. (2009). Medicine and management in English primary care: A shifting balance of power? *Journal of Social Policy, 38*(4), 627–647.

Singh, S., & Hamdy, S. (2005). The upper oesophageal sphincter. *Neurogastroenterology and Motility, 17*(s1), 3–12.

Singh, V., Berry, S., Brockbank, M. J., Frost, R. A., Tyler, S. E., & Owens, D. (2009). Investigation of aspiration: Milk nasendoscopy versus videofluoroscopy. *European Archives of Otorhinolaryngology, 266*, 543–545.

Stanley, B. M., Walters, D. J., & Maddern, G. J. (1998). Informed consent: How much information is enough? *Australian and New Zealand Journal of Surgery, 68*, 788–791.

Swigert, N. B. (2007). Update on current assessment practices for dysphagia. *Topics in Geriatric Rehabilitation, 23*(3), 185–196.

Terré, R., & Mearin, F. (2007). Prospective evaluation of oropharyngeal dysphagia after severe traumatic brain injury. *Brain Injury, 21*(13–14), 1411–1417.

Towfighi, A., Zheng, L., & Ovbiagele, B. (2010). Weight of the obesity epidemic: Rising stroke rates among middle-aged women in the United States. *Stroke, 41*, 1371–1375.

Wright, R. E., Boyd, C. S., & Workman, A. (1998). Radiation doses to patients during pharyngeal videofluoroscopy. *Dysphagia, 13*, 113–115.

Zammit-Maempel, I., Chapple, C. L., & Leslie, P. (2007). Radiation dose in videofluoroscopic swallow studies. *Dysphagia, 22*(1),13–15.

Chapter

2

ALTERNATIVE INVESTIGATIONS

Justin Roe

INTRODUCTION

Central to the comprehensive assessment and management of oropharyngeal dysphagia is a detailed instrumental swallowing evaluation. Although research has sought to establish a sensitive and specific comprehensive bedside assessment, patients who silently aspirate may not be detected until they present with respiratory compromise and are further examined using a technique such as videofluoroscopy (Logemann, 1993) or fiberoptic endoscopic evaluation of swallowing (FEES) (Langmore, Schatz, & Olsen, 1988). Research has shown that patient-reported symptoms may not be representative of findings from instrumental evaluation of swallowing (Jensen, Lambertsen, Torkov, Dahl, Jensen, et al., 2007). Silent aspiration is a phenomenon that has been highlighted across a range of medical conditions including those who have suffered strokes, or head injuries and following cardiothoracic surgery (Ramsey, Smithard, & Kalra, 2005; see

Chapters 9 and 10 for further information). While aspiration and aspiration pneumonia often receive much attention in the literature, other consequences of impaired swallowing function include compromised nutrition and hydration with subsequent impact on the individual's quality of life (Murray, 2009).

As well as evaluating the swallow it is important to understand the patient's perception of their swallowing difficulty and how it limits their activities and restricts their participation in everyday life. This can be achieved using a variety of measures that can be attributed to the International Classification of Functioning (ICF) framework for evaluating dysphagia (Threats, 2007).

In this chapter, the most commonly reported techniques used to evaluate swallow function are discussed along with their potential for improved understanding of oropharyngeal swallowing and optimizing rehabilitation. This is preceded by a description of the cornerstone of dysphagia assessment, the clinical swallowing evaluation (CSE).

CLINICAL SWALLOWING EVALUATION (CSE) AS A GUIDE TO INSTRUMENTAL EVALUATION

Patients may be referred to a speech-language pathologist (SLP) for instrumental swallowing evaluation due to a number reported symptoms or observed signs of difficulty. This is most likely to be in response to signs of difficulty such as coughing at mealtimes or a "wet" voice, suspected aspiration pneumonia or recurrent, unexplained chest infections. Alternatively, referral may be diagnosis driven, for example, referral of a head and neck cancer patient due to be treated with (chemo-)radiotherapy where a baseline functional evaluation is required. Another example may be a patient with a progressive neurologic disorder such as Parkinson's disease or multiple sclerosis who may be presenting with altered swallowing and may require further detailed assessment and amendment of their management plan.

Selection of the most appropriate instrumental evaluation technique should be preceded by a detailed clinical swallowing examination (CSE) carried out by a dysphagia specialist SLP. The CSE includes a full clinical history, detection of potential contributory factors, confirmation of the need for an instrumental evaluation, and identification of those who may need alternative evaluations prior to (or instead of) an assessment of oropharyngeal dysphagia (such as patients with suspected esophageal dysphagia). An oromotor evaluation is completed including assessment of cranial nerve function (see Chapter 5). This is usually followed by an assessment of swallowing on a range of textures. During this time, the SLP will observe the patient closely, gently palpating under the patient's chin to evaluate submandibular, hyoid and laryngeal movement on swallowing (Logemann, 1998). Observations and interpretation of the CSE can then be incorporated into a management plan and recommendations can be made. It is possible that a therapist may wish to trial compensatory strategies to minimize symptoms (for example texture modification or positional changes; see Chapters 1 and 9). However, without a detailed instrumental evaluation, it is would be impossible to accurately evaluate the nature and extent of any oropharyngeal dysphagia, implement appropriate therapy and ascertain the benefit of compensatory strategies.

The use of clinical assessments such as the 100ml and 3oz water swallow tests are valuable to highlight those who may benefit from an instrumental evaluation (DePippo, Holas, & Reding, 1992; Hughes & Wiles, 1996; Patterson, Hildreth, McColl, Carding, Hamilton, et al., 2010; Patterson, McColl, Carding, Kelly, & Wilson, 2009). This assessment also provides quantitative data for comparison with repeat assessment. Swallowing scales such as the Functional Oral Intake Scale (FOIS) (Crary, Mann, & Groher, 2005) and the Royal Brisbane Hospital Outcome Measure for Swallowing (RBHOMS) (Ward & Conroy, 1999) can also support the clinician in quantifying swallowing ability and recording outcomes.

The CSE will enable the clinician to establish appropriate candidacy for an instrumental assessment. This will include weighing the benefits in light of medical stability and cognitive status, plus psychosocial, environmental and behavioral factors; ultimately, the therapist needs to consider whether the instrumental assessment will change the patient's clinical management (American Speech-Language-Hearing Association, 2000).

EVALUATION OPTIONS

In clinical practice, the most commonly applied techniques for the evaluation of oropharyngeal dysphagia and implementation of rehabilitation strategies are videofluoroscopy and FEES. However, a range of methods are discussed in this section that have been developed to understand swallowing with each providing a unique insight in to specific features of the deglutition process. Imaging procedures being developed include cine magnetic resonance imaging (MRI) (Hartl, Albiter, Kolb, Luboinski, & Sigal, 2003; Hartl, Kolb, Bretagne, Bidault, & Sigal, 2010; Kreeft, Rasch, Muller, Pameijer, Hallo, et al, 2012) and advanced computed tomography (CT) techniques (Fujii, Inamoto, Saitoh, Baba, Okada, et al., 2011; Inamoto, Fujii, Saitoh, Baba, Okada, et al., 2011). However, their use is not widespread at this time and researchers have reported limitations and the need for further validation of these methods.

While much of the literature focuses on understanding swallowing physiology, functional MRI scanning has been employed to understand cortical activity during a range of swallowing and non-swallowing tasks associated with deglutition (Humbert & Robbins, 2007). More recently, use of this technology has been extended to understand cortical activation in response to swallowing rehabilitation maneuvers (Peck et al., 2010).

Barium Swallow

Although the focus of this chapter is oropharyngeal swallowing, it is important to bear in mind potential esophageal stage problems which may only be revealed to a limited degree by videofluoroscopy. To adequately evaluate motility and structural abnormalities of the upper gastrointestinal tract including the stomach and esophagus, a standard barium swallow may be required. Gas-producing granules with high density barium are used to evaluate potential mucosal irregularities and high-density liquid barium is used to evaluate esophageal motility with the patient exam-

ined upright and lying flat in lateral, anterior-posterior and oblique planes (Goldsmith, 2003). It differs from videofluoroscopy in the fact that during a standard barium swallow the image intensifier focuses on the hypopharynx and follows the bolus as it passes through the esophagus to the stomach. Although aspiration may be observed (and may signpost a referral to the SLP), the swallowing events leading to aspiration will not be clear without detailed observation of the oral and pharyngeal phases of swallowing (Goldsmith, 2003). Single or sequential plane films are usually generated for evaluation as opposed to videofluoroscopy where the entire swallowing process is captured to evaluate the oropharyngeal deglutition process.

For various reasons including time, finance, and staff specialties, not all institutions are able to offer a VFSS service. In this instance, many patients are (rightly or wrongly) referred for a standard barium swallow. However, although the purpose of the VFSS is to investigate the oropharyngeal and proximal esophageal swallowing function, a standard barium swallow may still highlight any structural abnormalities at the hypopharyngeal and cricopharyngeal stages of swallowing. Examples include a Zenker's diverticulum, postcricoid web, and (depending on patient positioning) cervical osteophytes (see Chapter 15, Structural Causes of High Dysphagia). This shows that although the standard barium swallow may not be the examination of choice, it still has the potential to reveal a structural cause of a high dysphagia. This examination is usually completed by a radiologist and/or a specialist radiographer, and therefore SLPs normally would not be involved.

Esophagoscopy

Additional techniques to evaluate the esophagus include sedated esophagoscopy conducted by gastroenterologists or increasingly, office-based transnasal esophagoscopy (TNE) which is easily repeatable and allows the endoscopist to directly evaluate the esophagus through to the proximal portion of the stomach (Aviv, 2006). It is reported that, although the technique was not initially embraced in the field of gastroenterology, it has a number of applications in the otolaryngology setting (Postma, 2006). These include the evaluation of dysphagia, globus, gastroesophageal or laryngopharyngeal reflux disease, suspected foreign body, and screening for Barrett's esophagus and second cancers (Andrus, Dolan, & Anderson, 2005). It is therefore a valuable tool for otolaryngologists involved in the comprehensive evaluation of dysphagia.

Manometry

Solid state manometry, and more recently High Resolution Manometry (HRM) have been utilised by SLPs in partnership with multidisciplinary colleagues to understand pharyngeal and esophageal pressures during swallowing. Pharyngeal manometry can be used independently or concurrently with either videofluoroscopy or FEES (Butler, 2009). It enhances these instrumental assessments by providing valuable quantitative information on swallowing physiology. This includes swallow coordination and pressures, pharyngeal strength, duration of the pharyngeal pressure and onset and extent of upper esophageal sphincter (UES) relaxation. A catheter with pressure transducers is passed transnasally with a sensors positioned at the level of the pharynx, hypopharynx and UES. Researchers have reportedly used catheters with 1 to 4 pressure sensors (McCulloch, Hoffman, & Cuicci, 2010). Studies have evaluated the impact of swallowing strategies on pharyngeal pressure and the timing and duration of UES relaxation (Hiss & Huckabee, 2005). The use of concurrent videofluoroscopy can confirm

correct positioning of pressure transducers and timing of swallowing events (Pauloski, Rademaker, Lazarus, Boeckxstaens, Kahrilas, & Logemann, 2009). It has been discussed that there are technological limitations with standard manometry and that assumptions are made regarding pressure events based on visual observations using videofluoroscopy (McCulloch, Hoffman, & Cuicci, 2010). Manometric techniques have developed further with the introduction of HRM. HRM has 36 circumferential sensors at 1cm intervals (Sierra Scientific Instruments, Los Angeles, CA) evolving from traditional esophageal manometry technology, allowing for significantly improved evaluation of pharyngeal, UES and esophageal physiology and pathophysiology (Fox & Bredenoord, 2008; Ghosh, Pandolofino, Zhang, Jarosz, & Kahrilas, 2006). Given this enhanced technology and the high level spatial and temporal resolution HRM provides, it is now being employed not only to understand swallowing physiology but also to evaluate the impact of swallow maneuvers on swallowing pressures (McCulloch, Hoffman & Ciucci, 2010).

Scintigraphy

Oropharyngeal scintigraphy is a nuclear medicine test whereby any bolus which can be labeled with a radionuclide marker (technetium) is given to the patient to swallow (Hamlet et al., 1997). The patient is positioned in front of a gamma camera that images radiation emitted from the bolus. The advantage of scintigraphy is the ability to accurately measure the precise amount of aspiration. However, it cannot determine the cause due to poor image resolution and definition of structures. As a result, scintigraphy is not a screening or diagnostic evaluation of oropharyngeal dysfunction (Shaw, Williams, Cook, Wallace, Weltman, et al., 2004). In addition, only a limited number of boluses can be presented given the radioactive nature of the materials required.

Accurate determination of oropharyngeal residue is not possible using videofluoroscopy as a two-dimensional image is used to quantify residue in a three-dimensional cavity (Shaw et al., 2004). However, scintigraphy is of particular interest as one can accurately determine bolus transit times; the percentage volume of the bolus swallowed; the amount remaining in the pharynx post swallow, and how much (if any) is aspirated. Oropharyngeal Swallowing Efficiency (OPSE) is a validated perceptual rating scale used by SLPs to estimate the percentage of the bolus swallowed and aspirated when analyzing videofluoroscopic images (Rademaker, Paulowski, Logemann, & Shanahan, 1994). Although it is not possible to concurrently evaluate patients using videofluoroscopy and scintigraphy due to the nature of the contrasts used in each examination, researchers have compared scintigraphically quantified residue with OPSE (Logemann et al., 2005). They found that, when compared with scintigraphy, oral residue defined on videofluoroscopy was underestimated and pharyngeal immobility was overestimated by an average of 6% and 10%, respectively.

The potential added value of using scintigraphy as a research tool and part of comprehensive swallowing management is the ability to collect an accurate measure of swallowing efficiency and measure therapeutic outcomes (Shaw et al., 2004). However, it is expensive and it has been recognized that in the absence of ready access to scintigraphy, a perceptual measure such as OPSE used by a trained rater allows for comparison of patient performance on subsequent videofluoroscopic examinations (Logemann et al., 2005).

Ultrasound

Ultrasound is an imaging procedure that can provide real-time two-, three-, and four-dimensional images of swallowing. Other developments include Doppler, duplex, and Time-Motion ultrasonic images. Detailed reviews of these techniques in relation to swallowing have been published (Chi-Fishman, 2005; Watkin, 1999). The process involves the placement of a probe, usually submentally, through which ultrasound signals are transmitted. The importance of a higher resolution probe has also been emphasized to obtain optimal images (Watkin, 1999). The transmitted sounds are then reflected from the internal structures of the body and monitored during swallowing. This information is then converted into video images.

Ultrasound is low cost, requires no radiation or contrast medium, and is repeatable. It has generated interest in the literature, particularly with reference to the infant and pediatric population (Geddes, Chadwick, Kent, Garbin, & Hartmann, 2010; Jadcherla et al., 2006; Yang, Loveday, Metreweli, & Sullivan, 1997). Given the placement of the probe, it has been of particular interest in the study of lingual function (Chi-Fishman, 2005). It has also been used to chart hyoid movement (Chi-Fishman & Sonies, 2002; Sonies, Wang, & Sapper, 1996; Yabunaka et al., 2011) and using ultrasound can have benefits in measuring cross-sectional area and tissue composition in the geniohyoid muscle in normal adults and head and neck cancer patients (Watkin et al., 2001). Other studies have examined the benefit of ultrasound in the analysis of lateral pharyngeal wall movement (Miller & Watkin, 1997). The potential to observe vocal fold closure has also been reported in the literature (Jadcherla et al., 2006).

While studies have highlighted that ultrasound has the potential to provide important instrumental information regarding anatomical changes following rehabilitation, a number of limitations have been reported. Although ultrasound is beneficial in the assessment of soft tissue, a limitation of this technique is that the ultrasound signal is subject to noise, and artifacts, and is reflected (Chi-Fishman, 2005). This is particularly relevant when the ultrasound signal comes into contact with bone and reaches air, and a limitation of the technique is that aspiration cannot be evaluated directly (Willging, Miller, Thompson Link, & Rudolph, 2001).

Videofluoroscopy

Videofluoroscopy is often led by an SLP working in close partnership with radiographers and radiologists. Its primary purpose is to evaluate the nature and extent of oropharyngeal dysphagia using a range of food and fluid consistencies in varying amounts. Foods and fluids are infused with contrast agents including barium sulfate or water-soluble nonionic isotonic agents (such as Omnipaque or Gastromiro). Water-soluble nonionic contrast should be used particularly where high levels of aspiration are anticipated (New Zealand Speech-Language Therapist's Association (NZSTA), 2011; Royal College of Speech and Language Therapists (RCSLT), 2006) as these are proven to cause no toxic effects to the lung tissue (Auffermann, Geisel, Wohlmann, & Günther, 1988). Patients are viewed both laterally and in the anterior-posterior (AP) plane. As a result of the observations of the assessing SLP, compensatory strategies can be implemented if necessary and radiologically evaluated. After close analysis, a targeted rehabilitation program can be designed based on the evaluation.

Although standardized procedures have been reported in the literature (Logemann, 1993), most centers adopt their own protocols. Validated rating scales can be employed to classify observations such as Oropharyngeal Swallowing Efficiency (OPSE) (Rademaker, Pauloski, Logemann, & Shanahan, 1994) and the Penetration-Aspiration Scale (Rosenbek, Robbins, Roecker, Coyle, & Wood, 1996).

More recently, there has been move towards improved standardized reporting of videofluoroscopic studies (Martin-Harris et al., 2008). The added benefit of videofluoroscopy is the ability to use the recorded images as a baseline upon which to re-evaluate swallowing performance as well as supporting patient education on the rationale for swallowing rehabilitation.

Although videofluoroscopy has become probably the most used instrumental swallowing evaluation, a number of issues have been raised in the literature. The term *instrumental* is used rather than *objective* as it has been highlighted that there are potentially issues around inter- and intrarater reliability when interpreting swallowing events (Kuhlemeier, Yates, & Palmer, 1998; Scott, Perry, & Bench, 1998). Videofluoroscopy suites vary in accessibility: non-ambulant patients may not be able to access the facilities or positioning may not be representative of "real-life" situations.

The number of personnel required to participate in the examination may vary. Professional guidelines highlight that it is best practice that in addition to the examining SLP and radiographer, a radiologist should be present for the examination where possible (American Speech-Language-Hearing Association [ASHA], 2004; New Zealand Speech-Language Therapist's Association [NZSTA], 2011; Royal College of Speech and Language Therapists [RCSLT], 2006). With pressure on radiology departments, procedures increasingly take place in the absence of a radiologist (who may be replaced by a second SLP with expertise in dysphagia). In the event that there is a highly unusual presentation or concerns beyond the SLP and radiographer's scope of practice such as severe esophageal stage problems, a radiologist's opinion should be sought to evaluate and advise on further investigations. As well as releasing radiologists to continue with other procedures, an evaluation of SLP-radiographer led clinics have led to reports of increased capacity, reduced waiting times, improved reporting procedures, and no adverse events relating to radiation dose (Newman & Nightingale, 2011).

Videofluoroscopy involves the use of x-rays and this can be of concern to patients and clinicians. Deterministic and nondeterministic effects have been described in the literature (Zammit-Maempel, Chapple, & Leslie, 2007). Deterministic effects are defined as detrimental effects that occur above a certain radiation dose. This is reported to be a rare incident in diagnostic radiology departments except in the case of lengthy interventional procedures. Nondeterministic effects are described as mutations arising at a cellular level and potentially leading to hereditary effects or cancer induction. In light of these potential effects, radiologists and radiographers in the United Kingdom are legally required to limit the radiation dose, adhering to the ALARP (as low as reasonably practicable) principle (IR[ME]R, 2000).

FEES

Practicalities such as patient suitability and lack of access to videofluoroscopy have highlighted the need for an examination which can detect pathological features of the swallow and allow for management decisions to be made and treatment to commence. Since 1988, FEES has emerged as an additional technique in evaluating patients with oropharyngeal dysphagia (Langmore, Schatz, & Olsen, 1988). FEES is a comprehensive evaluation which includes:

> an assessment of the anatomy and physiology of the pharyngeal and laryngeal muscles; an assessment of the swallowing function and a therapeutic examination to determine which of a variety postural, dietary, and behavioral strategies might facilitate safer and more efficient swallowing. (Langmore, 2001a, p. 2)

In 1997 a trademark was approved for the acronym FEES to ensure that the procedure was a comprehensive evaluation as described and not simply to identify dysphagia or aspiration (Langmore, 2001a).

A fiberoptic nasendoscope is passed transnasally allowing the SLP to directly view the laryngopharyngeal structures, and movements, and evaluate sensation (Langmore, 2003); see Figures 2–1 and 2–2 in grayscale below and in a more realistic, full-color view in the color insert. The FEES procedure has been documented in detail in the literature (Langmore & Aviv, 2001). The endoscope is connected

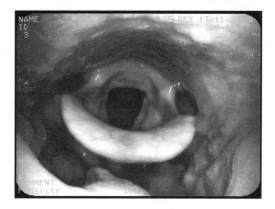

Figure 2–1. *Image showing the scope in the high position.*

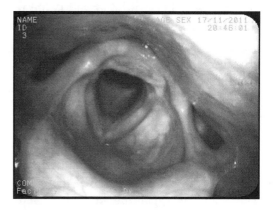

Figure 2–2. *Image showing the scope in the low position.*

to a camera, light source, and monitor with audiovisual recording equipment. When the scope has been positioned and prior to commencing swallowing trials, assessment of velar and laryngopharyngeal anatomy, movement and sensation is conducted. This includes an evaluation of the hypopharynx and larynx at rest, management of secretions and swallowing frequency. Tongue base, pharyngeal, and laryngeal function is also evaluated. Sensory testing can be achieved by touching the structures with the tip of the scope. It has been argued that, although FEES and videofluoroscopy assess the motor component of swallowing, neither directly evaluates sensation (Aviv, 2000). As a result, the FEES procedure has been adapted to include sensory testing by delivering pulses of air to the pharyngeal mucosa innervated by the superior laryngeal nerve. This has been achieved by the addition of an internal port a specially adapted endoscope. The procedure was first described in 1998 and is known as fiberoptic endoscopic evaluation of swallowing with sensory testing (FEEST) (Aviv et al., 1998).

On completion of the first section of the evaluation, the swallowing examination can commence. One of the advantages is that patients can be observed eating real food, and compensatory strategies can be implemented as required during the examination. Green or blue dye is added to food and liquid to clearly distinguish them from the pharyngeal mucosa. The clinician can report on a range of swallowing features including penetration, aspiration, and pharyngeal stasis. Given the placement of the scope, it is not possible to view the oral phase of the swallow. Although events prior to and post swallow are viewed using FEES, the pharyngeal swallow itself is not. Whiteout occurs during the swallow as the structures contract around the scope. This occurs when light emitted from the scope is reflected off the tissues back in to the lens of the scope. Depending on the height of

the scope, whiteout occurs during the swallow either due to the velum or the tongue base contacting the posterior pharyngeal wall (Murray, 2001).

The patient can view the examination in real time on a suitably positioned monitor, and can also be recorded for analysis by the clinician as part of rehabilitation planning as well as being shown to patients to enhance their understanding of their difficulties. Portability (particularly for those patients for whom positioning and medical status are issues) and repeatability in the absence of radiation risk are examples of the significant advantages of using FEES (Wu, Hsiao, Chen, Chang, & Lee, 1997). With equipment such as the Kay-Pentax Digital Swallowing Workstation (Kay Elemetrics, Lincoln Park), additional parameters can be evaluated such as respiration during the swallow and surface electromyography.

SLPs are specialists in the assessment and management of oropharyngeal dysphagia and after completion of specified training and a recognition of the practice as part of their role, they can carry out FEES independently (ASHA, 2005; RCSLT, 2005). As with any instrumental evaluation of swallowing, the patient's medical lead should be informed of the plan to carry out FEES. Concerns have been raised by otolaryngologists regarding the implementation of FEES by SLP services. Hiss and Postma (2003) state that these concerns include the potential diagnosis of anatomical disease by SLPs outside their scope of practice or a failure to recognize potential disease in the absence of an otolaryngologist. They also reiterate the importance of clarifying the purpose of the FEES evaluation and the development of local policies to reflect this. FEES and videofluoroscopy are assessments utilized as part of a multidisciplinary approach to comprehensive dysphagia management and where possible, FEES should be carried out with an otolaryngologist present. In the event that this is not possible, the recorded examination should be reviewed at a later time with both specialists offering their opinion in their area of expertise (Hiss & Postma, 2003). It is specified that in certain situations, an otolaryngologist should be present, for example in patients with movement disorders, skull base and facial fractures, and following skull base surgery (RCSLT, 2005).

A number of potential complications have been reported during FEES including vasovagal attack (overstimulation of the vagus nerve resulting in a drop in blood pressure and heart rate), epistaxis (bleeding from the nose) and laryngospasm (spasm of the vocal cords resulting in closure of the airway). In a study of 500 examinations in 253 patients over a 2½ year period, only 3 cases of epistaxis were noted and no airway compromise or significant change in heart rate was recorded (Aviv et al., 2000). In addition, 81% of patients rated their levels of discomfort as either "no discomfort" or "mild." When considering comfort of the patient, nasal decongestant and/or topical anesthesia may be used if required. Nasal decongestants constrict the small blood vessels and therefore induce shrinkage of the tissues (ASHA, 2005). However, routine use of local anesthesia is not recommended as it may impact on sensory features of the swallow (RCSLT, 2005). If topical anesthesia is to be used, it should only be applied to the nasal passages, and the use of aerosols rather than gels can increase the risk of the anesthetic reaching the pharynx (ASHA, 2005). While the evidence is reported to be unclear regarding the benefits of decongestants and anesthesia, it is suggested that their use may alleviate anxiety and improve comfort for those undergoing the procedure (ASHA, 2005). However, FEES can be performed safely without anesthesia, and in most cases the use of lubrication gel applied to the scope minimizes discomfort (RCSLT, 2005).

There are no restrictive screening times with FEES, therefore enabling clinicians to observe for potential fatigue effect. It also provides useful biofeedback for patients who are able to view examinations in real time thus supporting the rehabilitation process. This biofeedback is beneficial when trialing new compensatory techniques such as a supraglottic swallow, where research has shown that patients are not always successful in closing their vocal folds under instruction (Hirst, Sama, Carding, & Wilson, 1998; Figure 2–3 in grayscale below and in full color in the color insert). Viewing images has now been greatly improved with the introduction of chip-tip camera endoscopes.

FEES or VFSS?

A number of research studies and review articles have been published to establish the relative benefits of each procedure from a variety of perspectives (Aviv, 2000; Aviv, Sataloff, et al., 2001; Kidder, Langmore, & Martin, 1994; Langmore, Schatz, & Olson, 1991; Madden, Fenton, Hughes, & Timon, 2000; Périé et al., 1998; Wu, Hsiao, Chen, Chang, & Lee, 1997). High levels of sensitivity and specificity have been reported between the procedures. Crucially, few studies report on simultaneous evaluation of swallowing events with FEES

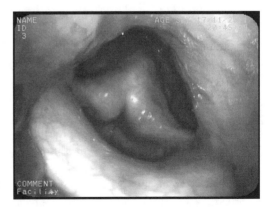

Figure 2–3. *Image showing a voluntary breathhold used in the supraglottic swallowing maneuver.*

and videofluoroscopy (Kelly, Drinnan, & Leslie, 2007; Kelly, Leslie, Beale, Payten, & Drinnan, 2006; Logemann, Rademaker, Pauloski, Ohmae, & Kahrilas, 1998; Rao, Brady, Chauduri, Donzelli, & Wesling, 2003).

An important factor for consideration in the FEES evaluation is the position of the scope as this potentially affects interpretation of the swallowing events. Important data have been reported on scope positioning during the swallow evaluation and its significance in relation to which areas of the pharynx the clinician wants to view (Logemann, Rademaker, Pauloski, Ohmae, & Kahrilas, 1998). They reported that the tip of the scope should be positioned just below the uvula to view the pharyngeal structures and below the tip of the epiglottis to view the laryngeal structures. Twelve features of the oropharyngeal swallow were analyzed, with two swallows on each with the scope repositioned to the high (see Figure 2–1) or low position (see Figure 2–2) for each one. This found that videofluoroscopy offered the most comprehensive view of the pharyngeal swallow as hyoid movement, laryngeal closure at the airway entrance, cricopharyngeal opening and tongue base to posterior pharyngeal wall contact can be observed. Conversely, the onset, extent, and completion of arytenoid movement and vocal fold closure were only observable on FEES. However, neither procedure was found to observe the duration of vocal fold closure during the swallow.

Standardized reporting procedures have been developed for videofluoroscopy and FEES (Langmore, 2001b; Logemann, 1993; Martin-Harris et al., 2008). Unlike videofluoroscopy, during FEES it is possible to view pharyngeal secretions, the presence of which may be an important predictor of aspiration, and a secretion rating scale has been developed to document this (Murray, Langmore, Ginsberg, & Dostie, 1996). Other scales have been validated for use with FEES and videofluoroscopic studies such as the Penetration-Aspiration Scale (PAS), an 8-point clinical scale used by SLPs to rate the depth of penetration and aspiration and airway clearance (Rosenbek, Robbins, Roecker, Coyle, & Wood, 1996; Colodny, 2002; see Chapter 16).

Two recent studies have compared videofluoroscopy and FEES simultaneously with respect to aspiration and penetration (Kelly et al., 2007) and pharyngeal residue (Kelly et al., 2006). Fifteen dysphagia specialist SLPs were required to score the examinations having been blinded to which examinations were paired. Fifteen adults with dysphagia of mixed etiology were assessed for pharyngeal residue and PAS scores. They found that FEES residue scores were consistently higher for FEES than videofluoroscopy. Similarly, penetration and aspiration were perceived to be more severe on FEES than videofluoroscopy. These studies have highlighted that FEES and videofluoroscopy should not be considered as interchangeable procedures, as observed features may suggest improvement or deterioration in swallowing function with different assessment modalities.

In addition to the relative benefits of each procedure, a preliminary study concluded that FEES (with sensory testing) was more cost-effective than videofluoroscopy (Aviv et al., 2001).

CONCLUSION

Although a number of imaging methods have been reported in the literature, videofluoroscopy and FEES continue to be the most commonly used assessments in the evaluation of swallowing physiology and rehabilitation planning. Following an evidence-based technical review, it was reported that each yields false-negative and false-positive results (Agency for Health Care Policy and Research, March 1999). Videofluoroscopy allows for a comprehensive evaluation of swallowing physiology which also enables the clinician to implement compensatory procedures and plan ongoing rehabilitation. FEES is a valuable addition and should complement rather than replace videofluoroscopy in the comprehensive assessment of swallowing disorders. However, given the practicalities of accessing videofluoroscopy for those patients with more extensive physical disability and precarious medical status, FEES offers the potential for an extensive, repeatable assessment of the pharyngeal swallow.

The evaluation of oropharyngeal dysphagia requires the SLP to understand the nature of the swallowing disorder using a variety of textures and bolus sizes. Furthermore, the purpose of the instrumental swallowing evaluation includes the option to implement swallowing strategies and design a targeted rehabilitation program. Other techniques have been developed to enhance our understanding of swallowing such as ultrasound and scintigraphy, each offering potential benefits as research tools and methods of evaluating rehabilitation outcomes. However, these techniques do not provide the breadth of information re-quired to understand the nature and extent of any oropharyngeal dysphagia and plan intervention.

Although clinicians and researchers work to consolidate existing instrumental evaluation methods and identify novel assessment techniques, assessment tools are only as good as the clinician interpreting them. Misdiagnosis of a swallowing disorder may result in inappropriate, potentially life-threatening management of patients and valuable therapeutic resources may be misdirected (Murray, 2009). In addition, swallowing evaluation needs to be multidimensional and tailored to the needs and wishes of the patient. There is a need for increased standardization of procedures and education programs to ensure that maximum benefit is derived from instrumental evaluation to inform the rehabilitation process. Although techniques such as ultrasound and scintigraphy offer additional insights into swallowing function, FEES offers its own particular advantages and should be available as a valuable adjunct to the evaluation and rehabilitation process. However, videofluoroscopy remains the most comprehensive evaluation of oropharyngeal dysphagia and can guide management to other evaluation techniques as necessary.

REFERENCES

Agency for Health Care Policy and Research. (March 1999). *Diagnosis and treatment of swallowing disorders (Dysphagia).* Rockville, MD: Author.

American Speech-Language-Hearing Association. (2000). *Clinical indicators for instrumental assessment of oropharyngeal dysphagia* [Guidelines]. Retrieved January 8, 2011, from http://www.asha.org/policy

American Speech-Language-Hearing Association (ASHA). (2004). *Guidelines for speech-language pathologists performing videofluoroscopic swallowing studies.* Retrieved January 8, 2011, from http://www.asha.org/policy

American Speech-Language-Hearing Association. (2005). *The role of the speech-language pathologist in the performance and interpretation of endoscopic evaluation of swallowing: Technical report.* Retrieved January 8, 2011, from http://www.asha.org/policy

Andrus, J. G., Dolan, R. W., & Anderson, T. D. (2005). Transnasal esophagoscopy: A high-yield diagnostic tool. *Laryngoscope, 115*(6), 993–996.

Auffermann, W., Geisel, T., Wohlmann, D., & Günther, R. W. (1988). Tissue reaction following endobronchial application of iopamidol and ioxithalamate in rats. *European Journal of Radiology, 8,* 13–17.

Aviv, J. E. (2000). Prospective, randomized outcome study of endoscopy versus modified barium swallow in patients with dysphagia. *Laryngoscope, 110*(4), 563–574.

Aviv, J. E. (2006). Transnasal esophagoscopy: State of the art. *Otolaryngology—Head and Neck Surgery, 135*(4), 616–619.

Aviv, J. E., Kaplan, S. T., Thomson, J. E., Spitzer, J., Diamond, B., & Close, L. G. (2000). The safety of flexible endoscopic evaluation of swallowing with sensory testing (FEESST): An analysis of 500 consecutive evaluations. *Dysphagia, 15*(1), 39–44.

Aviv, J. E., Kim, T., Sacco, R. L., Kaplan, S., Goodhart, K., Diamond, B., & Close, L. G. (1998). FEESST: A new bedside endoscopic test of the motor and sensory components of swallowing. *Annals of Otology, Rhinology, and Laryngology, 107*(5 Pt 1), 378–387.

Aviv, J. E., Sataloff, R. T., Cohen, M., Spitzer, J., Ma, G., Bhayani, R., & Close, L. G. (2001). Cost-effectiveness of two types of dysphagia care in head and neck cancer: A preliminary report. *Ear, Nose, and Throat Journal, 80*(8), 553–556, 558.

Butler, S.G. (2009, May 26). The role of pharyngeal and esophageal manometry in swallowing assessment. *ASHA Leader.*

Chi-Fishman, G. (2005). Quantitative lingual, pharyngeal and laryngeal ultrasonography in swallowing research: A technical review. *Clinical Linguistics and Phonetics, 19*(6–7), 589–604.

Chi-Fishman, G., & Sonies, B. C. (2002). Kinematic strategies for hyoid movement in rapid sequential swallowing. *Journal of Speech, Language, and Hearing Research, 45*(3), 457–468.

Colodny, N. (2002). Interjudge and intrajudge reliabilities in fiberoptic endoscopic evaluation of swallowing (FEES) using the penetration-aspiration scale: A replication study. *Dysphagia, 17*(4), 308–315.

Crary, M. A., Mann, G. D., & Groher, M. E. (2005). Initial psychometric assessment of a functional oral intake scale for dysphagia in stroke patients. *Archives of Physical Medicine and Rehabilitation, 86*(8), 1516–1520.

DePippo, K. L., Holas, M. A., & Reding, M. J. (1992). Validation of the 3-oz water swallow test for aspiration following stroke. *Archives of Neurology, 49*(12), 1259–1261.

Fox, M., & Bredenoord, A. (2008). Oesophageal high-resolution manometry: Moving research into clinical practice. *Gut, 57*, 405–423.

Fujii, N., Inamoto, Y., Saitoh, E., Baba, M., Okada, S., Yoshioka, S., . . . Palmer, J. B. (2011). Evaluation of swallowing using 320-detector-row multislice CT. Part I: single- and multiphase volume scanning for three-dimensional morphological and kinematic analysis. *Dysphagia, 26*(2), 99–107.

Geddes, D. T., Chadwick, L. M., Kent, J. C., Garbin, C. P., & Hartmann, P. E. (2010). Ultrasound imaging of infant swallowing during breast-feeding. *Dysphagia, 25*(3), 183–191.

Ghosh, S. K., Pandolfino, J. E., Zhang, Q., Jarosz, A., & Kahrilas, P. J. (2006). Deglutitive upper esophageal sphincter relaxation: A study of 75 volunteer subjects using solid-state high-resolution manometry. *American Journal of Physiology—Gastrointestinal and Liver Physiology, 291*, G525–531.

Goldsmith, T. (2003). Videofluoroscopic evaluation of oropharyngeal swallowing. In P. M. Som & H. D. Curtin (Eds.), *Head and neck imaging* (4th ed., Vol. 2, pp. 1727–1754). St. Louis, MO: Mosby.

Hamlet, S., Faull, J., Klein, B., Aref, A., Fontanesi, J., Stachler, R., . . . Simpson, M. (1997). Mastication and swallowing in patients with postirradiation xerostomia. *International Journal of Radiation Oncology, Biology, Physics, 37*(4), 789–796.

Hartl, D. M., Albiter, M., Kolb, F., Luboinski, B. & Sigal, R. (2003). Morphologic parameters of normal swallowing events using single-shot fast spin echo dynamic MRI. *Dysphagia, 18*(4), 255–262.

Hartl, D. M., Kolb, F., Bretagne, E., Bidault, F., & Sigal, R. (2010). Cine-MRI swallowing evaluation after tongue reconstruction. *European Journal of Radiology, 73*(1), 108–113.

Hirst, L. J., Sama, A., Carding, P. N. & Wilson, J. A. (1998). Is a "safe swallow" really safe? *International Journal of Language and Communication Disorders, 33*(Suppl.), 279–280.

Hiss, S. G., & Huckabee, M. L. (2005) Timing of pharyngeal and upper esophageal sphincter pressures as a function of normal and effortful swallowing in young healthy adults. *Dysphagia, 20*, 149–156.

Hiss, S. G., & Postma, G. N. (2003). Fiberoptic endoscopic evaluation of swallowing. *Laryngoscope, 113*(8), 1386–1393.

Hughes, T. A., & Wiles, C. M. (1996). Clinical measurement of swallowing in health and in neurogenic dysphagia. *Quarterly Journal of Medicine, 89*(2), 109–116.

Humbert, I. A., & Robbins, J. (2007). Normal swallowing and functional magnetic resonance imaging: A systematic review. *Dysphagia, 22*(3), 266–275.

Ionising Radiation (Medical Exposure) Regulations. (2000). London, UK: The Stationary Office.

Inamoto, Y., Fujii, N., Saitoh, E., Baba, M., Okada, S., Katada, K., . . . Palmer, J. B. (2011). Evaluation of swallowing using 320-detector-row multislice CT. Part II: Kinematic analysis of laryngeal closure during normal swallowing. *Dysphagia, 26*(3), 209–217.

Jadcherla, S. R., Gupta, A., Stoner, E., Coley, B. D., Wiet, G. J., & Shaker, R. (2006). Correlation of glottal closure using concurrent ultrasonography and nasolaryngoscopy in children: A novel approach to evaluate glottal status. *Dysphagia, 21*(1), 75–81.

Jensen, K., Lambertsen, K., Torkov, P., Dahl, M., Jensen, A. B., & Grau, C. (2007). Patient assessed symptoms are poor predictors of objective findings. Results from a cross-sectional study in patients treated with radiotherapy for pharyngeal cancer. *Acta Oncologica, 46*(8), 1159–1168.

Kelly, A. M., Drinnan, M. J., & Leslie, P. (2007). Assessing penetration and aspiration: How do videofluoroscopy and fiberoptic endoscopic evaluation of swallowing compare? *Laryngoscope, 117*(10), 1723–1727.

Kelly, A. M., Leslie, P. Beale, T., Payten, C., & Drinnan, M. J. (2006). Fibreoptic endoscopic evaluation of swallowing and videofluoroscopy: Does examination type influence perception of pharyngeal residue severity? *Clinical Otolaryngology, 31*(5), 425–432.

Kidder, T. M., Langmore, S. E., & Martin, B. J. (1994). Indications and techniques of endoscopy in evaluation of cervical dysphagia: Comparison with radiographic techniques. *Dysphagia, 9*(4), 256–261.

Kreeft, A. M., Rasch, C. R., Muller, S. H., Pameijer, F. A., Hallo, E., & Balm, A. J. (2012). Cine MRI of swallowing in patients with advanced oral or oropharyngeal carcinoma: A feasibility study. *European Archives of Otorhinolaryngology.* doi:10.1007/s00405-011-1861-y

Kuhlemeier, K. V., Yates, P., & Palmer, J. B. (1998). Intra- and interrater variation in the evaluation of videofluorographic swallowing studies. *Dysphagia, 13*(3), 142–147.

Langmore, S. E. (2001a). The role of endoscopy in the evaluation and treatment of swallowing disorders. In S. E. Langmore (Ed.), *Endoscopic evaluation and treatment of swallowing disorders.* New York, NY: Thieme.

Langmore, S. E. (2001b). Scoring a FEES examination. In S. E. Langmore (Ed.), *Endoscopic evaluation and treatment of swallowing disorders.* New York, NY: Thieme.

Langmore, S. E. (2003). Evaluation of oropharyngeal dysphagia: Which diagnostic tool is superior? *Current Opinion in Otolaryngology and Head and Neck Surgery, 11*, 485–489.

Langmore, S. E., & Aviv, J. E. (2001). Endoscopic evaluation of oropharyngeal swallowing. In S. E. Langmore (Ed.), *Endoscopic evaluation and treatment of swallowing disorders.* New York, NY: Thieme.

Langmore, S. E., Schatz, K., & Olsen, N. (1988). Fiberoptic endoscopic examination of swallowing safety: A new procedure. *Dysphagia, 2*(4), 216–219.

Langmore, S. E., Schatz, K., & Olson, N. (1991) Endoscopic and videofluoroscopic evaluations of swallowing and aspiration. *Annals of Otology, Rhinology, and Laryngology, 100*(8), 678–681.

Logemann, J. A. (1993). *Manual for the videofluorographic study of swallowing* (2nd ed.). Austin, TX: Pro-Ed.

Logemann, J. A. (1998). *Evaluation and Treatment of Swallowing Disorders.* Austin, TX: Pro-Ed.

Logemann, J. A., Rademaker, A. W., Pauloski, B. R., Ohmae, Y., & Kahrilas, P. J. (1998). Normal swallowing physiology as viewed by videofluoroscopy and videoendoscopy. *Folia Phoniatrica et Logopaedica, 50*(6), 311–319.

Logemann, J. A., Williams, R. B., Rademaker, A., Pauloski, B. R., Lazarus, C. L., & Cook, I. (2005). The relationship between observations and measures of oral and pharyngeal residue from videofluorography and scintigraphy. *Dysphagia 20*(3), 226–231.

Madden, C., Fenton, J., Hughes, J., & Timon, C. (2000). Comparison between videofluoroscopy and milk-swallow endoscopy in the assessment of swallowing function. *Clinical Otolaryngology and Allied Sciences*, *25*(6), 504–506.

Martin-Harris, B., Brodsky, M. B., Michel, Y., Castell, D. O., Schleicher, M., Sandidge, J., . . . Blair, J. (2008). MBS measurement tool for swallow impairment — MBSImp: Establishing a standard. *Dysphagia*, *23*(4), 392–405.

McCulloch, T. M., Hoffman, M. R., & Ciucci, M. R. (2010). High-resolution manometry of pharyngeal swallow pressure events associated with head turn and chin tuck. *Annals of Otolaryngology Rhinology and Laryngology*, *119*, 369–376.

Miller, J. L., & Watkin, K. L. (1997). Lateral pharyngeal wall motion during swallowing using real time ultrasound. *Dysphagia 12*(3), 125–132.

Murray, J. (2001). Endoscopic mechanics and technique. In S. E. Langmore (Ed.), *Endoscopic evaluation and treatment of swallowing disorders*. New York, NY: Thieme.

Murray, J. (2009). Food for thought: Self-criticism and raising the bar of dysphagia practice. *Perspectives on Swallowing and Swallowing Disorders (Dysphagia) — American Speech-Language-Hearing Association Division*, *18*(2), 68–77.

Murray, J., Langmore, S. E., Ginsberg, S., & Dostie, A. (1996). The significance of accumulated oropharyngeal secretions and swallowing frequency in predicting aspiration. *Dysphagia*, *11*(2), 99–103.

New Zealand Speech-Language Therapist's Association (NZSTA). (2011). *New Zealand Speech-Language Therapy clinical practice guideline on videofluoroscopic study of swallowing (VFSS)*. Author.

Newman, R. D., & Nightingale, J. (2011). Improving patient access to videofluoroscopy services: Role of the practitioner-led clinic. *Radiography*, *17*(4), 280–283.

Patterson, J. M., Hildreth, A., McColl, E., Carding, P. N., Hamilton, D., & Wilson, J. A. (2010). The clinical application of the 100-mL water swallow test in head and neck cancer. *Oral Oncology*, *47*(3), 180–184.

Patterson, J. M., McColl, E., Carding, P. N., Kelly, C., & Wilson, J. A. (2009). Swallowing performance in patients with head and neck cancer: A simple clinical test. *Oral Oncology*, *45*(10), 904–907.

Pauloski, B. R., Rademaker, A. W., Lazarus, C., Boeckxstaens, G., Kahrilas, P. J., & Logemann, J. A. (2009). Relationship between manometric and videofluoroscopic measures of swallow function in healthy adults and patients treated for head and neck cancer with various modalities. *Dysphagia*, *24*(2), 196–203.

Peck, K. K., Branski, R. C., Lazarus, C., Cody, V., Kraus, D., Haupage, S., . . . Kraus, D. H. (2010). Cortical activation during swallowing rehabilitation maneuvers: A functional MRI study of healthy controls. *Laryngoscope*, *120*(11), 2153–2159.

Périé, S., Laccourreye, L., Flahault, A., Hazebroucq, V, Chaussade, S., & St Guily, J. L. (1998). Role of videoendoscopy in assessment of pharyngeal function in oropharyngeal dysphagia: Comparison with videofluoroscopy and manometry. *Laryngoscope*, *108* (11 pt. 1), 1712–1716.

Postma, G. N. (2006). Transnasal esophagoscopy. *Current Opinion in Otolaryngology and Head and Neck Surgery*, *14*(3), 156–158.

Rademaker, A. W., Pauloski, B. R., Logemann, J. A., & Shanahan, T. K. (1994). Oropharyngeal swallow efficiency as a representative measure of swallowing function. *Journal of Speech and Hearing Research*, *37*(2), 314–325.

Ramsey, D., Smithard, D., & Kalra, L. (2005). Silent aspiration: What do we know? *Dysphagia*, *20*(3), 218–225.

Rao, N., Brady, S. L., Chauduri, G., Donzelli, J. J. & Wesling, M. W. (2003). Gold-standard? Analysis of the videofluoroscopic and fiberoptic endoscopic swallow examinations. *Journal of Applied Research*, *3*(1), 89–96.

Rosenbek, J. C., Robbins, J. A., Roecker, E. B., Coyle, J. L., & Wood, J. L. (1996). A penetration-aspiration scale. *Dysphagia*, *11*(2), 93–98.

Royal College of Speech and Language Therapists (RCSLT). (2005). *Fibreoptic endoscopic evaluation of swallowing (FEES): The role of speech and language therapy*. RCSLT Policy Statement.

Royal College of Speech and Language Therapists (RCSLT). (2006). *Videofluoroscopic evaluation of oropharyngeal swallowing disorders (VFS) in adults: The role of speech and language therapists.* RCSLT Policy Statement.

Scott, A., Perry, A., & Bench, J. (1998). A study of interrater reliability when using videofluoroscopy as an assessment of swallowing. *Dysphagia, 13*(4), 223–227.

Shaw, D. W., Williams, R. B., Cook, I. J., Wallace, K. L., Weltman, M. D., Collins, P. J., . . . Simula, M. E. (2004). Oropharyngeal scintigraphy: A reliable technique for the quantitative evaluation of oral-pharyngeal swallowing. *Dysphagia, 19*(1), 36–42.

Sonies, B. C., Wang, C., & Sapper, D. J. (1996). Evaluation of normal and abnormal hyoid bone movement during swallowing by use of ultrasound duplex-Doppler imaging. *Ultrasound in Medicine and Biology, 22*(9), 1169–1175.

Threats, T. T. (2007). Use of the ICF in dysphagia management. *Seminars in Speech and Language, 28*(4), 323–333.

Ward, E. C., & Conroy, A. (1999). Validity, reliability and responsiveness of the Royal Brisbane Hospital Outcome Measure for Swallowing. *Asia Pacific Journal of Speech, Language, and Hearing, 4*, 109–129.

Watkin, K. L. (1999). Ultrasound and swallowing. *Folia Phoniatrica et Logopaedica, 51*(4–5), 183–198.

Watkin, K. L., Diouf, I., Gallagher, T. M., Logemann, J. A., Rademaker, A. W., & Ettema, S. L. (2001). Ultrasonic quantification of geniohyoid cross-sectional area and tissue composition: A preliminary study of age and radiation effects. *Head and Neck, 23*(6), 467–474.

Willging, J. P., Miller, C. K., Thompson Link, D., & Rudolph, C. D. (2001). The use of FEES to assess and manage pediatric patients. In S. E. Langmore (Ed.), *Endoscopic evaluation and treatment of swallowing disorders.* New York, NY: Thieme.

Wu, C. H., Hsiao, T. Y., Chen, J. C., Chang, Y. C., & Lee, S. Y. (1997). Evaluation of swallowing safety with fiberoptic endoscope: comparison with videofluoroscopic technique. *Laryngoscope, 107*(3), 396–401.

Yabunaka, K., Sanada, H., Sanada, S., Konishi, H., Hashimoto, T., Yatake, H., . . . Ohue, M. (2011). Sonographic assessment of hyoid bone movement during swallowing: A study of normal adults with advancing age. *Radiological Physics and Technology, 4*(1), 73–77.

Yang, W. T., Loveday, E. J., Metreweli, C., & Sullivan, P. B. (1997) Ultrasound assessment of swallowing in malnourished disabled children. *British Journal of Radiology, 70*(838), 992–994.

Zammit-Maempel, I., Chapple, C. L., & Leslie, P. (2007). Radiation dose in videofluoroscopic swallow studies. *Dysphagia, 22*(1), 13–15.

Chapter

3

IMPROVING PATIENT EXPERIENCE AND MINIMIZING RISK

Julie M. Nightingale, Tracy Lazenby-Paterson, and Hannah Crawford

INTRODUCTION

VFSS examinations have traditionally been undertaken by a speech-language pathologist (SLP) working alongside a radiologist and a radiographer (ASHA, 2004). Historically, the radiologists have led the imaging procedure as practitioner/operator (as defined by IR[ME]R 2000 legislation), operating the fluoroscopy equipment and providing the definitive radiological report. The role of the radiographer was typically managing session workflow, fluoroscopy suite preparation, recording of patient identity, and preparation of appropriate contrast agents. They assisted the radiologist in appropriate image capture and were responsible for the monitoring/recording of radiation dose.

However, in many clinical centers, particularly in the UK, a lack of clarity has existed over which profession should take overall responsibility for videofluoroscopy patients, in some cases resulting in stagnation of the VFSS service. The knowledge and expertise of the nonmedical health professionals was often undervalued in this medically dominated setting, a finding not unique to radiology (Department of Health, 2000).

Radiologists and SLPs rarely received formal education in the conduct of the VFSS procedure or the detailed evaluation required to interpret the images (Gates et al, 2006; Power et al, 2006). Indeed, a U.K. questionnaire survey identified a lack of VFSS standardization with some evidence of dangerous practice (Power et al., 2006). Recognizing this concern, the United Kingdom RCSLT (2007) published a guidance document aimed at improving standards in videofluoroscopy. Similar guidance has been issued for SLP practitioners within the United States (ASHA, 2004). This increasing professional interest in VFSS, combined with reducing radiologist availability, opened up opportunities for radiographers and SLPs to develop practitioner-led services. Extensions of the traditional radiographer and SLP roles have been reported in the United Kingdom and the United States (ASHA, 2004), including VFSS image acquisition, protocol formation and selection, image interpretation, and clinical reporting. Following completion of relevant education, a range of practitioner-led VFSS clinic improvements have been reported, related to communication, protocols, safety, quality assurance and audit (Nightingale & Mackay, 2009). Longer term follow-up of a practitioner-led clinic has identified significantly improved patient access, reduced hospital stays, and improved report turnaround times (Newman & Nightingale, 2011).

With the introduction of new VFSS working practices and increased roles and responsibilities, comes a requirement to ensure that any service changes are ultimately introduced in the best interests of the patient. Although this requirement is paramount, any steps to secure and improve patient experience and outcomes will conversely also protect the medicolegal and professional interests of the health professionals involved in the service. This chapter explores the potential for patient physical or emotional distress within the VFSS examination, and identifies ways of improving patient and carer experience and minimizing medicolegal risk. Although the evidence reviewed is primarily from the United Kingdom, the principles discussed within this chapter are directly transferable to other health care systems.

THE PATIENT EXPERIENCE

Quality in health care consists of two related but distinct components. Technical or outcome quality is most frequently measured in health care, and in medical imaging in particular. However, the quality of service delivery, as perceived by the patient, is increasingly considered to be of value (Ondategui-Parra et al, 2006).

Analyzing and understanding the patient experience to improve the quality of care is now of paramount importance within the National Health Service (NHS), following a political steer to drive forward individualized patient-focused care (DoH, 2008). The NHS Constitution for England was published in January 2009, giving patients information regarding their rights within the health service, including choice, consent, confidentiality, dignity, and privacy (DoH, 2009). Increasingly, there has been recognition within government that one cannot measure heath care with targets and outcomes alone:

> Quality of care includes the quality of caring. This means how personal care is—the compassion, dignity and respect with which patients are treated. It can only be improved by analysing and understanding patient satisfaction with their own experiences. (High Quality Care for All: NHS Next Stage Review Final Report, 2008)

Traditionally, health outcomes have been defined by professionals and these may differ from those of importance to patients (Sitzia & Wood, 1997). Understanding the experiences of patients is important, as they are capable of "providing insights that complement or even "counterbalance" those of health professionals and researchers" (Mathers et al., 2006). There are several reasons for this growing interest in patient experience: patients are increasingly seen as consumers of health care (particularly so in many countries with a largely private health care system), with a greater emphasis on choices of provider. Growing access to private health care in the United Kingdom, as well as NHS patients experiencing NHS-purchased private health care, has led to increasing public expectations of health care delivery. Where expectations are not met, dissatisfied patients are increasingly more likely to make complaints or pursue legal action. The National Audit Office in 2008 estimated that over three years, 88% of adults in England had contact with the NHS, yet 13% were in some way dissatisfied with their experience. In 2006 to 2007, the NHS received 133,400 written complaints: the estimated cost of handling and review of these complaints was £89 million (NAO, 2008). The costs of handling health care complaints and subsequent litigation is spiraling in many countries.

CONSEQUENCES OF A POOR PATIENT EXPERIENCE

A complaint can be defined as "an expression of dissatisfaction, disquiet or discontent about the actions, decisions or apparent failings of service provision which requires a response" (NAO, 2008). The number of complaints about the NHS is rising each year, and in 2011 it reached over one million a year. The number of patients seeking independent review from the health ombudsman (independent adjudicator) has also risen (*Guardian*, 2011). There are several possible reasons for this rise, including worsening NHS care, increased demand for health care and better awareness of the complaints process.

Patients may be dissatisfied with their care, yet the majority of them do not make a formal complaint. They may complain informally to health care staff, or they may decide to do nothing, usually because they believe it will not make a difference (NAO, 2008). Scrutiny of local patient satisfaction and patient experience surveys can give some indication of the areas of the service that result in dissatisfaction, so that these can be addressed. However, there are several possible reasons for dissatisfaction to become a formal complaint:

- They believe that their care has fallen below the required standard;
- Their treatment was not explained thoroughly or in a way they could comprehend;

- They believe they were not treated with dignity, consideration and courtesy;
- Their reasonable requests were ignored or refused; and/or
- They were discharged from care before fully fit.

In some cases their complaint may not be upheld, often because they may have had unrealistic expectations. However, insufficient explanations and information offered as part of the informed consent process often underlie these raised expectations.

Although most complaints will be sent direct to a hospital, some complaints may be made direct to a professional registration body: for radiographers and speech and language therapists in the United Kingdom this would be the Health Professions Council, and for radiologists it would be the General Medical Council. Historically, the majority of complaints about professional suitability were made by employers, but for the first time in 2011 the majority of complaints against individual practitioners were from patients (Health Professions Council, 2011).

Complaints are not the only area of concern for health professionals, with the potential for legal action where a patient's concerns have not been addressed. The focus of legal actions against any health professional is more likely to be on the nature of the information given to, or withheld from a patient, prior to examination or treatment. Where a patient has suffered harm as a result of the procedure, they may pursue legal action under the tort of negligence. To succeed in a negligence case, a plaintiff has to prove (Jones, 2000) that:

- They were owed a duty of care;
- The standard of care was below that required;
- Harm has occurred;
- There was causation linking the standard of care and any harm caused; and
- There is a potential for damages

PATIENT EXPERIENCE AND THE VFSS SERVICE

There are a number of aspects of the VFSS service that have the potential to cause the patient and their carers/relatives distress, and thus provoke subsequent complaints or litigation.

The VFSS Service

Complaints within radiology often are associated with long referral to test waiting times, although in the United Kingdom all "nonurgent" patients should now be treated within a maximum waiting time frame. Waiting beyond appointment times while in the imaging department is also a cause of dissatisfaction. Many complaints relate to poor staff-patient communication, and a perceived loss of dignity and privacy, including patient confidentiality issues.

The VFSS Imaging Procedure

A substandard imaging procedure, even if not identified as such by the patient, has the potential to result in an incorrect report, and subsequent patient mismanagement. Evidence-based protocols linked with service audit reduce procedural variation and are likely to improve standards of performance. However, patients can experience distress and even harm within the VFSS procedure. Physical causes of potential harm include the risk of radiation and in women of child-bearing age the potential for exposure in utero. Physical injury may be caused by falls within the imaging room, or bruises and skin damage (particularly in the elderly) from banging limbs on inappropriately positioned equipment. Inap-

propriate referrals may also cause distress or even harm due to inability to appropriately position or secure the patient for imaging, for example due to immobility or obesity.

The imposing equipment and often dimly lit environment can seem threatening and create anxiety (Murphy 1999, 2001, 2006), particularly for children and patients with a learning disability. Experiences of claustrophobia while the head and neck is in close proximity to the imaging equipment are noted in many imaging examinations (McKenzie, Simms, Owens, & Dixon, 1995; Melendez & McCrank, 1993). This may be particularly noticeable within VFSS where a traditional under-couch x-ray tube configuration is used: the bulky exploratory/image intensifier mechanism can be very intimidating when positioned close to the face. Anxiety and discomfort have been shown to increase the likelihood of noncompliance and dissatisfaction in other complex imaging procedures (Loeken et al., 1997; MacKenzie et al., 1995). There is also a risk of potential coughing, choking, and aspiration associated with the ingestion of contrast agents, and subsequent hospitalization for aspiration pneumonia in rare cases.

The VFSS Reporting Procedure

According to Robinson (1997), "The weakest link in the chain of events which represents clinical imaging is the performance of the observer" (p. 1093). Errors of image interpretation and report-writing are the most common cause of litigation related to radiology. The Royal College of Radiologists (RCR) (2001) clearly defines three categories of mistakes made in reporting:

- An **error** occurs when there is a disagreement with the opinion of the "gold standard" body of experts.

- Most reporting errors come to light at a later date with the benefit of additional information, and they are then known as **discrepancies**. The RCR recommend that discrepancy meetings are held on a regular basis to learn from the experiences: where VFSS discrepancies are discussed, reporting radiographers and SLPs should have input into these department audit meetings. Most discrepancies are insignificant and may never come to light, but they may become significant where there is an impact on patient management.
- A **critical incident** occurs when an error results in mismanagement of the patient with resultant morbidity or mortality, requiring mandatory further investigation.

There are a range of reasons why mistakes in reporting are made, including insufficient education and training. However, the most significant is the quality of the images: the performance of the investigation may be substandard, for example where there was inadequate distension and coating in a barium swallow, where exposure factors were incorrect, or radiographic positioning was inappropriate. This can result in a failure to demonstrate a significant lesion or to be able to confirm normality. Technical quality of the examination undoubtedly will be optimal when the individual performing the examination is also issuing the report. Inadequate, incomplete or incorrect clinical information has also been implicated in reporting errors. Correct clinical information is essential to avoid wasting time looking for findings which are irrelevant.

Reporting errors may be categorized as follows:

- Overreporting (**false positives**): occurs when one diagnoses disease in an essentially normal case. Such errors are more common in the inexperienced, untrained observer, and may result in further unnecessary investigations or treatment
- Perception errors (**false negatives**): observational misses occur when pathology is present and visible on the image but it is not detected
- **Errors of interpretation**: occur when a pathology is spotted, but the disease is incorrectly identified
- **Errors of communication**: pathology may be spotted and correctly identified, but the communication of the findings to the referring clinician may be inadequate, misinterpreted, or even mislaid

Interobserver variation is noted to be high in many imaging procedures (Robinson, 1997), including chest reporting, barium enemas, and CT scans. The VFSS examination, similar to other fluoroscopic, dynamic procedures is also likely to have high interobserver variation. A well-documented standardized procedure and image capture, alongside appropriate training is likely to improve reporting accuracy and reduce variation. Many VFSS services incorporate some degree of peer reporting: true blind double reporting has been found in other imaging procedures to reduce perception errors (Leslie & Virjee, 2002).

Concerns may be raised by patients related to the wider VFSS service, the VFSS procedure, and the accuracy of the resultant report. The potential for a poor patient experience described above, and subsequent dissatisfaction and complaints, is vastly reduced by providing good patient preparation (written information and verbal explanations), working within agreed evidence-based protocols and procedures (including radiology-wide procedures such as data protection and confidentiality, checking identification and pregnancy status), and obtaining valid consent. The following sections explore the role of patient information, protocols, confidentiality, and consent.

PATIENT INFORMATION

Information about the procedure should be provided to the patient on a continuum, commencing with the referrer, and then backed up by good quality written information created by the radiology department in conjunction with patients and service users. On arrival, the patient has the opportunity to receive further explanations from the professionals undertaking the procedure, and an opportunity to ask questions, as part of the consent process.

The main tenet of patient information is that the right information should be delivered and received at the right time, and suited to personal needs (DoH, 2003). Written information, however, is no substitute for face-to-face discussions with staff.

Further information about a procedure such as VFSS is often provided through written information leaflets, produced jointly by the radiography and SLP teams. Although information leaflets are abundant in the NHS, the Audit Commission has noted that the quality and distribution is often patchy (National Audit Office, 2008). The reading age of the literature is often too high for the target population, and may not be widely accessible to people with reading difficulties, or where English is not their first language. Translation in a variety of languages appropriate to the local population can be very helpful. The Department of Health (2003) has produced an online toolkit for producing patient information leaflets, using templates that help to standardize information and raise it to a minimum level.

A recent study of patient experience of a complex imaging procedure identified that information leaflets were often praised by patients, even though when questioned the patients had poor knowledge of the procedure they were about to undergo. The researchers suggested that many imaging information leaf-

lets are more focused to gaining compliance from the patient, rather than truly informing them about the procedure (Nightingale et al., 2012). However the inclusion of visual aids within the leaflets (drawings, images, and photographs of equipment) can be very beneficial in informing the patient, particularly for children or patients with learning disabilities who are invited for VFSS.

Increasingly health care organizations and providers are using the internet to offer information to patients on their own Web sites, offering opportunities for incorporation of videos and podcasts to aid understanding. However the sheer volume and complexity of resources available at the click of a button can increase anxiety, especially if inaccurate information is accessed by the patient.

ROLE OF PROTOCOLS

Practitioners engaged in VFSS are strongly advised to develop (and work within) an agreed set of guidelines, commonly termed a protocol. However, this terminology is not universally applied across health care practice, and a number of terms are used interchangeably: practice guidelines, clinical protocols, clinical guidelines, operational policies, and schemes of work. Within health care the term "protocol" commonly refers to a set of "best practice" guidelines for performing a particular procedure. In simple terms, a protocol is an agreed and documented system which outlines how certain categories of patients are to be managed, and by whom (Nightingale, 2008; Owen, Hogg, & Nightingale, 2004).

The protocol is an official formula for practice, incorporating regulations, customs and etiquette to be observed by any group on any occasion, and it should encompass a degree of standardization, evidence-informed practice and risk-reducing strategies. This view is supported by the NHS Modernisation Agency (2002), stating that a protocol has the potential to drive up standards, and can improve care in almost any setting. The importance of protocols to support both existing and new practices is not to be underestimated, and is a requirement where advanced practices (moving outside the traditional scope of practice of a profession) are being introduced (BFCR, 1999; CoR, 1997; Paterson et al., 2004).

There is no one correct way of designing a protocol: every hospital will have its own requirements, with some offering standard templates to complete. Protocols will be required to be submitted for external scrutiny and approval (for example, via hospital Clinical Governance units), and will generally be made available as a public document via hospital Web sites. The most effective way of gaining approval and acceptance of the policy is to involve all relevant stakeholders in its creation from the outset (Table 3–1 suggests steps for developing a protocol).

The protocol may include a number of procedures (prescribed way of doing a task), including a step-by-step guide to performing the VFSS examination. However, the protocol should encompass much more than how to do the VFSS: it should also give clear guidance regarding staff requirements (qualifications, experience, and updating), the referral criteria, indications and contraindications, emergency procedures, reporting requirements and audit of the service. These suggested elements are listed in Table 3–2; further detail can be obtained from Nightingale (2008). Although detailed protocols offer an inexperienced practitioner a supportive framework within which to work, there is a danger that some protocols can be overly prescriptive. This prevents staff from being able to use their experience to adapt their practice to an individual situation, and may inadvertently work against patient care rather than improve it (Crawley et al., 1998). As practitioners gain experience

Table 3–1. *Key Steps to Developing Protocols*

Stage in Protocol Development Cycle	Description
Stage 1	Select and prioritize a topic
Stage 2	Set up a team
Stage 3	Involve patients and service users
Stage 4	Agree on objectives
Stage 5	Build awareness and commitment
Stage 6	Gather information
Stage 7	Baseline assessment
Stage 8	Produce the protocol
Stage 9	Approve and pilot the protocol
Stage 10	Implement the protocol
Stage 11	Monitor variation (audit)
Stage 12	Review the protocol

Source: Adapted from the NHS Modernisation Agency, 2002.

and their professional scope of practice widens, there is a danger they may begin to stray from the boundaries of the protocol. Review at least annually will identify when the professional latitude within the protocol needs to be revisited.

A well-designed evidence-based protocol has the potential to be used to defend against a future complaint, investigation, or medico-legal claim, as it documents the normal course of patient management undertaken by practitioners. However, the protocol must be written, agreed by all relevant parties (including hospital management) and must have been

Table 3–2. *Key Elements of a Protocol*

Section of Protocol	Content and Purpose	VFSS Examples
Title	Clearly identifies the contents	Protocol for practitioner-led videofluoroscopic swallowing examinations
Background	Documents current evidence base to support the practice Historical development of the role at the hospital—explores service need	May include key professional body guidance (e.g., RCSLT, 2007) and research articles, and may describe local/regional practice
Education and training	Minimum staff requirements (formal and in-house education) to perform or report the examinations Special requirements for those in training	Completion of dysphagia / swallowing disorders courses Completion of mandatory training (e.g., CPR / moving and handling
Scope of practice	Particular examinations and patient categories that can be managed within this protocol Degree of autonomy enabled by protocol	Inclusion / exclusion criteria e.g., exclude pediatrics/exclude postoperative Scope for adapted technique—e.g., further images, proceed to barium swallow, recommend further imaging
Procedure(s) for performing or reporting examinations	Steps involved in performing or reporting the procedure, and standards to which practitioners should conform May refer to other department procedures (e.g., checking identification, consent, pregnancy checks) Minimum facilities (and staffing) required for safe practice Contraindications and unusual/emergency scenarios when the normal protocol is not followed	Contrast agents used (quantities, preparation); imaging sequences; recording mechanisms; potential maneuvers and trials; recording of dose and screening time. Adverse events—when to stop procedure/action in event of significant aspiration, etc. Skills for Health publish working competences and core skills for professionals involved in VFSS
Reporting mechanism	Report process (e.g., preliminary/definitive reports), report verification. Elements of the report, including possible reporting codes used	Role of SLP, radiographer, and radiologist. Storage and communication (e.g., PACS)
Clinical audit	What, why, when, how, and to what standard to audit Procedure in event of not reaching standard required	Possible audits to be undertaken: Radiation dose and screening time; No images taken; Waiting times; Report turn-around times; Report accuracy

Table 3–2. *continued*

Section of Protocol	Content and Purpose	VFSS Examples
CPD requirements	Minimum (and recommended) CPD expectations of staff to maintain and document their competence	Registering body requirements (e.g., HPC in the UK) Examples of suitable CPD—e.g., observation and peer review of practice
Verification	Approval of the protocol at all levels (individual/department /hospital) Verification information should include: version numbers, dates, signatures, designations, and expected date of next review	Approval on initial review, and then at subsequent intervals (usually annual). May include service managers of SLP and Radiology, Clinical Directors and Clinical Governance/Hospital Boards
References	Key recent references to demonstrate practices are evidence based.	May include peer-reviewed and professional body/Department of Health literature

Source: Adapted from Nightingale, 2008.

regularly updated and reviewed. Even where no changes are made, the review must be noted, and all earlier copies of the protocol archived. This is essential, as many legal claims and investigations occur many months or even years after the initial imaging examination when a practitioner is unlikely to remember in detail the protocol used.

CONFIDENTIALITY

Patients should expect that their medical or personal details should only be shared with those health professionals who are directly concerned with their medical care. Similarly, a patient's consent should be gained before sharing information with their relatives or carers (SCoR, 2008). Although health professionals have a clear understanding of confidentiality, confidentiality is often inadvertently broken. For example: discussing patient details within earshot of other patients; accidentally leaving patient data in a public place; leaving a "logged on" computer unattended; sending patient information or invitations for appointments to an incorrect address; or leaving messages on telephone answering machines regarding appointments or results (SCoR, 2008).

The need for maintaining confidentiality is clearly set out within professional body and registration codes of practice (e.g., Health Professions Council, 2008). However, there is concern about the inherent dangers posed to confidentiality as we move toward a more IT-driven health care system. In particular, the advent of Picture Archiving and Communications Systems (PACS) in radiology has introduced additional challenges regarding data security, with images and reports being made more widely available across (and beyond) a hospital network. For this reason, the Royal College of Radiologists (2008) published a document setting standards regarding maintaining confidentiality with regard to a PACS environment. They reaffirm that information held within PACS is subject to the same confidentiality restraints as any other electronic information.

The Society and College of Radiographers (2009) have also issued guidance to their members regarding the inherent dangers for health professionals posed by the proliferation of social networking sites, and the trend for informal and frequent communication. They express concern that the use of this modern media raises potential dangers for breaches of patient confidentiality and consent. They remind members to never reveal or share any information inappropriately. Images are not to be used for entertainment purposes and extreme care must be taken in posting any work related comments on any social networking site.

CONSENT

Importance of Consent

It is a general legal and ethical principle that valid consent must be obtained before starting treatment or physical investigation, or providing personal care, for a patient (DoH, 2001). It is a common courtesy and helps to establish a convincing and appropriate trust relationship between the health professional and patient. For consent to be deemed valid, it must be given voluntarily by an appropriately informed person who has the capacity to consent to the intervention in question: acquiescence where the person does not know what the intervention entails is not "consent."

Obtaining valid consent is of prime importance, as touching a patient (or indeed delivering a dose of radiation to them) without consent may constitute, under English law, an allegation of battery under the tort of trespass to the person. Battery is defined as "intentionally bringing about a harmful

or offensive contact with the person" (Fleming, 1998). Although legal actions for battery against health professionals are relatively rare and unlikely to succeed (Dimond, 2001), traditionally, the importance of gaining consent was to protect a doctor against an allegation of battery. If the patient subsequently suffers harm from the procedure, a lack of valid consent may be a factor in a negligence claim, or in fitness to practice or employer action against an employee. Lack of valid consent is the largest factor in patient complaints in the NHS. The health professional carrying out the procedure is ultimately responsible for ensuring that the patient is genuinely consenting to what is being done: it is they who will be held responsible in law if this is challenged later (DoH, 2001).

Voluntary Consent

In order for consent to be valid, it must be given voluntarily. This means that there must be no pressure (coercion) or undue influence (duress) to accept or refuse treatment. Pressure may be applied by health professionals, and this is of particular concern when consenting patients for research studies, where the patient may receive payments and there may be no direct benefit to them as an individual (RCR, 2005). Radiographers and SLPs may have influence over their patients and should therefore refrain from consciously, or subconsciously manipulating the patient's decision-making process. Similarly, they must take steps to ensure that consent is not sought when the patient is in a vulnerable state, for example already undressed, or lying on the imaging table: "The differential power relationship between professional and patient may make it difficult for a patient to make a rational, considered decision and might be construed as duress" (SCoR, 2007).

Partners or relatives may also be a source of pressure to proceed (or not) with examination or treatment; for this reason it is advisable to consent patients alone where possible.

Informed Consent

For a patient to consent, they must be in possession of "sufficient information." This includes the nature and purpose of the examination/treatment, information about related anesthesia where relevant, and information regarding significant risks. Significant risks, as established within seminal case law (*Sidaway v. Board of Governors of the Bethlem Royal and the Maudsley Hospital*, 1985), includes serious or frequently occurring risks of the treatment (or lack of it), and any alternatives to the treatment. The patient also expects to know who is conducting the procedure (including whether it is a student), and to receive answers to their questions. However, where information is offered and declined, this should be recorded in the patient's medical records.

Patients attending for VFSS should be informed of the benefits of the procedure, and are entitled to know about potential risks, including radiation dose. Some patients, upon being made aware that radiation is involved in their examination, may ask pertinent questions about potential risks to themselves or future offspring. The College of Radiographers (2007) advises radiographers to respond in an appropriate way using their own judgment to decide on the ability of the patient to understand a risk-benefit approach (see Chapter 8). However, health professionals are cautioned to avoid using the term "safe" in favor of terms that outline radiation risk compared with other risks in society. For example, in 2001 the National Radiological Protection Board (now the Health Protection Agency, or HPA) offered helpful suggestions for explaining to the public the level of radiation risk associated with imaging investigations, using comparisons such as "equivalent period of natural background radiation" and "lifetime additional risk of cancer per examination" (SCoR, 2007). Radiographers are advised to ensure that they are familiar with these figures and can provide patients with the appropriate risk equivalents for common imaging examinations, but they should also be aware of the potential harm that information on risk could cause.

The variation in radiation dose and screening time in any fluoroscopy examination makes it difficult to accurately categorize the radiation risk, but using the HPA guidelines, the risk arising from a VFSS examination (centered on oropharynx) would be likely to be equivalent to a few weeks of background radiation, with negligible additional risk of cancer. Converting the examination to a barium swallow and meal (with further imaging of the abdominal cavity and increased exposure factors) would raise the risk level.

Other risks of the procedure should also be discussed with the patient—for the VFSS this may include the risk of significant aspiration, weighed up against the risks of not having the procedure (and potential for undiagnosed conditions). The Royal College of Radiologists (2005) issued guidance for radiology departments on levels of risk: only procedures with a known potential risk of complications greater than 1 in 2,000 should be mentioned to patients when seeking consent. However, the College of Radiographers (2007) highlights a study undertaken by Mayberry and Mayberry (2002) which found that 83% of their patient sample only wanted to be told of any procedural risks greater than 1 in 1,000. This would be unlikely to include significant aspiration.

The Consent Process

The clinician providing the treatment or investigation should normally be responsible for seeking consent, but this activity may be delegated to another professional if suitably trained and qualified, but they must know the procedure in depth including risks. Obtaining consent should be seen as a **process** as opposed to a one-off event, with consent being sought well in advance if possible, and again immediately prior to the examination. The SLP is well placed to engage in the consent-seeking process for VFSS, as often they are working with the patient over a period of time, having undertaken an appropriate clinical assessment of swallowing beforehand. The clinical evaluation enables candidate suitability for the procedure to be assessed (including cognition, feeding arrangements, role of carer, physical ability, and anxiety), and allows the opportunity for full explanations. The referring SLP has often built a relationship with the patient, and may accompany the patient to the VFSS appointment. The consent continuum is strengthened further, with further explanations and continuing consent being established by the practitioner undertaking the procedure. However, the most fundamental right regarding the consent process is that the patient is free to withdraw their consent at any time, without fear of creating offence or their continuing medical care being affected. The right to withdraw is also a central tenet in research where participants may be undergoing investigations with arguably little benefit to the individual.

Types of Consent

Consent for examination or treatment may be offered in several ways. Nonverbal (implied) consent is experienced when a patient acquiesces, for example, in research, by completing and returning a questionnaire, or by offering an arm for a blood test. However, professional body advice urges radiographers to distinguish between patient compliance and implied consent, both signaled through behavior. Implied consent requires that the patient is provided with sufficient information on which to proceed with the examination or treatment (SCoR, 2007; RCR, 2005).

However for "noncomplex" medical imaging procedures that may involve discomfort or even risk, express consent (verbal) is a prerequisite. VFSS procedures would be expected to fall under this category. The College of Radiographers advise radiographers to always ask a patient to confirm in his or her own words their understanding of the procedure, and to seek the patient's explicit verbal affirmation to proceed (SCoR, 2007). The law, however, does not require that consent is given in written form.

Written consent may be advised for certain cases dependent on the employing authority's policies (SCoR, 2007) and/or as advised by the U.K. General Medical Council (1998), and these may include:

- The procedure involves a significant risk and/or side effects.
- The procedure is part of a research project.
- There may be significant consequences for a patient's personal life or employment.

The written consent form is not a legal waiver: it is an aide-memoire offering a checklist of information to be given to patient. It is increasingly used to record the discussions that have taken place between the patient and the health professional, with both having a written record of discussions and outcomes. However, it is essential to note that from a legal and moral perspective, a signature on a written consent form does not mean that valid consent has actually been given. The patient must have received sufficient information to make a decision, must have capacity to consent, and must have given this consent voluntarily. It is important to remember that some patients may be able to consent, yet have difficulty in communicating their decision in writing; in this case it is important to have an independent witness to the consent decision.

Capacity to Consent

One of the most difficult aspects of obtaining valid consent is the issue of "capacity" to consent. To give valid consent, patients must be able to comprehend and retain relevant information about the procedure (especially related consequences and risks), and be able to weigh this information and come to a decision. Patients may have capacity to consent to some examinations and not others; for example, an adult with a learning disability may be able to consent to a simple procedure, but may not have the required understanding to consent to a complex operation. Some patients may have a temporary incapacity to consent, for example after a head injury, or under the influence of anesthetics, recreational drugs, or alcohol. Similarly, illnesses such as an acute stroke may render a patient unable to understand the required information, yet their ability to consent may return over time. Where possible, their procedure should be delayed until capacity returns. Patients, however, may have capacity even if their ability to communicate is impaired, and every effort must be made to provide them with alternative means of expressing their wishes. A patient may have capacity to consent even if their decision is seen as "irrational" to the health professional: this can be challenging to staff, but they should attempt to seek an understanding of the patient's choices.

Adults Without Capacity

Everyone age 16 and over, including those with learning disabilities, is presumed competent to consent, unless proven otherwise. In the United Kingdom, the Adults with Incapacity (Scotland) Act (2000), The Adult Support and Protection (Scotland) Act (2007), and the Mental Capacity (England) Act (2005) guide clinical practice, stating that individuals should be supported to make their own decisions wherever possible, and given all practicable help to make these decisions. Good practice dictates that the referring clinician is best placed to determine whether their client is able to make and communicate decisions about videofluoroscopy assessment and its potential outcomes. Where possible these decisions should be made with the rest of the multidisciplinary team and family. If the client is able to make his or her own decision and provide consent, then the intervention should be discussed, negotiated, and planned with the patient.

Adults are deemed not competent to consent if they are unable to comprehend and retain relevant information, and/or are unable to weigh and use this information to come to a decision. If capacity to consent is under debate, then the team should attempt all means to help the adult with learning disabilities understand the assessment and intervention. Many clients with learning disabilities may be deemed not to have capacity: in this case English law states that where something must be done to someone who cannot consent, it must be done in their best interests, and should be the least restrictive of their basic rights and freedom.

The aforementioned Acts of Law provide guidance for carrying out procedures in the best interests of the individual. The Acts state that decisions should not be based on age, appearance, condition or behavior, and that if there is potential for capacity to return, to wait until this time to make a decision. If the individual cannot consent then they should be encouraged to participate in decision making, and this can include taking into account past and present wishes, beliefs, and values. Guidance also dictates that all important and/or involved parties should be consulted and all relevant circumstances considered. Following this, the least restrictive options should be chosen. Similar practice is followed in the

United States and Canada (Buchanan, 2004). The College of Radiographers (2007) also advises that acting in the best interests of the patient may involve the radiographer delaying or postponing the procedure if, in their opinion, more time needs to be taken to obtain consent. In these circumstances the referrer should be informed and discussions may include possible alternative procedures if relevant. Where valid consent is not achievable, the radiographer must ensure that by proceeding they are acting in the best interests of the patient. These decisions must be recorded and archived in patient medical records.

In cases where a client lacks the ability to consent, it is essential to pay due regard to a solid framework of evidence-based practice (Sackett, Rosenberg, & Gray, 1996) alongside the guidance of the aforementioned Acts. Once lack of capacity has been established, a multidisciplinary meeting should be convened with all relevant parties (including the medical team, the family, carers, and client, if appropriate), to ensure that three essential elements of evidence-based practice are considered: **patient preference** (discuss patient concerns, behavior, wishes and values), **clinical experience** (discuss past experience of clinicians, colleagues and caregivers), and **best available evidence** (discuss anecdotal and graded evidence) (Figure 3–1).

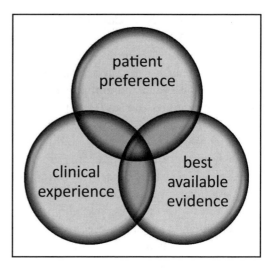

Figure 3–1. *Conceptualized model of evidence-based practice. Adapted from Sackett (1996).*

Children and Young People

Under U.K. guidelines, a young person aged 16 or 17 can consent to procedures themselves, but they may wish a parent to countersign. However, they may not refuse treatment if it is for a life-threatening condition. For many children under 16 (including children and infants attending for VFSS), they may not be able to fully understand the procedure/treatment and associated risks. Consent therefore relies on parental responsibility, and a separate consent form is completed. In the VFSS examination, parents should be fully informed, not only about the procedure, which can be distressing for some children, but potentially also about the VFSS outcomes (for example where decisions are being made regarding instigation of nonoral feeding).

However, under some circumstances children under the age of 16 are able to consent for themselves if they have "sufficient understanding and intelligence to enable him or her to understand fully what is proposed." This is known in England as "Gillick competence," following a landmark court ruling (*Gillick* v. *West Norfolk and Wisbech Area Health Authority*, 1985). The Gillick ruling does not apply in Scotland, where young people have a statutory right to give their own consent to treatment provided that, in the opinion of a qualified medical practitioner, he/she is capable of understanding the nature and possible consequences of the treatment. The parents are still involved in any decisions.

Speech-language pathologists and radiographers should be aware of the issues surrounding consent for procedures and consent to disclosure where children are involved, and helpful guidance has been issued for radiographers (SCoR, 2005).

PATIENT ADVOCACY

The SCoR 2008 Code of Conduct and Ethics states that in their relationships with service users, radiographers should demonstrate respect for individual dignity, belief, culture, and autonomy through a commitment to the principles of consent and confidentiality and, when deemed appropriate, to act as a patient advocate. These principles are reflected for radiographers and SLPs in many nations.

Not all patients attending for imaging procedures, including the VFSS, have the desire or ability to be assertive. Patients attending for imaging or radiotherapy are often vulnerable for a variety of reasons, and this vulnerability may prevent patients (or parents/guardians in the case of children) from expressing their requirements or their wishes. These vulnerable people may need a person to "speak on their behalf," acting in a capacity as an advocate. Radiographers and SLPs must ensure that they are objective in their advocacy, and that they do not knowingly or accidentally manipulate patients decisions (SCoR, 2009).

Five elements of patient advocacy have been presented by SCoR (2009) to enlighten radiographers about the advocacy roles that they may use to empower their patients:

1. Guarding patients' rights and conserving the patients' best interests;
2. Protecting/maintaining patients' autonomy;
3. Protecting patients against any type of malpractice: suspected or blatant;
4. Championing ethical and social justice in the provision of health care; and
5. Referring patients to the most appropriate service.

SUMMARY

Health professionals providing a VFSS service should be competent to perform the investigation to a high standard, and should be working within approved evidence-informed protocols to ensure best practice is followed. Health professionals should be mindful of ensuring patients in their care are treated with dignity and respect, and are afforded assurances of confidentiality and informed consent. Protecting the patient in this way has undoubted benefits in also ensuring protection of the practitioners, who should be guided by advice from professional organizations and registration bodies, which aim to preserve the highest standards of integrity and ethical principles. These include the following codes which should guide practitioners working within the VFSS service:

- Code of Ethics (ASHA, 2010)
- Standards of Conduct, Performance, and Ethics (HPC, 2008)
- ARRT Standards of Ethics (2011)
- GMC Good Medical Practice 2006 (updated 2009)
- RCSLT Code of Ethics and Professional Conduct (2011)

REFERENCES

American Registry of Radiologic Technologists. (2011). *Standards of ethics.* Retrieved from https://www.arrt.org/pdfs/Governing-Documents/Standards-of-Ethics.pdf

American Speech-Language-Hearing Association. (2004). Guidelines for speech-language pathologists performing videofluoroscopic swallowing studies. *ASHA Supplement, 24,* 77–92.

American Speech-Language-Hearing Association. (2010). *Code of ethics.* Retrieved February 20,

2012, from http://www.asha.org/docs/html/ET2010-00309.html

Board of the Faculty of Clinical Radiology. (1999). *Skills mix in clinical radiology.* London, UK: The Royal College of Radiologists Ref BFCR(99)3.

Buchanan, A. (2004). Mental capacity, legal competence and consent to treatment. *Journal of the Royal Society of Medicine, 97,* 415–420.

College of Radiographers. (1997). *Reporting by radiographers: A vision paper.* London, UK: Author.

Crawley, M. T., Shine, B., & Booth, A. (1998). Radiation dose and diagnosticity of barium enema examinations by radiographers and radiologists: A comparative study. *British Journal of Radiology, 71,* 399–405.

Department of Health. (2000). *Meeting the challenge: A strategy for the allied health professions.* Retrieved March 24, 2011, from http://www.publications.doh.gov.uk/pdfs/meetingthechallenge.pdf

Department of Health. (2001). *Reference good practice in consent implementation guide: Consent for examination or treatment.* London, UK: TSO Nov 2001.

Department of Health. (2003). *Toolkit for producing patient information.* Retrieved March 24, 2011, from http://www.dh.gov.uk/en/PublicationsandstatisticsPublications/Publications/PolicyAndGuidance/DH_4070141

Department of Health. (2008). *High quality care for all: NHS next stage review final report,* June 2008.

Department of Health. (2009). *Reference guide to consent for examination and treatment.* Retrieved March 23, 2010, from http://www.dh.gov.uk/prod_consum_dh/groups/dh_digitalassets/documents/digitalasset/dh_103653.pdf

Dimond, B. (2001). *Legal aspects of radiography and radiology.* London, UK: Blackwell.

Fleming, J. G. (1998). *The law of torts* (9th ed.). North Ryde, NSW: Law Book Co.

Gates, J., Hartnell, G. G., & Gramigna, G. D. (2006) Videofluoroscopy and swallowing studies for neurologic disease: A primer. *RadioGraphics,* e22. Retrieved March 20, 2010, from http://radiographics.rsna.org/content/26/1/e22.full,2006;26

General Medical Council. (1998). *Seeking patient's consent: The ethical considerations.* London, UK: Author.

General Medical Council. (2006). *Good medical practice* (updated 2009). London, UK: Author.

Gillick v. West Norfolk and Wisbech Area Health Authority. (1985). 3 All ER 402 (HL).

Guardian. (2011). NHS patients' complaints procedure must be reviewed "immediately." Retrieved June 28, 2011, from http://www.guardian.co.uk

Health Professions Council. (2008). *Standards of conduct, performance and ethics.*

Health Professions Council. (2011). *Fitness to practice annual report 2011.*

Ionising Radiation (Medical Exposure) Regulations. (2000). London, UK: The Stationary Office.

Jones, B. (2000). Legal aspects of consent. *British Journal of Urology International, 86,* 275–279.

Leslie, A., & Virjee, J. P. (2002). Detection of colorectal carcinoma on double contrast barium enema when double reporting is routinely performed: An audit of current practice. *Clinical Radiology, 57,* 184–187.

Loeken, K., Steine, S., SandviK, L., & Laerum, E. (1997). A new instrument to measure patient satisfaction with mammography: Validity, reliability and discriminatory power. *Medical Care, 35*(7), 731–741.

MacKenzie, R., Simms, C., Owens, R. G., & Dixon, A. K. (1995) Patients' perceptions of magnetic resonance imaging. *Clinical Radiology, 50,* 137–143.

Mathers, S. A., Chesson, R. A., Proctor, J. M., McKenzie, G. A., & Robertson, E. (2006). The use of patient-centered outcome measures in radiology: A systematic review. *Academic Radiology, 13,* 1394–1404.

Mayberry, M. K., & Mayberry, J. F. (2002). Consent with understanding: A movement towards informed decisions. *Clinical Medicine, 2*(6), 523–526.

Melendez, J. C., & McCrank, E. (1993). Anxiety-related reactions associated with magnetic resonance imaging examinations. *Journal of the American Medical Association, 270,* 745–747.

Mental Capacity (England) Act. (2005). Retrieved March 25, 2012, from http://www.legislation.gov.uk/ukpga/2005/9/contents.

Murphy, F. J. (1999, July). How was it for you? Imaging technology and the patient experience. *Synergy—Imaging and Therapy Practice*, pp. 4–5.

Murphy, F. (2001). Understanding the human interaction with medical imaging technology. *Radiography, 7,* 193–201.

Murphy, F. J. (2006). The paradox of imaging technology: A review of the literature. *Radiography, 12,* 169–174.

National Audit Office. (2008). *Feeding back? Learning from complaints handling in health and social care.* London, UK: The Stationary Office.

NHS Modernisation Agency, National Institute for Clinical Excellence. (2002). A step-by-step guide to developing protocols. Retrieved March 30, 2008, from http://www.nodelaysachiever.nhs.uk/Resources/ResourceGuideItems/AþStepþbyþStepþGuideþtoþDevelopingþProtocols.htm

Newman, R. D., & Nightingale, J. (2011). Improving patient access to videofluoroscopy services: Role of the practitioner-led clinic. *Radiography, 17*(4), 280–283.

Nightingale J. (2008) Developing protocols for advanced and consultant practice. *Radiography, 14*(Suppl. 1), e55–e60.

Nightingale, J., & Mackay, S. (2009). An analysis of changes in practice introduced during an educational programme for practitioner-led swallowing investigations. *Radiography, 15,* 63–69.

Nightingale, J., Murphy, F. & Blakeley, C. (2012). "I thought it was just an x-ray": The expectation-reality divide experienced in cardiac SPECT CT imaging. *Nuclear Medicine Communications, 33*(3), 246–254.

Ondategui-Parra, S., Erturk, S. M., & Ros, P. R. (2006). Survey of the use of quality indicators in academic radiology departments. *American Journal of Roentgenology, 187,* W451–W455.

Owen, A., Hogg, P., & Nightingale, J. (2004). A critical analysis of a locally agreed protocol for clinical practice. *Radiography, 10,* 139–144.

Paterson, A. M., Price, R. C., Thomas, A., & Nuttall, L. (2004). Reporting by radiographers: A policy and practice guide. *Radiography, 10,* 205–212.

Power, M., Laasch, H. U., Kasthuri, R. S., Nicholson, D. A., & Hamdy, S. (2006). Videofluoroscopic assessment of dysphagia: A questionnaire survey of protocols, roles and responsibilities of radiology and speech and language therapy personnel. *Radiography, 12,* 26–30.

Robinson, P. (1997). Radiology's Achilles' heel: Error and variation in the interpretation of the roentgen image. *British Journal of Radiology, 70,* 1085–1098.

Royal College of Radiologists. (2001.) *To err is human . . . The case for review of reporting discrepancies.* London, UK: Author.

Royal College of Radiologists. (2005). *Standards for patient consent particular to radiology.* London, UK: Author.

Royal College of Radiologists. (2008). *Standards for patient confidentiality and PACS.* London, UK: Author.

Royal College of Speech and Language Therapists. (2007). *Videofluoroscopic evaluation of oropharyngeal swallowing disorders (VFS) in adults: The role of speech and language therapists* [RCSLT policy statement]. London, UK: Author.

Royal College of Speech and Language Therapists. (2011). *Code of ethics and professional conduct.* Retrieved January 12, 2012, from http://www.rcslt.org/members/welcome/CQ3_chapter_1.pdf

Sackett, D. L., Rosenberg, W. M. C., & Gray, J. A. M. (1996). Evidence-based medicine: What it is and what it isn't. *British Medical Journal, 312,* 71–72.

Scottish Parliament. (2000). *Adults with incapacity (Scotland) act 2000,* asp 4.

Scottish Parliament. (2007). *The adult support and protection (Scotland) act 2007.* Retrieved November 13, 2011, from http://www.opsi.gov.uk/legislation/scotland/acts2007/asp_20070010_en_1

Sidaway v. *Board of Governors of the Bethlem Royal and the Maudsley Hospital.* (1985). 1 All ER, 643–666.

Sitzia, J., & Wood, N. (1997). Patient satisfaction: A review of issues and concepts. *Social Science and Medicine, 45*(12), 1829–1843.

Society and College of Radiographers. (2005). *The child and the law: The roles and responsibilities of the radiographer.* London, UK: Author.

Society and College of Radiographers. (2007). *Consent to imaging and radiotherapy treatment examinations.* London, UK: Author.

Society and College of Radiographers. (2008). *Code of conduct and ethics.* London, UK: Author.

Society and College of Radiographers. (2009). *Patient advocacy.* London, UK: Author.

Society and College of Radiographers. (2009). *Patient identification, confidentiality and consent: Further guidance.* London, UK: Author.

Society and College of Radiographers. (2010). *Consent and adults with impaired capacity.* London, UK: Author.

Chapter
4

ANATOMY AND PHYSIOLOGY OF SWALLOWING

Claire Butler and Paula Leslie

INTRODUCTION

Before beginning to investigate the abnormal or disordered swallow, an appreciation is needed of how normal swallowing function occurs. This requires an examination of the anatomy and physiology of the normal swallow.

In this chapter current thinking about the events of the normal swallow is presented, from food or drink first being placed in the mouth to it entering the esophagus, as well as a brief mention of the passage of food through the esophagus to the stomach. A detailed examination of the structures involved in each step of the process and how these structures work together to create a swallow is presented, following the path of the bolus as it travels from the mouth to the stomach.

Every muscle that is mentioned in the text is indicated in bold the first time it appears, and more information about the positioning and action of each of these can be found in Table 4–1. Similarly, many of the anatomical structures mentioned in the text are also marked in bold when first mentioned to indicate that more information about them and their muscle attachments can be found in Table 4–2. The figures that accompany these tables, orientating readers to the anatomical position of key structures and attachment points for muscles, are presented in grayscale throughout the chapter, but the same images in valuable and informative color format can also be found in the color insert. Due to their positioning or functional nature, some of the muscles and structures are difficult to illustrate, and therefore are not shown in the images, but their names, locations, and actions remain listed in the tables.

Table 4–1. *The Muscles Involved in Swallowing*

Muscle Name	Description	Action in Relation to Swallowing	Image(s)
Anterior belly of the digastric	One of the suprahyoid muscles. Arises from the inner surface of the mandible and extends below the mandible to join the **posterior belly of the digastric** via an intermediate tendon	With the hyoid fixed, contraction causes mandibular depression or jaw opening. Not used in chewing. With the mandible fixed, co-contraction with the posterior belly of the digastric raises the hyoid bone.	Figure 4–2
Aryepiglottic	Extends from the apex of the arytenoid cartilages to blend with the interarytenoid fibers and extend into the epiglottis.	May be involved in movement of the arytenoid cartilages for ventricular fold adduction.	Figure 4–7
Buccinator	Fibers extend from both the **maxillae** and mandible, at the level of the molars, to meet and insert into the **oral angles**. The muscle effectively fills the space between the maxilla and mandible to form the cheeks.	Contraction pulls back the angle of the mouth. Works with the risorius muscle to increase tension in the cheeks, helping to prevent food pooling in the lateral sulci and to hold food in place during chewing.	Figure 4–2
Cricopharyngeus	Forms the **inferior pharyngeal constrictor** with the thryopharyngeus muscle and is also one part of the upper esophageal sphincter. A pair of muscles which originate from either side of the cricoid cartilage and join at the **pharyngeal raphe** to create a complete loop of cartilage and muscle.	Tonically closed at rest, creating a seal between the pharynx and esophagus. Pulled open during the pharyngeal stage of the swallow to allow passage of the bolus.	Figure 4–3
Depressor anguli oris	Extends from the mandible to the oral angle.	Contraction lowers the oral angle, contributing to the lip movements required during chewing.	Figure 4–2

Table 4–1. *continued*

Muscle Name	Description	Action in Relation to Swallowing	Image(s)
Depressor labii inferioris	Extends from the mandible into the inferior orbicularis oris of the lower lip.	Lowers the bottom lip to open the mouth. Helps to coordinate lip movement with the jaw and tongue during chewing.	Figure 4–2
Digastric	One of the suprahyoid muscles. Consists of an anterior and posterior belly joined by an intermediate tendon. This tendon passes through the **stylohyoid** muscle and links the digastric to the hyoid bone via a fibrous loop.	With the mandible fixed, contraction acts to lift the hyoid bone.	Figure 4–2
Genioglossus	Originates from the mental symphisis of the mandible and attaches to intrinsic muscles along the length of the tongue dorsum with the longest fibers inserting into the hyoid.	Contraction of various fibers of the genioglossus can cause depression of the tongue tip; lateral movement of the tongue tip; creation of a channel along the length of the tongue surface, which is useful in swallowing liquids and in sucking; and pulling the hyoid up and forward. In coordination with styloglossus, the genioglossus determines the position of the tongue within the mouth.	Figure 4–2, Figure 4–4
Geniohyoid	One of the suprahyoid muscles. Originates from the mental symphisis of the mandible and attaches to the anterior hyoid.	Contraction raises the hyoid bone and pulls it anteriorly. Contraction with the hyoid fixed causes mandibular depression or jaw opening.	Figure 4–2, Figure 4–3
Hyoglossus	Extends from the hyoid to the sides of the rear of the tongue.	Contraction with the hyoid in a fixed position causes lowering and retraction of the tongue.	Figure 4–2
Incissivus labii	Small muscles running parallel to the orbicularis oris muscles of the lips.	Assist in formation of lip seal during the oral stages of the swallow.	

continues

Table 4–1. continued

Muscle Name	Description	Action in Relation to Swallowing	Image(s)
Inferior longitudinal fibers of the tongue	Originate at the hyoid and root of the tongue and form the underside of the tongue to the tongue tip.	Contractions shorten the tongue and lower the tongue tip. Useful for removing material from the anterior sulcus.	Figure 4–4
Inferior pharyngeal constrictor	Consists of the thryopharyngeus and cricopharyngeus muscles. Fibers extend from the **thyroid** and cricoid cartilages on either side to form a loop of muscle.	Contraction causes constriction of the lower pharynx. These muscles also contribute to the upper esophageal sphincter.	Figure 4–5
Intrinsic tongue muscles	Made up of **inferior longitudinal fibers**, **superior longitudinal fibers**, transverse fibers, and vertical fibers.	Contractions lead to changes in the basic shape of the tongue. Useful for general bolus formation and control.	
Lateral cricoarytenoid	Extends from the cricoid cartilage to the arytenoid cartilage.	Contraction causes rotation of the arytenoid cartilages resulting in adduction of the vocal folds.	Figure 4–7
Lateral pterygoid	Originates from the **sphenoid bone** and inserts into the anterior portion of the condyle of the mandible.	Contraction causes mandibular depression or jaw opening. Co-contraction with medial pterygoid causes jaw protrusion. Required for chewing.	Figure 4–2
Levator anguli oris	Extends from the maxillae to the oral angles.	Contraction lifts the oral angle, contributing to the lip movements required during chewing.	Figure 4–2
Levator labii superioris	Extends from several origin points below the eye, with the majority inserting into the superior orbicularis oris of the upper lip.	Raises the upper lip to open the mouth. Helps to coordinate lip movement with the jaw and tongue during chewing.	Figure 4–2
Levator veli palatini	Forms the bulk of the velum. Originates in the base of skull and inserts into the **palatal aponeurosis.**	Contraction causes the velum to lift toward the posterior pharyngeal wall.	Figure 4–5

Table 4–1. continued

Muscle Name	Description	Action in Relation to Swallowing	Image(s)
Masseter	A wide muscle with fibers originating from the maxillae and zygomatic bone and inserting into a large area of the ramus and angle of the mandible.	Creates the mandibular sling with the medial pterygoid, contraction of which causes the mandible to rise, closing the jaw.	Figure 4–2
Medial pterygoid	Originates predominantly from the sphenoid bone, inserting into the ramus and angle of the mandible.	Creates the mandibular sling with the masseter, contraction of which causes the mandible to rise, closing the jaw.	Figure 4–2
Middle pharyngeal constrictor	One of the three pharyngeal constrictor muscles. Originates from the hyoid bone and inserts into the posterior pharyngeal raphe just below the superior pharyngeal constrictor.	Relaxation during the early part of the pharyngeal stage of the swallow assists in opening the pharynx to accept the bolus. Contraction behind the tail of the bolus helps to push the bolus through the pharynx both directly and by impacting on the pressure differentials within the structure.	Figure 4–5
Musculus uvulae	Extends from the palatine bone to the uvula.	Contraction causes the uvula to rise, improving contact between the velum and posterior pharyngeal wall.	Figure 4–5
Mylohyoid	One of the suprahyoid muscles. Fibers running from the anterior portion and from either side of the inside of the mandible to join at the center. Posterior fibers attach to the hyoid.	Forms the floor of the oral cavity. Contraction assists with upward and anterior movement of the hyoid.	Figure 4–2
Oblique interarytenoid	Also called the oblique arytenoid muscle. Extends from one arytenoid to the other.	Contraction causes adduction of the vocal folds and ventricular folds.	Figure 4–7

continues

Table 4-1. continued

Muscle Name	Description	Action in Relation to Swallowing	Image(s)
Orbicularis oris	Composed of a combination of orbicularis oris fibers with insertions of fibers from many other facial muscles.	Contraction creates the lip seal required to hold food or drink in the mouth during the oral preparatory stage of the swallow. It also acts to squash the anterior sulcus, helping to eliminate any food residue.	Figure 4–2
Palatoglossus	Originates from the palatal aponeurosis, extending down into the sides of the tongue. Forms the anterior faucial arch.	Contraction pulls the velum toward the tongue.	
Palatopharyngeus	Originates from the velum, with some fibers extending horizontally into the pharynx wall and the remainder extending down to combine with the stylopharyngeus and insert into the back of the thyroid cartilage. Forms the posterior faucial arch.	Contraction of the horizontal fibers moves the lateral walls of the pharynx inward to meet with the rising velum at the beginning of the pharyngeal stage of the swallow. Contraction of the vertical fibers causes elevation of the larynx and pharynx.	Figure 4–5
Pharyngeal constrictor muscles	Consist of three semicircular muscles, the superior, **middle,** and inferior **pharyngeal constrictors**	Contraction causes reduction of the diameter of the pharynx, which assists in moving the bolus through.	Figure 4–5
Posterior belly of the digastric	One of the suprahyoid muscles. Originates from the mastoid process, extending down to join the anterior belly of the digastric via an intermediate tendon.	With the mandible fixed, co-contraction with the anterior belly of the digastric raises the hyoid bone.	Figure 4–2
Risorius	Extends from the masseter muscle to the oral angles on either side.	Contraction pulls the corners of the mouth laterally. Works with the buccinator muscle to increase tension in the cheeks, helping to prevent food pooling in the lateral sulci and to hold food in place during chewing.	Figure 4–2

Table 4–1. continued

Muscle Name	Description	Action in Relation to Swallowing	Image(s)
Salpingopharyngeus	Originates in the eustachian tube in the nasal cavity and extends down to blend with the palatopharyngeus muscle.	Contraction causes elevation of the larynx and shortening and lifting of the pharynx.	Figure 4–5
Styloglossus	Originates from the **styloid process** and inserts into the side of the dorsum of the tongue.	In coordination with the genioglossus, determines the position of the tongue within the mouth. Contraction pulls the tongue into the mouth if stuck out or causes the rear of the tongue to lift.	Figure 4–2
Stylopharyngeus	Originates in the styloid process and extends between the superior and middle pharyngeal constrictors to insert into the pharynx and the thyroid cartilage.	Contraction causes elevation of the larynx and shortening and lifting of the pharynx.	Figure 4–5
Superior longitudinal fibers of the tongue	Originate at the tongue root and form the top layer of the tongue almost to the tongue tip. This muscle also has fibers running laterally across the top surface of the tongue.	Contraction of the longitudinal fibers pulls the tongue tip upward. Contraction of the lateral fibers creates a channel along the length of the tongue when swallowing a liquid bolus.	
Superior pharyngeal constrictor	Consists of fibers originating from four areas, including the sphenoid, the mandible and the sides of the tongue root. These join to insert in a wide band on the upper part of the posterior pharyngeal wall	Contraction acts to create Passavant's pad during the oral stage of the swallow. Contraction during the pharyngeal stage of the swallow helps to move the bolus through the pharynx.	Figure 4–5
Suprahyoid muscles	Consist of the digastric, geniohyoid, and mylohyoid muscles.	Contractions cause lifting and forward movement of the hyoid and opening of the upper esophageal sphincter.	

continues

Table 4–1. continued

Muscle Name	Description	Action in Relation to Swallowing	Image(s)
Temporalis	Has fibers originating from a wide area in the region of the temporal bone and inserting into the coronoid process of the mandible.	Contraction causes rapid elevation and retraction of the mandible which is useful in the oral preparatory stage of the swallow.	Figure 4–2
Tensor veli palatini	Extends from the sphenoid bone to the palatal aponeurosis.	Contraction causes increased tension in the front section of the velum which assists the levator veli palatini muscles in lifting the velum toward the posterior pharyngeal wall.	Figure 4–5
Thyroarytenoid	Extends from the thyroid cartilage to the arytenoid cartilage.	Contraction causes adduction of the vocal folds.	Figure 4–7
Thyrohyoid	Extends from the thyroid cartilage to the hyoid bone.	Contraction assists in raising the larynx relative to the hyoid.	Figure 4–5, Figure 4–6
Thyropharyngeus	Forms the inferior pharyngeal constrictor muscle with the cricopharyngeus and is also one part of the upper esophageal sphincter. A pair of muscles which originates from either side of the thyroid cartilage and join at the pharyngeal raphe to create a complete loop of cartilage and muscle.	Contraction causes constriction of the pharynx.	
Zygomatic	Extends from the zygomatic bone to the edge of the superior orbicularis oris and the oral angle.	Contraction contributes to the lip movements required during chewing.	Figure 4–2

Table 4–2. *The Structures Involved in Swallowing*

Structure	Description	Muscle Attachments or Interactions Relevant to Swallowing (see Table 4–1)	Image(s)
Anterior sulcus	The space in the oral cavity between the lip and anterior portion of the gum.	Orbicularis oris	Figure 4–3
Arytenoid cartilage	Part of the larynx, which forms an attachment point for the vocal folds.	Aryepiglottic Lateral cricoarytenoid Oblique interarytenoid Thyroarytenoid Thyromuscularis	Figure 4–6, Figure 4–7
Cricoid cartilage	Part of the larynx, which forms an attachment point for various muscles.	Cricopharyngeus Inferior pharyngeal constrictor Lateral cricoarytenoid	Figure 4–1, Figure 4–3, Figure 4–4, Figure 4–6
Epiglottis	A flap of cartilage, attached to the thyroid cartilage and hyoid bone via the thryoepiglottic and hyoepiglottic ligaments respectively. At rest it lies almost vertically against the tongue base, directly posterior to the hyoid bone. During the pharyngeal stage of swallowing, the epiglottis tips over the entrance to the airway, helping to protect it from the passing food or drink.	Aryepiglottic	Figure 4–1, Figure 4–3, Figure 4–6, Figure 4–7
Hard palate	Forms roof of the mouth and separates the oral and nasal cavities. Anterior three-quarters formed by the maxilla. Posterior one-quarter formed of palatine bones that merge with the palatal aponeurosis. Forms attachment point for the upper teeth.		Figure 4–3

continues

Table 4–2. continued

Structure	Description	Muscle Attachments or Interactions Relevant to Swallowing (see Table 4–1)	Image(s)
Hyoid bone	A "floating" C-shaped bone situated between the base of the mandible and the C3 vertebra. The hyoid does not articulate with any other bones and is supported by a network of muscle attachments.	Digastric Genioglossus Geniohyoid Hyoglossus Inferior longitudinal fibers of the tongue Middle pharyngeal constrictor Mylohyoid Palatopharyngeus Salpingopharyngeus Stylopharyngeus Thyrohyoid	Figure 4–1, Figure 4–2, Figure 4–3, Figure 4–4, Figure 4–6, Figure 4–7
Laryngeal vestibule	The area at the top of the larynx, extending from the entrance from pharynx to airway to the vocal folds.		Figure 4–4
Laryngopharynx	Also called the hypopharynx. Extends from below the level of the epiglottis to the upper esophageal sphincter where it blends directly into the esophagus at about the level of the C6 vertebra.	Inferior pharyngeal constrictor	Figure 4–3
Larynx	A structure in the anterior neck at the level of the C3-C6 vertebrae in adults or the C2-C3 vertebrae in children. Extends from the epiglottis to the cricoid cartilage and incorporates the arytenoid, cricoids, and thyroid cartilages, the vocal folds, and ventricular folds. Connects the pharynx to the trachea with an important role in both speech production and airway protection during swallowing.	Digastric Geniohyoid Mylohyoid Thyrohyoid	Figure 4–6, Figure 4–7
Lateral sulci	The spaces in the oral cavity between the cheeks and teeth on each side.	Buccinator Risorius	

Table 4–2. *continued*

Structure	Description	Muscle Attachments or Interactions Relevant to Swallowing (see Table 4–1)	Image(s)
Lips	Formed of the inferior and superior orbicularis oris muscles, which meet laterally at the oral angles, or corners of the mouth. Lightly closed in their neutral position.	Depressor anguli oris Depressor labii inferioris Incissivus labii Levator anguli oris Levator labii superioris Orbicularis oris Zygomatic	Figure 4–3
Mandible	The bone forming the lower jaw. This is a horseshoe shaped bone, with the bend of the horseshoe forming the chin. The angle of the mandible marks the point where the bone turns by almost 90 degrees upward forming the ramus, which further subdivides posteriorly into the condylar and anteriorly into the coronoid process.	Anterior belly of the digastric Buccinator Depressor anguli oris Depressor labii superioris Genioglossus Geniohyoid Lateral pterygoid Masseter Medial pterygoid Mylohyoid Superior pharyngeal constrictor Temporalis	Figure 4–1, Figure 4–2, Figure 4–3
Maxillae	A U-shaped alveolar ridge at the front, leading into the hard palate and forming the roof of the mouth.	Buccinator Levator anguli oris Masseter	Figure 4–1, Figure 4–3
Median raphe	Longitudinal groove along the center of the hard palate.		Figure 4–3
Nasopharynx	Sits at the back of the nasal cavity, extending from the skull base to the velum.	Levator veli palatini Salpingopharyngeus Superior pharyngeal constrictor Tensor veli palatini	Figure 4–3
Oral angles	The corners of the mouth, where the superior orbicularis oris muscles meet the inferior orbicularis oris muscles.	Buccinator Depressor anguli oris Levator anguli oris Orbicularis oris Risorius Zygomatic	

continues

Table 4–2. continued

Structure	Description	Muscle Attachments or Interactions Relevant to Swallowing (see Table 4–1)	Image(s)
Oropharynx	Also called the mesopharynx. Sits at the back of the oral cavity, extending from the velum to level of the hyoid bone. Anterior portion consists of the entrance from the pharynx to the oral cavity at the top and the valleculae at the bottom.	Middle pharyngeal constrictor Superior pharyngeal constrictor	Figure 4–3
Palatal aponeurosis	Forms the connective tissue link between the bones of the hard palate and the muscles of the velum.	Levator veli palatini Palatoglossus Tensor veli palatini	
Passavant's pad	A bulging of the posterior pharyngeal wall, created through contraction of the superior pharyngeal constrictor muscle at the beginning of the pharyngeal stage of swallowing. This assists in creating contact between the velum and pharynx, which in turn prevents nasal regurgitation during swallowing.	Superior pharyngeal constrictor	
Pharyngeal raphe	A longitudinal structure running the length of the posterior pharynx and acting as an insertion point for the pharyngeal constrictor muscles	Cricopharyngeus Pharyngeal constrictor muscles Thyropharygneus	Figure 4–3
Pharynx	A tubelike structure, open at the front, that links the base of the skull to the upper esophageal sphincter. Separated into the **nasopharynx**, oropharynx, and laryngopharynx.	Palatopharyngeus Pharyngeal constrictor muscles Salpingopharyngeus Stylopharyngeus	Figure 4–3

Table 4–2. continued

Structure	Description	Muscle Attachments or Interactions Relevant to Swallowing (see Table 4–1)	Image(s)
Pyriform sinuses	Also called the pyriform fossae. Located in the laryngopharynx, to the sides of the thyroid cartilage and immediately superior to the upper esophageal sphincter, these recesses are formed when fibers of the inferior pharyngeal constrictor wrap around the thyroid cartilage to insert on the anterior side.		Figure 4–4
Salivary glands	Consist of submandibular glands, below the mandible, parotid glands in the cheeks, and the sublingual glands in the floor of the mouth. Produce saliva which is a combination of serous fluid, mucus, and enzymes to break down food.		
Styloid process	A protrusion from the temporal bone of the skull, which acts as an attachment point for various muscles.	Styloglossus Stylopharyngeus	Figure 4–1
Sphenoid bone	A bat-shaped bone sitting centrally in the head at the base of the skull. A portion of the front surface of this bone forms the posterior section of the orbit of the eye.	Lateral pterygoid Medial pterygoid Superior pharyngeal constrictor Tensor veli palatini	Figure 4–1
Thyroid cartilage	The most prominent cartilage in the larynx, which protects the vocal folds.	Inferior pharyngeal constrictor Palatopharyngeus Stylopharyngeus Thyroarytenoid Thyrohyoid Thryomuscularis Thyropharyngeus	Figure 4–1, Figure 4–3, Figure 4–4, Figure 4–6

continues

Table 4–2. *continued*

Structure	Description	Muscle Attachments or Interactions Relevant to Swallowing (see Table 4–1)	Image(s)
Tongue	A muscular structure, consisting of four intrinsic tongue muscles. The tongue tip sits at rest behind the lower teeth, with the tongue blade forming the bulk of visible tongue in the mouth, the dorsum toward the back of the mouth and the tongue root extending into the pharynx to attach to the hyoid.	Genioglossus Hyoglossus Intrinsic tongue muscles —inferior and superior longitudinal, transverse, and vertical muscles. Palatoglossus Styloglossus Superior pharyngeal constrictor	Figure 4–3
Upper esophageal sphincter	A high-pressure area that separates the pharynx from the esophagus and is made up of muscle, cartilage, and aponeuroses rather than being a true sphincter. Consists of fibers from the inferior pharyngeal constrictor muscles as well as the upper cervical esophagus muscle.	Cricopharyngeus Thyropharyngeus	Figure 4–3
Valleculae	A pair of recesses located between the base of the tongue and the epiglottis and separated by the hyoepiglottic ligament.		Figure 4–3
Velum	Also called the soft palate. Muscular structure forming the rearmost part of the roof of the mouth and terminating in the uvula. Connected to the hard palate via the palatal aponeurosis.	Levator veli palatini Musculus uvulae Palatoglossus Palatopharyngeus Tensor veli palatini	Figure 4–3
Ventricular folds	Also called the false vocal folds or vestibular folds. Situated immediately above the true vocal folds and formed of mucous membrane stretched across the larynx, extending from the thyroid to arytenoid cartilage.	Aryepiglottic Oblique interarytenoid	Figure 4–4, Figure 4–7

Table 4–2. *continued*

Structure	Description	Muscle Attachments or Interactions Relevant to Swallowing (see Table 4–1)	Image(s)
Vocal folds	Also called **vocal cords**. Formed of mucous membrane with a few muscular fibers stretched across the larynx, the vocal folds mark the lower boundary of the laryngeal vestibule.	Lateral cricoarytenoid Oblique interarytenoid Thyroarytenoid	Figure 4–4 Figure 4–7
Zygomatic bones	The cheekbones of the face.	Masseter Zygomatic	Figure 4–1

Why Do We Swallow?

The human body has evolved in such a way that we breathe, speak, and eat using the same structures. We rapidly switch tasks requiring perfect timing and co-ordination. This increases the risk that food or drink might enter the airway and pass below the level of the vocal folds: *aspiration*. The act of swallowing helps to protect the lungs from the entry of food or drink and works to assist gravity in guiding the food or drink successfully through the oral and pharyngeal cavities and into the esophagus.

What Happens When We Swallow?

The traditional approach is to divide the act of swallowing into four stages:

Oral preparatory: breaking food down and creating a bolus which can be easily swallowed.

Oral: transporting the bolus into the **pharynx** in readiness for the swallow response.

Pharyngeal: the passage of the bolus through the pharynx, past the entrance to the airway and through the **upper esophageal sphincter**. This stage includes a series of protective mechanisms to prevent entry of food or drink into the lungs.

Esophageal: the passage of the bolus from the upper esophageal sphincter to the stomach.

Definitions

To understand anatomical positioning and physiological movements it is useful to have a basic awareness of the terminology.

Superior: toward the top of a structure or upper

Inferior: toward the bottom of a structure or lower

Posterior: toward the back of a structure

Anterior: toward the front of a structure

Lateral: toward the sides of a structure

Levator: pulling up

Depressor: pulling down

Abduction: pulling away from the midline

Adduction: pulling toward the midline

THE ANATOMY AND PHYSIOLOGY OF THE SWALLOW

Oral Preparatory Stage

The key aspect of this stage of the swallow is preparation of the food or drink for swallowing: creation of a bolus. The first physical step of swallowing involves food entering the mouth. Figures 4–1 and 4–2 illustrate many of the muscles involved in the oral preparatory and oral stages of the swallow.

To open the mouth the **mandible** is lowered by combined contraction of the **lateral pterygoid**, **anterior belly of the digastric**, **geniohyoid,** and **mylohyoid** muscles. For smaller items, the **lips** can be opened in isolation from the jaw through contraction of the **levator labii superioris** (lip raising) and **depressor labii inferioris** (lip lowering). Contraction of the **temporalis** muscle results in the powerful up, back, and lateral movements of the mandible required for biting and tearing of solid food.

When ready to swallow the mouth is closed through raising of the mandible by contraction of the **masseter** and **medial pterygoid** muscles working in tandem as the mandibular sling. The lips form a light seal anteriorly, through contraction of the **orbicularis oris** and to a lesser degree the parallel **incissivus labii** muscles.

In the oral cavity food is broken down and combined with saliva to form a bolus for swallowing through a combination of action of the teeth, **tongue**, lips, and cheeks. The teeth are set into the jaw and are moved through contraction of the same muscles used for general jaw movement. Repeated rhythmical contractions of the temporalis, masseter, medial pterygoid, and lateral pterygoid muscles act to produce the powerful up, down, protruding, retracting and rotational jaw movements required for grinding, biting, and chewing of the bolus by the teeth.

Movements of the jaw are coordinated with movements of the tongue and lips. The tongue is controlled by contractions of the **styloglossus**, **hyoglossus**, **genioglossus,** and **intrinsic tongue muscles.** The lips are controlled by contractions of the **levator anguli oris**, **depressor anguli oris**, levator labii superioris, depressor labii inferioris, and **zygomatic** muscles.

The cheeks are tensed by contraction of the **buccinator** and **risorius** muscles and assist the tongue in holding food in position for chewing.

Bolus formation also requires saliva which contains enzymes to break down the food and add moisture. Saliva is produced by the **salivary glands** and the mucus within the saliva lubricates the oral and pharyngeal passageways for easier swallowing.

During the oral preparatory stage of the swallow the **velum** (soft palate) often rests against the tongue at the back of the mouth, although there is some evidence that this is not always the case (Hiiemae & Palmer, 1999).

Oral Stage

The key aspect of the oral stage of the swallow is the movement of the newly formed bolus into position for swallowing.

Figures 4–3 and 4–4 illustrate lateral views of the head and neck which are useful when examining the anatomy and physiology of the oral stage of the swallow.

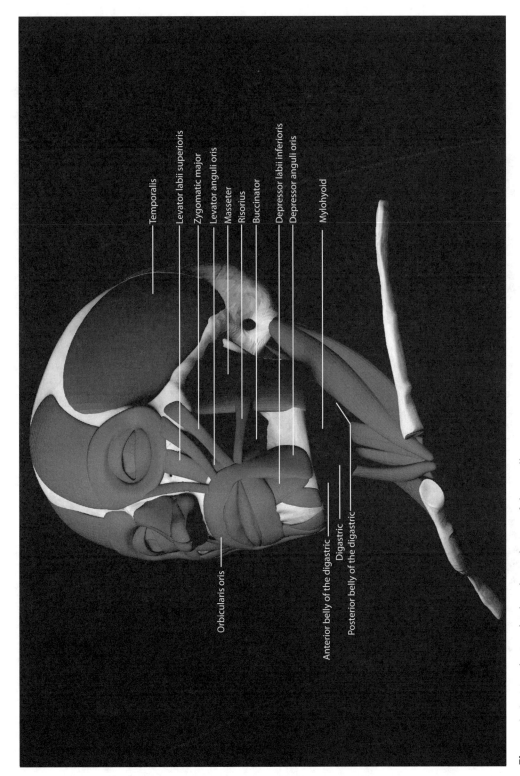

Temporalis

Levator labii superioris

Zygomatic major

Levator anguli oris

Masseter

Risorius

Buccinator

Depressor labii inferioris

Depressor anguli oris

Mylohyoid

Orbicularis oris

Anterior belly of the digastric

Digastric

Posterior belly of the digastric

Figure 4–1. Muscles involved in the oral stage of the swallow.

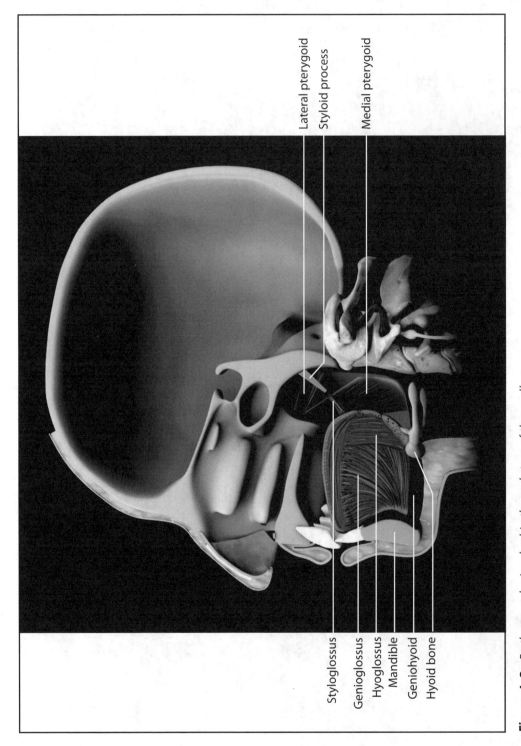

Lateral pterygoid
Styloid process

Medial pterygoid

Styloglossus
Genioglossus
Hyoglossus
Mandible
Geniohyoid
Hyoid bone

Figure 4–2. *Further muscles involved in the oral stage of the swallow.*

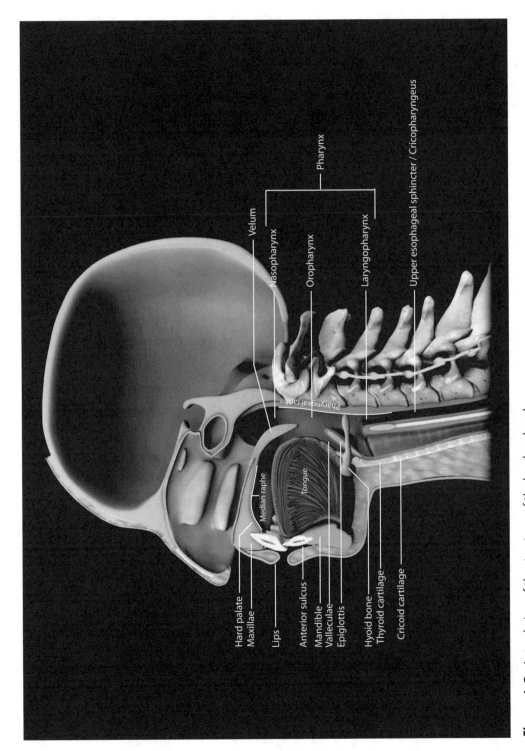

Figure 4–3. *Lateral view of the structures of the head and neck.*

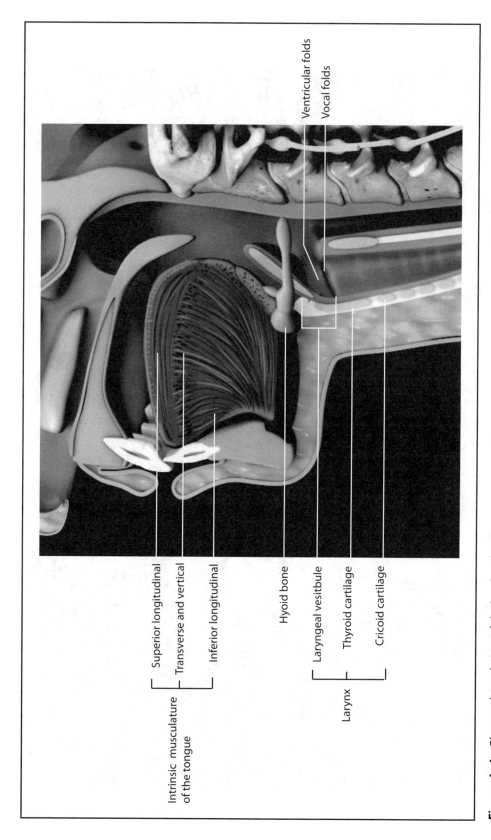

Figure 4–4. *Close-up lateral view of the head and neck.*

Intrinsic musculature of the tongue
- Superior longitudinal
- Transverse and vertical
- Inferior longitudinal

Hyoid bone

Larynx
- Laryngeal vesitbule
- Thyroid cartilage
- Cricoid cartilage

Ventricular folds

Vocal folds

Once the bolus is ready to be swallowed it is moved back in the oral cavity through coordinated movements of the tongue. The tongue tip initially raises to contact the **hard palate**, followed by the tongue blade working from the outside to the center and front to back, pushing the bolus behind it toward the back of the tongue (Hiiemae & Palmer, 1999). These movements are achieved through contraction of the **intrinsic tongue muscles** along with contraction of the **genioglossus** to raise the tongue tip and blade.

As the tongue works to push the bolus to the back of the mouth contraction of the orbicularis oris helps to clear material from the **anterior sulcus.** Contraction of the buccinator and risorius muscles help clear the **lateral sulci.**

Pharyngeal Stage

The key aspects of the pharyngeal stage of the swallow are airway protection and efficient movement of the bolus between the oral cavity and the esophagus. When the bolus leaves the oral cavity and enters the pharynx the pharyngeal stage of the swallow is said to have begun.

Figures 4–5 and 4–6 illustrate many of the muscles involved in the pharyngeal stage of the swallow. When sufficient bolus has accumulated to swallow, the velum is raised toward the posterior pharyngeal wall through contraction of the **levator veli palatini** and **tensor veli palatini** muscles and the **musculus uvulae.** As the velum elevates, the lateral walls of the pharynx are pulled in by contraction of the **palatopharyngeus** muscle and the posterior pharyngeal wall is pulled forward by contraction of the **superior pharyngeal constrictor** muscle. This creates a prominence known as **Passavant's pad**. Both actions help to form closer contact between the velum and posterior pharyngeal wall and together with

the velar movement act to block off the nasal cavity and prevent regurgitation of food or drink into the nose.

As the bolus moves farther into the pharynx the swallow response is initiated. The swallow response involves up and forward motion of the **larynx** and adjustments to the shape of the pharynx combined with three levels of airway protection. The timing of the triggering of this swallow response has been the subject of some debate and it is now acknowledged that there is huge variability among normal swallowers. Recent studies (Martin-Harris, Brodsky, Michel, Lee, & Walters, 2007; Matsuo & Palmer, 2008; Saitoh et al., 2007) have shown that the highest level at which **hyoid** movement may trigger in a healthy swallower is when the bolus head is at the level of the angle of the mandible. There is no clearly defined lowest level as the authors describe triggering of hyoid movement when the bolus head is at the level of the **laryngopharynx,** an area that extends from the lower border of the **epiglottis** to the upper esophageal sphincter.

Figure 4–7 illustrates the anatomy of the larynx and Figure 4–8 highlights those structures and muscles which are essential to airway protection. The first two of the three levels of airway protection are initiated by the closure of the true **vocal folds** and **ventricular (false vocal) folds** within the larynx. This marks the beginning of a brief period of swallow apnea, which is thought to always commence in healthy people before hyoid movement occurs (Martin-Harris et al., 2007). Adduction of the vocal folds is controlled by contraction of the **lateral cricoarytenoid, oblique interarytenoid,** and **thyroarytenoid** muscles. Adduction of the ventricular folds is due to contraction of the oblique interarytenoid muscles with possible additional involvement of the **aryepiglottic** muscle acting on the **arytenoid cartilages** to which the ventricular folds are attached.

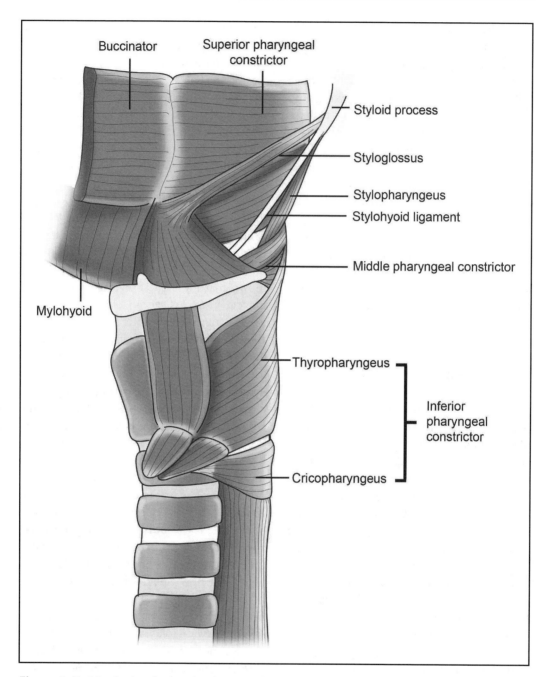

Figure 4–5. *Muscles involved in the pharyngeal stage of the swallow.*

The pharynx is shortened and lifted by contraction of the longitudinal **stylopharyngeus, salpingopharyngeus,** and palatopharyngeus muscles. As this occurs the diameter of the pharynx is increased through relaxation of the three levels of **pharyngeal constrictor muscle**. This elevation and dilatation allows the pharynx to lift up and meet the bolus in

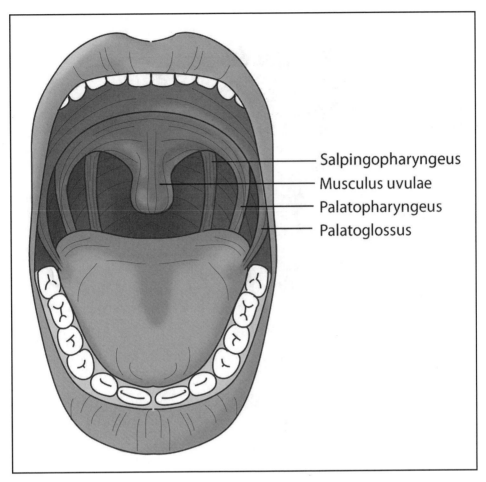

Salpingopharyngeus

Musculus uvulae

Palatopharyngeus

Palatoglossus

Figure 4–6. *Anterior-posterior view of the oral cavity showing further muscles involved in the pharyngeal stage of the swallow.*

the manner of a snake engulfing its prey (Leslie & McHanwell, 2008).

Concurrent with the movement of the pharynx, the larynx is pulled up and forward by movement of the hyoid, which is controlled by contractions of the **digastric**, geniohyoid, and mylohyoid muscles. This is partially caused by the contractions of the **thyrohyoid** muscle and the longitudinal muscles of the pharynx.

The final level of airway protection is movement of the epiglottis to cover the entrance to the airway. The up and forward movement of the hyoid during the pharyngeal swallow response pulls on the lower portion of the epiglottis via the hyoepiglottic ligament. This causes the body of the epiglottis to tip over the top of the larynx creating a loose seal at the entrance to the airway. The bolus then passes over the epiglottis or to either side of it via the **pyriform sinuses** in order to reach the entrance to the esophagus. The more solid and cohesive the bolus the more likely it is to pass the epiglottis centrally rather than laterally (Dua, Ren, Bardan, Xie, & Shaker, 1997).

The bolus movement through the pharynx is facilitated by a "wave" of contractions, beginning with the superior, then middle,

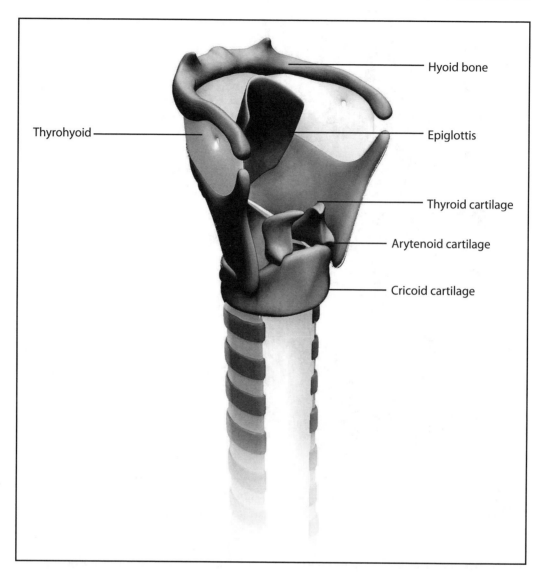

Figure 4–7. *Structures of the larynx.*

then inferior pharyngeal constrictor muscles. These contractions follow the tail of the bolus as it moves through the pharynx. Although to some degree the bolus is squeezed through the pharynx by the pharyngeal constrictors, a much greater part is played by the pressure differentials which these contractions, along with movements of other structures within the pharynx, create. This is discussed in more detail in Chapter 6, Biomechanical Analysis.

The final element of the pharyngeal stage of the swallow is the movement of the bolus through the upper esophageal sphincter. This high pressure area separating the pharynx from the esophagus is predominantly made up of fibers from the **cricopharyngeus** and **thyropharyngeus** muscles and at rest is held under tonic closure. Opening of the upper esophageal sphincter occurs predominantly due to the movement of the hyoid and larynx that

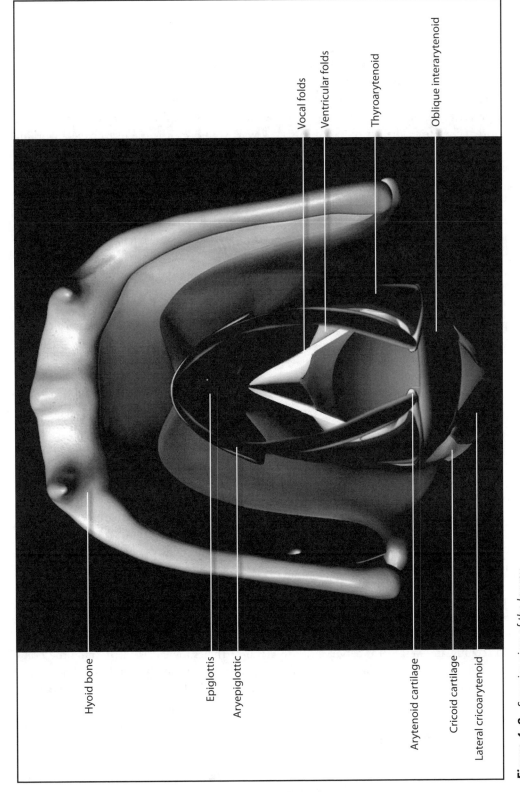

Figure 4–8. *Superior view of the larynx.*

Vocal folds

Ventricular folds

Thyroarytenoid

Oblique interarytenoid

Hyoid bone

Epiglottis

Aryepiglottic

Arytenoid cartilage

Cricoid cartilage

Lateral cricoarytenoid

are referred to collectively as the hyolaryngeal complex. These structures pull the **cricoid cartilage** up and forward, in turn pulling the cricopharyngeus up and forward. The posterior portion of the cricopharyngeus is attached to the prevertebral fascia and is unable to move anteriorly. Therefore, the cricopharyngeus is stretched open as the hyolaryngeal complex moves upward (Singh & Hamdy, 2005). The cricopharyngeus must relax to allow opening of the upper esophageal sphincter. Direct pressure of the bolus weight also helps to open the upper esophageal sphincter. Movement of the **suprahyoid muscles** has the most significant impact on this opening (Singh & Hamdy, 2005; Sivarao & Goyal, 2000).

Breakdown of swallowing into the oral preparatory, oral, and pharyngeal stages is particularly artificial when we consider swallowing of solids (Dua et al., 1997; Hiiemae & Palmer, 1999; Matsuo & Palmer, 2008) and continuous drinking of liquids (Daniels & Foundas, 2001). The Process Model of swallowing (Hiiemae & Palmer, 1999; Matsuo & Palmer, 2008) describes a gradual accumulation of the bolus on the pharyngeal surface of the tongue while chewing continues to take place in the oral cavity. A cycle of chewing followed by propulsion of chewed material to the **oropharynx** may be repeated several times for a single mouthful of food. As more material is propelled into the pharynx the bolus is gradually accumulated on the pharyngeal surface of the tongue. In some cases this extends as far as the **valleculae** before all material is removed from the mouth. In continual straw drinking, liquid accumulates in the oropharynx prior to swallowing in more than 50% of cases (Daniels & Foundas, 2001).

Esophageal Stage

The key aspect of the esophageal stage of the swallow is movement of the bolus between the pharynx and the stomach.

The esophageal stage of the swallow has traditionally fallen outside of the scope of the videofluoroscopic examination (RCSLT, 2006) and is not routinely included. In recent years there has been an increased understanding of esophageal conditions relative to the swallow and so it is useful to have a working knowledge of the basic esophageal anatomy and physiology. This enables a better understanding of what is normal versus abnormal when this area is included within the procedure.

The esophagus is a vertical tube of muscle approximately 23 cm long that is collapsed at rest. It is continuous with the laryngopharynx at the top and separated from the pharynx by the upper esophageal sphincter. The esophagus travels the length of the thoracic cavity within the superior and posterior mediastinum curving immediately anterior to the vertebral column. It passes through the diaphragm to the abdominal cavity, entering the cardiac orifice of the stomach via the lower esophageal sphincter. The esophagus can thus be considered to have arbitrary divisions known as the cervical, thoracic, and abdominal portions. As the esophagus traverses through these regions of the body, the highly complex anatomical relations, blood supply, venous return, innervations, and lymphatic drainage will change accordingly (Nightingale, 2010). Within radiological reports the esophagus is often delineated into upper, middle, and lower thirds.

Once the bolus has entered the esophagus the upper esophageal sphincter returns to its tonic resting state. This essentially seals the top of the esophagus and prevents the bolus from returning to the pharynx. The hyoid, larynx, and pharynx return to their resting positions and breathing usually recommences with an exhalation (Leslie, Drinnan, Ford, & Wilson, 2005).

Movement of the bolus through the esophagus is controlled by an involuntary peristaltic wave, or sequential contraction of smooth muscle, that acts to squeeze the bolus through the lumen. The primary peristaltic wave moves through the esophagus in 6 to 8 seconds, with the lower esophageal sphincter relaxing simultaneously. If a food bolus sticks, or moves slower than the primary wave, stretch receptors initiate a secondary peristaltic wave. Tertiary or nonperistaltic waves may occasionally be seen to occur spontaneously or during swallowing; these may be associated with structural or motility disorders (Nightingale, 2010). When the bolus passes into the stomach, the lower esophageal sphincter tonically closes and acts as a one-way valve preventing stomach contents from entering the esophagus.

CONCLUSION

We have presented here the most current evidence-based view of swallow anatomy and physiology. Due to the inherent difficulties with imaging parts of the sequence and in separating them out, new evidence may well emerge that realigns our thoughts on the process. As we study increasing numbers of healthy adults and children, our range of "normal" is also increasing. This suggests that the swallow mechanism can cope with a huge variety of conditions in the state of health—perhaps ill health is more to do with the system having a reduced capacity for variability?

Acknowledgments. Many thanks to Matt Briggs, Medical Artist from Lancashire Teaching Hospitals, for the design and production of all images for this chapter.

REFERENCES

Daniels, S. K., & Foundas, A. L. (2001). Swallowing physiology of sequential straw drinking. *Dysphagia, 16,* 176–182.

Dua, K. S., Ren, J., Bardan, E., Xie, P., & Shaker, R. (1997). Coordination of deglutitive glottal function and pharyngeal bolus transit during normal eating. *Gastroenterology, 112,* 73–83.

Hiiemae, K. M., & Palmer, J. B. (1999). Food transport and bolus formation during complete feeding sequences on foods of different initial consistency. *Dysphagia, 14,* 31–42.

Leslie, P., Drinnan, M. J., Ford, G. A., & Wilson, J. A. (2005). Swallow respiratory patterns and aging: Presbyphagia or dysphagia? *Journal of Gerontology, 60A*(3), 391–395.

Leslie, P., & McHanwell, S. (2008). Physiology of swallowing. In M. Gleeson (Ed.), *Scott-Browns otorhinolaryngology: Head and neck surgery* (Vol. II, 7th ed.). London, UK: Hodder & Staughton.

Martin-Harris, B., Brodsky, M. B., Michel, Y., Lee, F.-S., & Walters, B. (2007). Delayed initiation of the pharyngeal swallow: Normal variability in adult swallows. *Journal of Speech, Language, and Hearing Research, 50*(3), 585–594.

Matsuo, K., & Palmer, J. B. (2008). Anatomy and physiology of feeding and swallowing—normal and abnormal. *Physical Medicine and Rehabilitation Clinics of North America, 19*(4), 691–707.

Nightingale, J. (2010). Applied anatomy and physiology of the gastrointestinal tract (GIT). In J. Nightingale & R. L. Law (Eds.), *Gastrointestinal imaging: An evidence-based practice guide* (pp. 45–78). Edinburgh, UK: Churchill Livingstone.

RCSLT. (2006). *Videofluoroscopic evaluation of oropharyngeal swallowing disorders (VFS) in adults: The role of speech and language therapists.* RCSLT Policy Statement.

Saitoh, E., Shibata, S., Matsuo, K., Baba, M., Fujii, W., & Palmer, J. B. (2007). Chewing and food consistency: Effects on bolus transport and swallow initiation. *Dysphagia, 22,* 100–107.

Singh, S., & Hamdy, S. (2005). The upper esophageal sphincter. *Neurogastroenterology and Motility, 17*(Suppl. 1), 3–12.

Sivarao, D. V., & Goyal, R. K. (2000). Functional anatomy and physiology of the upper esophageal sphincter. *American Journal of Medicine, 108*(4A), 27S–37S.

Chapter

5

THE NEUROPHYSIOLOGY
OF SWALLOWING

Maggie-Lee Huckabee and Sebastian H. Doeltgen

INTRODUCTION

No instrumental assessment can be complete without a clear understanding and interpretation of the substrates of swallowing: structural and functional anatomy and neurophysiology. Referral for instrumental assessment of swallowing predicates that a clinician has first identified the potential for pathophysiology. The phenomenon of silent aspiration can easily be observed once the patient gets to instrumental assessment; however, by its very nature, it is elusive on clinical observation. Thus, patients are at risk of not making it past clinical screening to the point of diagnostic clarity. The astute clinician will possess a keen eye and ear for observation that is steadfastly paired with a working knowledge of the underlying substrates of swallowing. By applying knowledge of how peripheral innervation patterns and central processing may be impaired by known site of lesion, the clinician is able to infer what cannot be observed, thereby increasing sensitivity for further assessment.

A tool is only as valuable as the clinician who provides the interpretation. A videofluo-roscopic swallowing study (VFSS) arguably provides the most comprehensive imaging of deglutitive biomechanics. Very critically, this instrumental method provides a coordinative image of multiple phases of swallowing. However, instrumental imaging in the absence of sound clinical understanding is incomplete and can be misleading. The visualization of incomplete bolus transfer through the upper esophageal sphincter is a valuable diagnostic observation with significant clinical implications. However, the underlying pathophysiology that causes this is not discernible with this technique. Once again, working knowledge of the substrates of swallowing can facilitate differential diagnosis. Instrumentally observed pyriform sinus residue would lead a clinician toward a hypothesis of non-compliance of the cricopharyngeus muscle when paired with vocal dysphonia from vagal nerve damage. However, reduced traction from hyolaryngeal excursion may be more strongly suggested from clinically observed damage to the trigeminal nerve, assessed through resistance to jaw opening.

Chapter 4 presented an overview of swallowing anatomy and physiology. In this chapter, relevant neurological substrates are defined. However, separating neurology from physiology and covering this in isolation discourages carryover to clinical practice. As instrumental assessment is predicated on sound neurophysiologic understanding, this chapter will presents the underlying neural substrates of swallowing in their functional context, rather than anatomical location. Although swallowing should be seen as a single, continuous event, from mouth to stomach, paradigms have been used to classify phases of swallowing to facilitate discussion. This chapter uses the paradigm covered by Daniels and Huckabee (2009) that incorporates pre-oral parameters, as well as the oral, pharyngeal, and esophageal phases of swallowing. Within each phase, an association is made between biomechanical features of swallowing and their sensory and motor substrates at both a central and peripheral level. Figures are provided to schematically depict brain areas involved in various sensory and motor components of swallowing for each phase. By nature, these can only be indicative, based on previous research, and do not claim completeness. Figures 5–1 and 5–2 are included to orientate the reader regarding the relative anatomical location of the cranial nerves involved in swallowing. The four quadrants in Figures 5–3 to 5–10 depict: left lateral view (top left panel), anterior coronal section (top right panel), median-sagittal section (bottom left panel), and median-sagittal section of brainstem (bottom right panel).

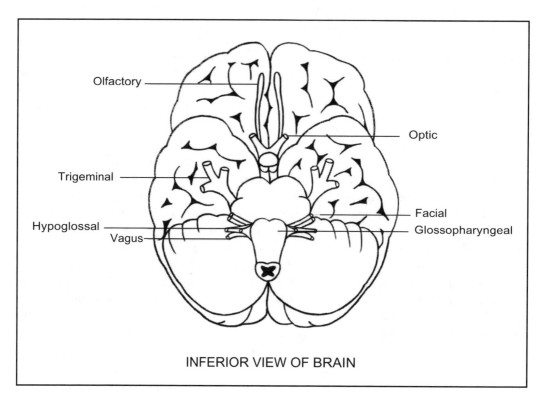

Figure 5–1. *Inferior view of the underside of the brain. Depicted are the cranial nerves relevant for swallowing as they emerge from the inferior surface of the brain (CN I [Olfactory], CN II [Optic]), pons (CN V [Trigeminal], CN VII[Facial]), and medulla oblongata (CN IX [Glossopharyngeal], CN X [Vagus], CN XII [Hypoglossal]).*

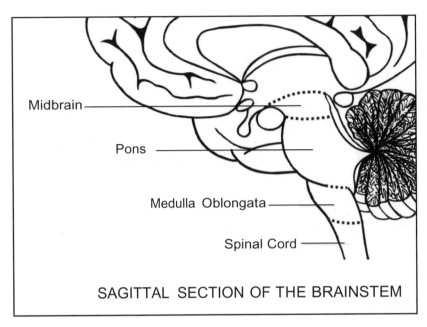

Midbrain

Pons

Medulla Oblongata

Spinal Cord

SAGITTAL SECTION OF THE BRAINSTEM

Figure 5–2. *Schematic definition of brainstem levels, including midbrain, pons, and medulla oblongata.*

PRE-ORAL PARAMETERS OF SWALLOWING

Although not visualized through instrumental assessment, inclusion of pre-oral features of swallowing is considered critical with rapidly emerging data regarding the importance of cortical modulation of the pharyngeal swallowing response. It is "deliciously" tempting to expand the discussion of preoral parameters well beyond the scope of a small section of a defined tutorial on neuroanatomy of swallowing. Our perception and enjoyment of food is heavily influenced by what we see and smell. Anecdotal evidence of this is clear if you smell a bakery, and the wafting smell of freshly baked bread propels you toward your destination. The consequent physiologic response is difficult to ignore. The proliferation of cooking programs on television, where key features of taste and smell are excluded, makes a persuasive, albeit anecdotal, argument for the impor-

tance of visual input to the ingestive process. "You eat with your eyes first" is the mantra of experienced chefs and perhaps is an increasing principle in dysphagia management. The literature in food science, and increasingly in dysphagia management, provides substantive and fascinating investigation of these issues. For this chapter, we adhere to a tutorial of neural substrates. Sensory information relevant to the pre-oral phase of swallowing includes visual cues regarding bolus size, shape, and consistency, and as importantly, its smell. Both the olfactory and optic nerves are not true peripheral nerves and are anatomically different and remote from many of the other peripheral nerves that govern swallowing.

Peripheral Sensory Reception

It is fitting that the first recognition of a bolus through smell, often well before reaching close proximity, is mediated through the first cranial nerve (CN). Odor is detected via sensory receptors of the olfactory nerve (CN I). As odorant molecules are inhaled nasally, or enter the oral cavity retronasally, they come in contact with the peripheral processes, or dendrites, of the bipolar primary olfactory neurons. These are embedded in the surface epithelium of the nasal cavity, which is coated with specialized odor binding proteins to facilitate transmission of olfactory information. With sensory information reaching the cell bodies, the activated neurons then send action potentials via the axons, through the cribriform plate where they synapse on second order neurons in the olfactory bulb.

Visual information about bolus size, color, texture, and shape is mediated peripherally through the optic nerve (CN II). Light enters the primary sensory organ for sight, the eye, and is transformed into a neural signal in the photoreceptors of the retina. The neural signal is detected by the bipolar first-order neurons which then promptly synapse with the ganglion cells that consequently leave the eye, develop myelin covering, and become the optic nerve. This nerve exits the optic canal and, with the optic nerve from the other eye, becomes part of the optic chiasm, from which consequent neural information containing visual information communicates with central brain regions.

Central Sensory Processing and Perception

Information regarding smell is projected to specialized cortical processing centers in the olfactory cortex on the pyriform lobe (Figure 5–3). The central processing of smell is a highly complex, and little understood process.

The bilateral olfactory bulbs present as bulbous outgrowths on the end of the olfactory tracts, positioned on the inferior surface of the frontal lobes. These second-order neurons send their long axons ipsilaterally to communicate with various higher cortical and subcortical regions, including the thalamus and olfactory cortex on the pyriform lobe via the olfactory tract. Interestingly, unlike other sensory information, the olfactory bulb also has direct connections to cortical olfactory cortices, without relaying through the thalamus. In addition, olfactory information is distributed to cortical areas involved in emotion, motivation, and memory. For example, connections exist to the entorhinal cortex (BA 28/BA 34)[1] and amygdala, which are thought to be involved in memory formation and emotional processing (Bear et al., 2007).

The amygdala sends olfactory information to the hypothalamus, the entorhinal cortex sends it to the hippocampus, and the pyriform cortex sends it to the hypothalamus and the orbitofrontal cortex (BA 10, 11, 47) via the dorsomedial nucleus of the thalamus (Carlson, 2001). The olfactory pathway in the medial thalamus is important in "learning behaviors based on olfactory cues" (Levine, 2000, p. 469). Information about taste and olfaction combine in the orbitofrontal cortex, to produce the complex sense of flavor (Carlson, 2001). Imaging studies have also identified activation in the insula and cerebellum following olfactory stimulation (Cerf-Ducastel & Murphy, 2003; Kettenmann et al., 1997).

Visual processing occurs in many occipital, temporal, and parietal brain regions (see Figure 5–3). Visual information is initially projected onto receptive fields in the striate cortex in the posterior lobe (BA 17), before

---

[1]In the early 20th century, German neurologist Korbinian Brodmann created very detailed maps of human and animal brains based on their histological characteristics (Brodmann & Garey, 2006). Brodmann's topographical maps, referred to as Brodmann's areas (BA), are still being used today to denote topographical and functional arrangements of cortical brain areas.

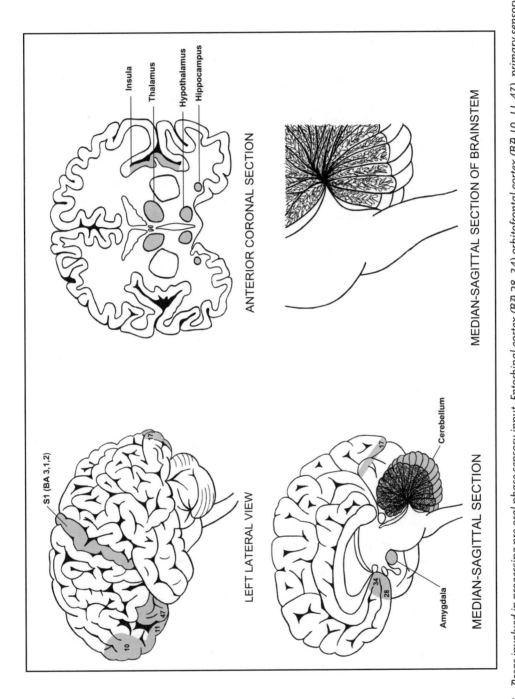

Insula
Thalamus
Hypothalamus
Hippocampus

ANTERIOR CORONAL SECTION

MEDIAN-SAGITTAL SECTION OF BRAINSTEM

S1 (BA 3,1,2)

17

11
47

10

LEFT LATERAL VIEW

Cerebellum

47

34
28

Amygdala

MEDIAN-SAGITTAL SECTION

Figure 5–3. *Areas involved in processing pre-oral phase sensory input. Entorhinal cortex (BA 28, 34) orbitofrontal cortex (BA 10, 11, 47), primary sensory cortex (S1, BA 3, 1, 2), visual cortex (BA 17), insula, thalamus, hypothalamus, hippocampus, amygdala, and cerebellum. Note: CN I (Olfactory) and CN II (Optic) not depicted.*

85

being further processed in several visual association areas that are considered part of the extrastriate system. Two distinct pathways, the dorsal and ventral streams, project visual information from BA 17 to these areas, which are involved in the detection of motion and recognition of objects, respectively.

Central Mechanisms of Motor Contribution

Sensory information processed by the primary olfactory and visual cortical systems projects to a variety of cortical, subcortical and limbic regions for further processing and neural adaptation. For example, following cortical processing, odor information is sent back to the olfactory bulb to allow online modulation of afferent input (Wilson, Kadohisa, & Fletcher, 2006). In addition, olfactory information from the olfactory bulb, insula and mediofrontal cortex travels to the *nucleus tractus solitarius* (NTS) (Neafsey, Hurley-Gius, & Arvanitis, 1986; Terreberry & Neafsey, 1983) for presumed adaptation of the pharyngeal swallowing response. Importantly, the olfactory cortex is not merely involved in the perception of the type of odor and its intensity, but its processing is also modulated by previous experience (plasticity), which in turn allows the neural gating of olfactory information (Wilson et al., 2006). As such, the olfactory cortex can modulate the perceived intensity of a persisting odor through suppression of synaptic excitability within seconds of odor onset (Wilson et al., 2006). Likewise, visual information is projected to several parietal and temporal regions concerned with the contextual interpretation of visual information and initiation of consequent motor actions. As such, visual information can modulate cortical activation relevant for movement execution. For example, presentation of swallowing-related visual biofeedback revealed blood-oxygen-level-dependent (BOLD) activation foci

in frontal regions that was accompanied by a decrease in primary sensory cortex activation, suggesting an activation shift toward regions that are primarily associated with motor planning (Humbert et al., 2012).

Together, the widespread connections to other cortical areas enable cortical olfactory and visual (and taste) systems to contribute significantly to the modulation of sensory and motor areas. Finally, at the transition from the pre-oral to the oral phase, all the sensory information processed and evaluated in the preoral phase triggers a number of precisely timed motor commands that initiate the opening of the mouth, control and modify hand, arm, and body movements, and modulate respiratory control in the anticipation of the arrival of a bolus. These voluntary movements are planned, executed and monitored by cortical and subcortical motor networks primarily in precentral motor areas (BA 4, 6), the basal nuclei, and the cerebellum, as discussed in more detail in the section elaborating on "Central motor preparation and planning" in the oral phase of swallowing. Concurrently, modification of respiratory movements of the intercostal musculature and the diaphragm is orchestrated by *central pattern generators* (CPG) in the medulla of the brainstem, which are also thought to incorporate voluntary commands from higher cortical networks.

Peripheral Motor Output

A number of preparatory processes occur in the pre-oral phase, and they rely on the central control of efferent oropharyngeal pathways (Figure 5–4). The range of these processes, when broadly defined, can include any number of voluntary, parasympathetic, and reflexive actions and depend on the nature of the bolus. This discussion is limited to two key actions: one parasympathetic and one reflexive.

Anticipation of a tasteful bolus can stimulate the parasympathetic nervous system to

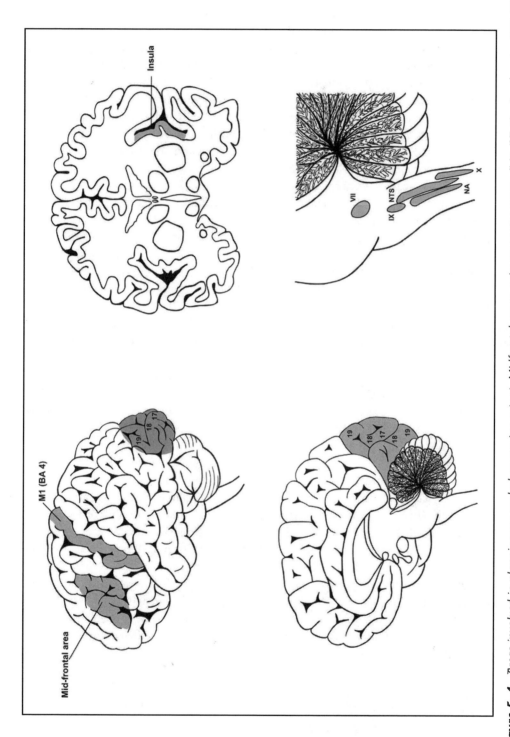

Figure 5-4. *Areas involved in planning pre-oral phase motor output. Midfrontal areas, primary motor cortex (M1, BA 4), visual cortex (BA 17) and visual association areas (BA 18, 19), insula, efferent nuclei of CN VII, IX, X, nucleus tractus solitarius (NTS), and nucleus ambiguus (NA).*

activate salivary glands. These include the submandibular and sublingual glands, innervated by the facial nerves (CN VII) and the paired parotid glands, innervated by the glossopharyngeal nerve (CN IX). Saliva plays an important role in preparation of the bolus during the oral phase of swallowing. For example, saliva contains salivary amylase that begins the breakdown of ingested starches, and lubricates both the bolus and oropharyngeal structures. In addition, saliva serves as a solvent for chemical stimulants in the ingested material that facilitate the perception of taste.

The region of the pons known as the *pontine tegmentum* houses the cell bodies for the parasympathetic division of the facial nerve (CN VII). These cell bodies, which subserve salivary flow, are collectively referred to as the superior salivary nuclei, and receive information directly from the limbic system and the hypothalamus. Long axons leave the nuclei as the chorda tympani branch of the facial nerve for innervation of salivary flow.

In addition to saliva production, the recurrent laryngeal branch of the vagus nerve (CN X) may initiate early onset of vocal adduction for airway protection, which occurs through contraction of the interarytenoid and cricoarytenoid muscles. The cell body for the vagus nerve is the *nucleus ambiguus* (NA), which lies in the ventral medulla. The central processes underlying this anticipatory reflex are not completely understood. It is likely that early adduction of the vocal cords assists airway protection and this process is thought to utilize similar central mechanisms as those that orchestrate vocal fold adduction in the pharyngeal phase of swallowing.

ORAL PARAMETERS OF SWALLOWING

Voluntary control of oral swallowing movements is heavily modulated by input from primary sensory cortices. This is particularly true for swallowing, given the multimodal characteristics of deglutition. Safe pharyngeal swallowing is highly dependent on oral sensory information about the qualities of an ingested bolus (size, consistency, temperature, taste, smell) and proprioceptive feedback about position and movement of the tongue, jaw, cheek, velum, and larynx.

Peripheral Sensory Reception

Within the oral phase, recognition of the bolus within the oral cavity is subserved primarily by two sensory systems, taste and touch, that are mediated through three cranial nerves, the trigeminal (CN V), facial (CN VII), and glossopharyngeal (CN IX), the nuclei for which are housed in two locations within the central nervous system. Although this may seem complex, a move from front to back in the oral cavity and top to bottom in the brainstem, corresponds for both types of sensory input with an increased number for the cranial nerve (V, VII, IX).

Starting at superior and anterior aspects of the oral cavity, several branches of the maxillary division of the trigeminal nerve (CN V: alveolar and palatine branches) supply tactile sensation for the palate and teeth. Neural fibers travel from peripheral sensory receptors to join fibers from the mandibular branch before entering the trigeminal ganglion. Moving posteriorly and laterally, the mandibular branch of the trigeminal (CN V) provides sensory innervation for the mucous membranes of the mouth and gums (buccal nerve), and the anterior two-thirds of the tongue (the lingual nerve). Sensory axons of the nerves pair with those from the maxillary division and enter the trigeminal ganglion, which penetrates the pons on its lateral border. They then synapse on one of three nuclei, dependent on functional consequence. The *mesencephalic trigeminal nucleus* (MTN) mediates proprioceptive and reflex information critical for mastication. The pontine trigeminal nucleus mediates touch, which then communicates with cortical regions via contralateral and ipsilateral pathways through the thalamus. The spinal trigeminal nucleus mediates pain and temperature, which decussates in the lower pons for contralateral projections to the thalamus via the spinal trigeminal pathway. Very importantly, sensory information that is critical for deglutitive purposes also synapses with the *nucleus tractus solitarius* (NTS) in the brainstem. Taste receptors for the anterior two-thirds of the tongue send sensory information via the axons of the chorda tympani branch of the facial nerve to enter the brainstem at the pontomedullary junction. First-order neurons then synapse at the NTS, which is the primary sensory nucleus associated with swallowing.

Moving posteriorly in the oral cavity, the glossopharyngeal nerve (CN IX) provides sensory innervation for the posterior third of the tongue, the tonsils, soft palate, fauces, uvula, and proximal (adjacent) pharyngeal wall. This input synapses directly on the NTS for contribution to the swallowing motor plan before decussating within the medulla, and then merges with the spinal trigeminal tract as it transcends to the cortex. Taste for the posterior tongue is also mediated by the glossopharyngeal nerve (CN IX), whose first-order neurons synapse at the NTS. Secondary fibers then project ipsilaterally to the thalamus. Quite critically, cumulative sensory information transfers either directly from the facial and glossopharyngeal nerves or indirectly from the trigeminal sensory nucleus in the pons to the NTS of the dorsal medulla to contribute to motor planning for the pharyngeal swallow.

Central Sensory Processing and Perception

As in the pre-oral phase, sensory information from all kinds of oropharyngeal receptors is processed by the relevant cortical sensory areas and is integrated by premotor areas into a suitable motor plan (Figure 5–5). The layered structure of the somatosensory cytoarchitecture, especially in the primary sensory cortex (BA 3), allows efficient and fast interconnections with other areas of the brain, in particular those concerned with the integration of sensory information for complex, coordinated movements (e.g., BA 6).

It is noteworthy that somatosensory networks display similar capability for neuroplastic adaptation as has been demonstrated in many other brain regions. For example, studies in the adult owl monkey have shown that increased sensory input through increased use of a certain digit resulted in an expansion of the relevant sensory map representation at the expense of the unused digits (Jenkins, Merzenich, Ochs, Allard, & Guic-Robles, 1990). Importantly, changes in the excitability of somatosensory circuits can have significant flow-on effects on motor output. Studies in animals and humans have demonstrated a link between changes in sensory input and motor cortical excitability, for example, in response to exercise (Classen et al., 1998), peripheral nerve stimulation (Doeltgen et al., 2010; Ridding et al., 2000) and amputation of limbs (Chen et al., 1998). Likewise, in the swallowing motor system, flavored liquids, presented concurrently with an image representing their taste and the matching olfactory stimulus, resulted in increased BOLD activation in the sensory cortices (BA 1, 2, and 3) as well as motor and supplementary motor areas (BA 4 and 6) compared to control saliva or water swallows (Babaei et al., 2010). The close link between sensory input and motor output is thought to be an important mechanism in the generation of a swallowing motor plan that rapidly adapts to the properties of the ingested bolus. In addition, the functionally relevant interactions between sensory input and motor output may provide promising avenues for modulating swallowing biomechanics through the use of rehabilitative interventions.

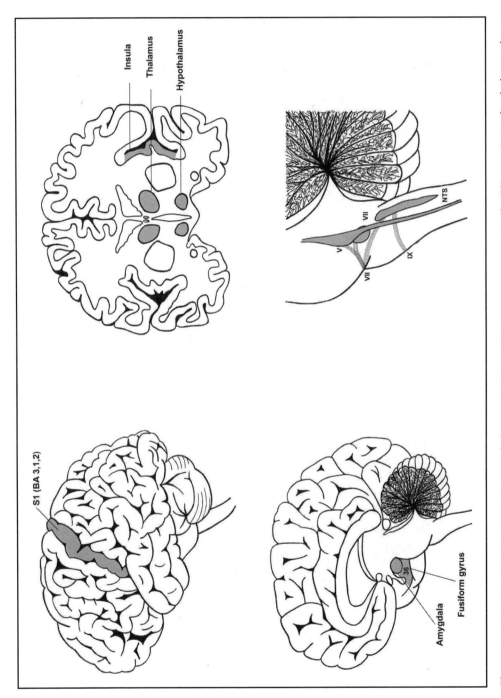

Figure 5–5. *Areas involved in processing oral phase sensory input. Primary sensory cortex (S1, BA 3, 1, 2), insula, thalamus, hypo-thalamus, amygdala, fusiform gyrus (BA 36), sensory nuclei of CN V, VII, IX, and nucleus tractus solitarius (NTS).*

In addition to the information provided about mechanical bolus properties (size, consistency, temperature), information regarding its *taste* is a critical component in the sensory feedback provided to cortical and subcortical swallowing sensorimotor control networks in preparation of a swallow. Unpleasant tastes are key evolutionary survival mechanisms that protect from the ingestion of hazardous, usually poisonous materials. In contrast, pleasant tastes and smells are usually associated with nutritious foods and often trigger an anticipatory response, such as increased salivation. At a cortical level, sensory input from the taste buds is first gated through the thalamus, specifically the *ventral posterior medial* (VPM) nucleus, before being received in the sensory receptor fields for taste in the cerebral cortex, specifically in the primary gustatory cortex (BA 36 and insula). Gustatory information projected from the brainstem is also distributed to other cortical and subcortical networks involved in deglutition, for example, the hypothalamus or amygdala, involved in food preference selection and drive to eat.

Central Motor Preparation and Planning

Biomechanically, the oral phase of swallowing is characterized by volitionally controlled movements of the tongue, jaw, cheeks, and lips in order to achieve bolus preparation (breakdown of solid foods, mixing with saliva, formation of a smooth bolus) before pharyngeal phase swallowing. Masticatory movements of the orofacial structures are under the control of voluntary cortical motor networks, similar to those engaged in voluntary movements of the limbs and torso. The cortical region most heavily involved in the control of volitional movements is the primary motor cortex, also referred to as BA 4 or M1 (Figure 5–6). Within BA 4, the muscles of the body are represented

topographically, with distinct but overlapping muscle representations commonly depicted as the *motor homunculus*. The motor representations of the orofacial musculature are located on the lateral aspects of the precentral gyrus, in close proximity to those of the hands and fingers. They play a critical role in the initiation and control of voluntary orofacial movements during the oral phase of swallowing. The key orofacial muscles for swallowing, all receive neural input from motor output cells located in BA 4. The axons of these output cells, which are also known as *upper motor neurons*, descend bilaterally along the corticobulbar motor pathway through the *corona radiata, internal capsule,* and *cerebral peduncle* toward the brainstem. There, they synapse onto the cell bodies of the *lower motor neurons*, which are located in clusters known as *cranial nerve nuclei*. The axons of the lower motor neurons project from these motor nuclei to the muscle.

Neural commands from cortical motor output cells in BA 4 are the final result of a myriad of preceding motor planning processes that occur at cortical and subcortical levels. For the successful execution of a voluntary movement, an optimal motor plan must be generated and executed in a precisely timed manner. In fact, even during motor execution, the descending motor command is continuously monitored and, if necessary, modified. A number of cortical regions contribute to the planning, initiation, and monitoring of voluntary movements, including: (a) parietal and frontal areas (e.g., BA 4, 6), (b) networks including the basal nuclei and ventral lateral nucleus of the thalamus, and (c) the cerebellum.

It is generally accepted that BA 6, located just anterior to BA 4, plays a key role in movement planning. BA 6 receives extensive axonal input from prefrontal and parietal areas, which are involved in abstract thinking and anticipating consequences, and somatosensory processing, respectively. There are also

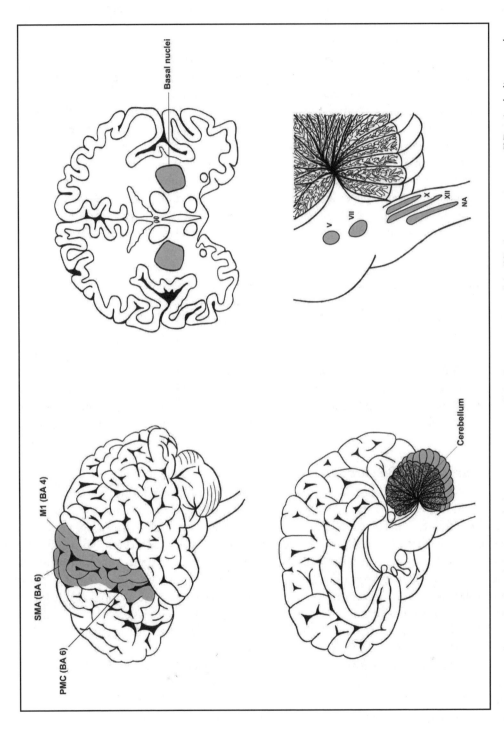

Figure 5–6. *Areas involved in planning oral phase motor output. Primary motor cortex (M1, BA 4), premotor areas (BA 6, including supplementary motor area [SMA] and premotor cortex [PMC]), basal nuclei, cerebellum, motor nuclei of CN V, VII, X, XII, and nucleus ambiguus (NA).*

considerable interconnections between these prefrontal and parietal areas, creating neural networks that are capable of generating movement intentions and anticipating their consequences. This ultimately allows these networks to make a decision about the optimal motor plan for the movement that is to be executed. Support for the role of parietal and frontal areas in movement planning is provided by research showing that finger movement performed from memory activates primary sensory, posterior parietal areas, and BA 6 and BA 4, all of which are implicated in movement planning and execution (Roland, Larsen, Lassen, & Skinhof, 1980). Interestingly, thinking about performing the same movements activates the same cortical areas, except for BA 4, underscoring the "executive" role of this cortical region in motor control.

Within BA 6, activation of the supplementary motor area, or SMA, has been shown to increase approximately one second before movement onset, suggesting that this region plays an important role in premotor planning. Unilateral damage of the SMA often results in impairment of coordination of complex tasks, a condition also known as *apraxia*. The topographical organization of BA 6 neighboring on BA 4 reflects the functional connectivity of these two brain regions and it is thought that these interconnections enable the translation of movement intention to motor commands that specify how this will be achieved.

Once the movement plan has been created, it is ready to be executed. In other words: it is ready to be transferred from BA 6 to the motor output neurons in BA 4 for execution. BA 6 receives the command to "transfer" from a subcortical region referred to as the *basal nuclei* (BN). The BN are a network of subcortical nuclei that receive input from many cerebral areas, in particular the parietal, frontal, and prefrontal cortices. In turn, the BN project onto BA 6 via the ventral lateral nucleus of the thalamus. Together, these neu-

ral connections form a loop, from cortical regions to the BN and the thalamus, back to the cortex, in particular BA 6. It is thought that input from the BN plays a key role in the selection, and initiation, of the movement plan held in BA 6. In short, cortical input to the BN results in a boost of excitation of the SMA (located in BA 6), which in turn facilitates the transfer of the motor plan held in BA 6 to BA 4. The neurotransmitter dopamine plays an important role in the functioning of the BN. Clinically, Parkinson's disease is an example of a disorder of the BN that is related to a lack of dopaminergic excitation of BN cells, which ultimately results in pathological inhibition of the BN pathway that helps initiate voluntary movements.

Finally, the cerebellum also plays a critical role in the successful execution of voluntary movements. Although neocortical areas provide information about movement intention, the optimal motor plan and ultimately its initiation, the cerebellum is thought to be involved in the precise sequencing of muscle contractions in order to achieve the desired movement. Disorders of the cerebellum result in uncoordinated movements, also referred to as *ataxia*.

Peripheral Motor Output

Coordinated inhibition and excitation of several muscle groups are required for bolus entry into the oral cavity. Inhibition of fibers of the buccal branch of the facial nerve (CN VII) that contract orbicularis oris must occur to allow mouth opening. There may be activation of other fibers of the buccal branch and some from the zygomatic branch of the facial nerve (CN VII) to retract accessory facial muscles (such as risorius, zyomaticus, and levator labii superioris), allowing greater spread of the lips for larger food boluses. These muscles receive only contralateral innervation from upper motor neurons, with decussation in the pons just superior to the facial motor nucleus. Upper motor neurons for the trigeminal motor nuclei are bilaterally, ipsilaterally, and contralaterally innervated again with decussation in the pons just above the primary nuclei. The lower motor neurons of the pons consist of five separate nerves. The mylohyoid nerve of the mandibular branch of the trigeminal nerve (CN V) controls active contraction of the jaw openers (anterior belly of digastric and mylohyoid); this movement is further facilitated by activation of the ansa cervicalis (CN VII, and first two nerves exiting the cervical spine C1, C2) for contraction of geniohyoid. Concurrent relaxation of the antagonist jaw closers (temporalis, masseters) is facilitated via the masseteric and deep temporal nerves of the mandibular branch of the trigeminal. As jaw opening is dependent on stabilization of the hyoid bone to resist anterior pull, ansa cervicalis (CN XII, C1, C2) will provide increased tone in the collective anterior strap muscles.

An important feature of airway protection that is easily visualized on VFSS is glossopalatal approximation. Upon bolus entry to the oral cavity, the base of tongue approximates the palate to contain the bolus orally. The neural substrates of this movement provide an excellent example of redundancy in the neuromuscular system that facilitates airway protection even at this very early stage in the swallowing process. Glossopalatal approximation is accomplished primarily via excitation of the pharyngeal plexus contracting the palatoglossus muscle. The pharyngeal plexus is formed by the pharyngeal branches of both of the glossopharyngeal and vagus nerves with contributions from the superior cervical sympathetic ganglion. The lower motor neuron cell bodies of the glossopharyngeal and vagus nerves are positioned in the shared NA of the medulla and nerves of both exit the medulla between the olive and inferior cerebral peduncle. As with many other cranial nerves, there are both contra- and ipsilateral innervations with decussation of fibers within the pons. Additional contributors to glossopalatal approximation are motor fibers of the facial nerve (CN VII) controlling contraction of stylohoid and posterior belly of digastric and the hypoglossal nerve (CN XII) via innervation and subsequent contraction of the styloglossus. The hypoglossal nerve rootlets emerge from the anterior face of the medulla between the pyramids and the olive.

With the airway secured via glossopalatal approximation, the bolus can safely enter the oral cavity. The hypoglossal nerve (CN XII) activates the intrinsic lingual muscles (verticalis, transverse, and longitundinal) to facilitate contouring of the tongue surface for bolus acceptance, and the extrinsic muscles (genioglossus, hyoglossus, and styloglossus) to change the position of the tongue within the oral cavity. Unlike many other swallowing-related biomechanical movements, bolus manipulation is heavily dependent on a single cranial nerve for neural control; all muscles that change the configuration of the lingual surface are innervated by the hypoglossal nerve (CN XII). Upper motor neurons that feed this nerve decussate in the pons for contra- and ipsilateral innervations, and synapse on the hypoglossal nucleus, which is located in the tegmentum of the medulla and emerges as peripheral nerves from the anterior medullary surface in the ventrolateral sulcus. Lingual position in the oral cavity may be secondarily facilitated by facial nerve (CN VII) innervation of posterior belly of digastric and stylohyoid to provide some compensatory function in the event of injury.

Throughout bolus preparation, the base of tongue is relatively more elevated than the tongue tip primarily through activation of the pharyngeal plexus (CN IX, X) that maintains tone in the palatoglossus muscle for glossopalatal approximation. Once the bolus is ready for transfer, the tongue base must drop to allow bolus transfer; this is accomplished passively via terminated activation of pharyngeal plexus for palatoglossal relaxation, paired with excitation of fibers of the hypoglossal nerve (CN XII) for active contraction of the genioglossus and hyoglossus, which pulls the base of tongue inferiorly. As the tongue base drops, the hypoglossal nerve (CN XII) also transmits the command to the collective intrinsic lingual muscles to pull the tip of the tongue toward the palate and then "squeeze the bolus" from the oral cavity.

PHARYNGEAL PARAMETERS OF SWALLOWING

Peripheral Sensory Reception

Onset of the pharyngeal swallow for deglutitive purposes requires three types of input into the NTS: cognitive cortical processing of the food to be ingested via descending corticobulbar pathways, sensory perception of bolus characteristics via trigeminal, facial, and glossopharyngeal nerves, and perhaps some component of deep muscle receptor input linked to depression of the tongue base for bolus transfer. This information converges on the NTS as a series of graded potentials, which summate until breaching an electrochemical threshold to trigger an action potential, which presents as the pharyngeal swallow. The dorsal nucleus (NTS) then sends the motor command to the ventral nucleus or the NA for execution. Inconsistency in the onset of the pharyngeal swallow may represent variable contributions from these three sources of sensory input. Post-swallow pharyngeal residue is detected in normal swallowing via mucosal sensory recep-

tors that initiate glossopharyngeal nerve fibers (CN IX). This information relays back to the NTS and subsequently results in initiation of a clearing swallow to manage such pharyngeal residue (Figure 5–7).

Central Sensory Processing and Perception

Sensory information relevant to the pharyngeal phase of swallowing is processed at the brainstem level, as well as in several cortical processing centers associated with various bolus properties (BA 3, 2, 1; gustatory cortex and olfactory cortex; see Figure 5–7). This sensory information is thought to play a role in modulating the brainstem generated motor response. At the brainstem level, the NTS, receiving input from vagal afferent fibers, in particular the superior laryngeal nerve (SLN), as well as from trigeminal (CN V), facial (CN VII), and glossopharyngeal (CN IX) nerves, constitutes the main sensory hub involved in swallowing. Animal stimulation studies have shown that afferent fibers of the SLN play a key role in the triggering of the patterned swallowing response, whereas stimulation of the glossopharyngeal nerve (CN IX) facilitates, but does not elicit, a swallowing response (for an excellent review, see Jean, 2006). Experimentally lesioning the NTS abolishes swallowing in response to SLN stimulation, underscoring its critical role in the initiation of swallowing (Doty et al., 1967). Peripheral sensory input is not only critical for swallowing initiation, but also for the execution of the swallowing motor response. For example, the patterned contraction of the oropharyngeal musculature is highly dependent on bolus properties, suggesting that peripheral sensory feedback modulates the centrally generated motor plan. For this to occur, excitatory and inhibitory modulation of the swallowing motor plan is

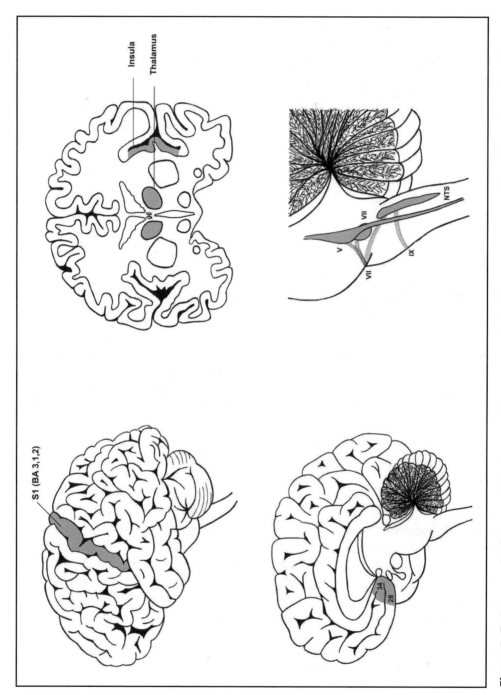

Figure 5–7. *Areas involved in processing pharyngeal phase sensory input. Primary sensory cortex (S1, BA 3, 1, 2), insula, thalamus, entorhinal cortex (BA 28, 34), sensory nuclei of CN V, VII, IX, and nucleus tractus solitarius (NTS).*

necessary to accommodate bolus requirements and coordinate the precisely timed swallowing motor sequence. At the brainstem level, such neural modulation is thought to occur via interneurons between the NTS and swallowing-related *central pattern generators* CPGs (Jean, 2001).

Swallowing-related CPGs also receive input from cortical and subcortical areas that participate in the modulation of the final swallowing motor sequence. Therefore, cortical sensorimotor excitability facilitated by input from pharyngeal sensory receptor fields is, for obvious reasons, of major relevance for swallowing sensorimotor control. In this context, research has shown that short lasting anesthesia of the pharyngeal mucosa leads to a decrease in cortical activation of both sensory and motor cortical areas as observed with magnetoencephalography (MEG) (Teismann et al, 2007). Functionally, pharyngeal anesthesia was associated with increased floor-of-mouth muscle activation during swallowing, suggesting a compensatory mechanism for decreased sensory feedback (Teismann et al., 2007). Interestingly, anesthesia-induced disruption of sensory input can result in disordered swallowing, but does not completely abolish swallowing, suggesting that sensory processing plays a modulatory role rather than being an absolute prerequisite for swallowing (Mansson & Sandberg, 1974). In contrast, increasing sensory feedback from the pharynx by electrically stimulating the pharyngeal mucosa has been shown to modify cortical sensory processing approximately 80 ms following the pharyngeal electrical stimulus, an effect that was accompanied by increased motor cortical excitability (Gow et al., 2004). Thus, processing of swallowing-related pharyngeal sensory input influences the central pattern generated motor plan both directly via sensory afferents targeting the NTS, and more indirectly via descending cortical input that is mediated by sensory-driven changes in cortical excitability.

Central Motor Preparation and Planning

It is generally accepted that the motor plan for the pharyngeal phase of swallowing is generated by networks of swallowing-related neurons, also known as *central pattern generators* (CPGs) in the medulla of the brainstem (Jean 2001, 2006). There are two main CPGs relevant for pharyngeal swallowing pattern generation: a group of neurons in the dorsal part of the medulla, known as the dorsal swallowing group (DSG) and a second group of neurons in the *ventrolateral* part of the medulla, known as the ventral swallowing group (VSG). In general, the DSG is thought to be primarily responsible for the triggering and timing of patterned oropharyngeal muscle contractions, whereas the VSG distributes this motor plan to the various CN motor neuron pools involved in the contraction. Topographically, the DSG is closely associated with the NTS, the main sensory nucleus in the medulla. Conveniently, the VSG has close associations with the NA, an important motor circuitry of the efferent fibers of the vagus (CN X) and glossopharyngeus (CN IX) nerves. Importantly, both the DSG and the VSG have connections with cortical sensorimotor networks that modulate their excitability through excitatory and inhibitory connections, thus influencing their output and ultimately the patterned motor response.

This notion is supported by a growing body of research indicating that a number of cortical neuronal networks are active during swallowing. For example, *functional magnetic resonance imaging* (fMRI) studies have demonstrated swallowing-related activation in a number of distinct cortical areas, including motor areas on the lateral precentral gyrus, sensory areas on the postcentral gyrus, and the right insula (Martin et al., 2001). Interestingly, differential cortical activation has been reported for saliva and water swallows, indicating that the sensory and biomechanical characteristics of each swallow type may, at least in part, have a cortical origin. Plasticity studies have shown that increasing the excitability of pharyngeal M1 representations of the swallowing dominant hemisphere using pharyngeal electrical stimulation facilitates motor cortical excitability, which functionally is accompanied by a reduction in pharyngeal transit time and aspiration risk in dysphagic patients (Fraser et al. 2002). Likewise, increasing pharyngeal corticobulbar excitability using facilitatory *repetitive transcranial magnetic stimulation* (rTMS) was able to counteract motor cortical inhibition following inhibitory rTMS (Jefferson, 2009) and, clinically, was associated with reduced aspiration, improved feeding status and shorter stays in hospital (Jayasekeran, 2010). Together, these studies support the notion that M1 excitability is functionally relevant for pharyngeal swallowing neuromotor control. Further evidence for an involvement of cortical areas in the control of swallowing can be derived from studies analyzing the associations of cortical lesion locations and dysphagic symptoms. For example, Gonzalez-Fernandes et al. (2008) identified a significant association between internal capsule lesions and dysphagia. In addition, Daniels and Foundas (1999) documented that anterior lesions and lesions in subcortical periventricular white matter sites are commonly associated with risk of aspiration than posterior lesions.

Together, current research suggests that the patterned motor plan for pharyngeal phase swallowing is generated by CPG's in the brainstem and is modified through input from higher subcortical and cortical centers. Thus, swallowing appears to rely on highly distributed neural networks involving neuronal networks on all levels of the brain.

Peripheral Motor Output

The peripheral nerves involved in pharyngeal swallowing are all housed within the brainstem and are all linked either directly (CN IX, X, XI) or indirectly (CN V, VII, XII) to the NA (Figure 5–8). This ensures that motor control for the pharyngeal phase of swallowing produces a cascade of rapid and overlapping, complex biomechanical movements that can adapt quickly to bolus conditions.

Anterior hyoid movement is the most consistently observed initial marker of the pharyngeal swallow. Neuromuscular forces acting on the hyoid must maintain a delicate balance to allow for anterior movement required for epiglottic deflection and upper esophageal sphincter (UES) opening. Anterior hyoid movement requires excitation of the mylohyoid nerve, a component of the mandibular branch of the trigeminal nerve (CN V; located in the pons and receives input from NA). This stimulates ipsilateral contraction of the anterior belly of digastric and mylohyoid muscles and the ansa cervicalis (CN VII, C1, C2 with nuclei in the brainstem and spinal cord; also synapsing with NA) for contraction of the geniohyoid muscle. This redundancy in neural input is of significance, as anterior hyoid movement is critical for consequent biomechanical events associated with bolus transfer and airway protection. Concurrent with anterior movement, the facial nerve (CN VII motor nucleus in the pons) activates the posterior belly of digastric and the stylohyoid muscles, whereas the pharyngeal plexus (CN IX, X arising from NA in the medulla) initiates activation of the middle pharyngeal constrictor which bilaterally inserts into the cornu of the hyoid bone to biomechanically pull the hyoid back and up and facilitates pharyngeal shortening. The integrated swallowing motor plan, with all motor output ultimately initiating at the NA, allows for a balance in degree of contraction. Velopharyngeal closure is another early event in the pharyngeal swallow. Activation of the pharyngeal plexus (CN IX, X) emerging from the NA in the ventral medulla results in innervation of the levator veli palatini to facilitate velopharyngeal closure.

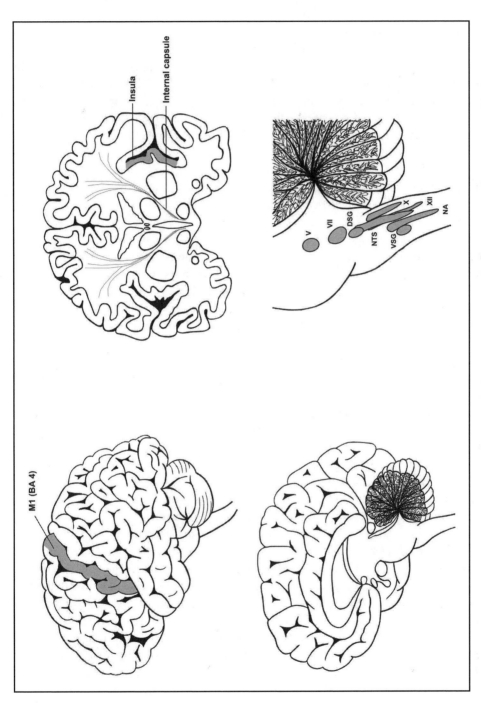

Figure 5–8. Areas involved in planning pharyngeal phase motor output. Primary motor cortex (M1, BA 4), internal capsule, insula, motor nuclei of CN V, VII, X, XII, nucleus tractus solitarius (NTS) and associated dorsal swallowing group (DSG, and nucleus ambiguus (NA) and associated ventral swallowing group (VSG). Note: Nerves of cervical section of spinal cord (C1, C2) not depicted. Motor fibers of CNIX arising from NA.

Once again, neural redundancy is in place to provide multiple levels of closure for deglutitive airway protection. External forces must act on the non-muscular epiglottis to ensure deflection. Anterior hyoid movement effectively pulls the base of the epiglottis anteriorly, resulting in a functional deflection. This anterior movement, innervated by trigeminal (CN V) and ansa cervicalis (CN XII, C1, C2), is key to offset the posterior pull of the middle pharyngeal constrictors (CN IX, X) and the posterior suprahyoids including the stylohyoid and posterior belly of digastrics (CN VII). In the absence of anterior movement, the epiglottis will simply elevate and thus fail to occlude the airway entrance. Airway protection is further facilitated through excitation of fibers of the ansa cervicalis (CN XII, C1, C2), which results in contraction of the anterior strap muscles, particularly the thyrohyoid. Both the infrahyoid and suprahyoid muscle groups result in supraglottic shortening, which consequently allows supraglottic compression of quadrangular membrane over the anterior aspect of the airway entrance. The recurrent laryngeal branch of the vagus nerve (CN X) innervates the interarytenoid and cricoarytenoid muscles to facilitate vocal adduction.

Airway protection is further facilitated by sensory feedback systems within the pharynx and larynx. The pharyngeal plexus (CN IX, X with cell bodies housed in the NTS of the dorsal medulla) provides sensory innervation to the oropharynx and hypopharynx. The superior laryngeal nerve of the vagus (CN X arising from NTS) provides sensory input to the larynx and trachea, whereas the recurrent laryngeal nerve of the vagus accepts afferent information from the carina, or tracheal bifurcation. As an important mechanism for eliciting a rapid cough response, sensory input from the superior laryngeal nerve transmits not only to the NTS as the primary sensory nuclei, but also transfers directly to the NA,

the motor nucleus controlling CN X, such that a reflexive cough can be elicited within milliseconds of sensory receptor activation at the larynx.

The pharyngeal plexus (CN IX, X), the hypoglossal (CN XII) and the facial (CN VII) nerves all contribute to bolus propulsion through the pharynx. In order to transfer the bolus into the oropharynx, CN X innervates the styloglossus muscles and CN VII receives input from NA to elicit activation of the stylohyoids and posterior belly of digastrics to retract and elevate the tongue base. The pharyngeal plexus (CN IX, X) innervates the glossopharyngeus muscles, part of the superior pharyngeal constrictor, which pulls the tongue base directly back to the posterior pharyngeal wall for positive pressure on the bolus. These same nerves and muscles contribute to pharyngeal shortening and are further facilitated in this movement by the glossopharyngeal (CN IX) activation of the stylopharyngeus, and pharyngeal plexus activation of the salpingopharyngeus and palatopharyngeus muscles. The pharyngeal plexus innervates the superior, middle, and inferior constrictor muscles sequentially to clear the tail of the bolus from the pharynx by providing not only positive pressure on the bolus, but also shortening the pharynx to elevate the UES to meet the oncoming bolus.

The rostral branch of the superior laryngeal nerve of the vagus (CN X) maintains a state of excitation at rest which results in tonic contraction of the cricopharyngeus muscle. Bolus transport through the UES requires inhibition of this activation to allow the UES to be pulled open. The trigeminal nerve (CN V) activates the anterior belly of digastric and mylohyoid, while the ansa cervicalis (CN XII, C1, C2) innervates the geniohyoid to exert the external traction force to open the UES. As all pharyngeal structures are elevating, anterior hyoid movement is critical for opening. As the bolus passes through the UES, the pharyngeal plexus (CN IX, X) innervates the inferior pharyngeal constrictor to squeeze the tail of the bolus into the esophagus.

ESOPHAGEAL PARAMETERS OF SWALLOWING

Peripheral Sensory Reception

Sensory osmo-, chemo-, mechano-, and thermoreceptors in the mucosa of the esophagus detect changes in the esophageal lumen. Additionally, stretch receptors contained within the smooth muscle layer of the esophagus are sensitive to distention (Fass, 2004). These first-order viscerosensory neurons of the vagus nerve (CN X), along with fibers from the heart and lungs, then converge with abdominal visceral fibers traveling up from the stomach. With their cell bodies in the nodose ganglion in the peripheral nervous system, they ultimately enter the medulla and synapse on the NTS. Other sensory information is received from spinal afferents, with cell bodies in the dorsal root ganglia. Fibers of these nerves terminate in the spinal column and in the nucleus gracilis and cuneatus in the brainstem. They then project to cortical regions for perception of pain and discomfort.

Central Sensory Processing and Perception

Similar to the sensory processing of pharyngeal sensory input, esophageal afferent input is processed both at a brainstem and cortical level. Vagal afferent input projects to cell clusters in the NTS (Fass, 2004), before projecting to cortical sensory centers including (BA3,2,1 [also known as S1]) and the insula via the thalamus (Aziz & Thompson, 1998) (Figure 5–9). Studies investigating the cortical processing of esophageal sensory input following esophageal acid perfusion using fMRI or *positron emission tomography* (PET) scanning have demonstrated activation of sensory association areas, including the anterior and posterior cingulate cortex, prefrontal cortexes and the insula (Aziz et al., 1997; Kern et al., 1998). These areas are generally associated with the perception of nonspecific pain. Interestingly, cortical activation in response to acidification occurred even at subthreshold levels, suggesting that chemical stimulation of esophageal receptors activates widespread cortical sensory areas.

Central Motor Preparation and Planning

Unlike the pharyngeal swallowing motor response, which can be volitionally modified through descending cortical input, the esophageal motor response is exclusively driven by brainstem generated motor plans. Esophageal motor control is orchestrated by parasympathetic and sympathetic nervous systems. It has been proposed that a relatively direct circuitry may exist between afferent sensory fibers from the esophagus, linking neurons in the DSG with motor neurons in the NA or vagal dorsal motor nucleus via direct interneurons or via the VSG (Jean, 2006).

Peripheral Motor Output

The esophageal musculature is predominantly innervated by efferent fibers of the vagus nerve (CN X). Vagal nerve fibers originating in the NA in the medulla project to the proximal, striated esophageal musculature, includ-

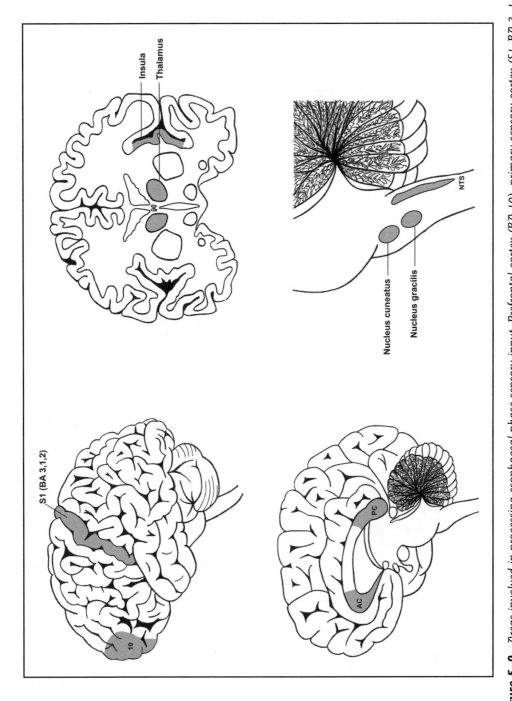

Figure 5-9. *Areas involved in processing esophageal phase sensory input. Prefrontal cortex (BA 10), primary sensory cortex (S1, BA 3, 1, 2), insula, thalamus, anterior cingulate (AC), posterior cingulate (PC), nucleus cuneatus, nucleus gracilis, and nucleus tractus solitarius (NTS).*

ing the upper esophageal sphincter. The more distal, smooth muscle segments and the lower esophageal sphincter receive motor commands from the dorsal motor nucleus of the vagus nerve. Parasympathetic nerves from the NA and dorsal motor nucleus of the vagus (also in the medulla) innervate glands within the esophagus (Figure 5–10). Peristaltic activity and blood vessel constriction of the outer esophagus are innervated through sympathetic fibers from the spinal nerve segments T1 to T10. Innervation of intrinsic muscle fibers of the esophagus is dependent on two interconnected plexi that lie within layers of the esophagus. Myenteric plexus regulates contraction of the outer muscle layers, whereas submucosal plexus regulates secretion and the peristaltic contractions of the mucosa.

CONCLUSION

The physiological processes of swallowing, as assessed by VFSS and other imaging and clinical assessment tools, are the functional result of a myriad of neurophysiological processes that occur in the peripheral and central nervous systems in a precisely timed and staggeringly rapid manner. As outlined in this chapter, a number of neurophysiological processes contribute to unimpaired swallowing function at various levels of the nervous system, with some neural redundancies controlling certain key aspects of the oropharyngeal swallowing response ensuring additional robustness and adaptability of this vital neuromotor system. Careful interpretation of visually observed swallowing (dys)-function paired with a sound knowledge of the underlying neural impairment enables the clinician to derive a differentiated and clinically meaningful diagnosis. This, in turn, is critical for designing a suitable rehabilitation program tailored to the individual patient and will ultimately improve rehabilitative outcomes. In addition, sound knowledge of the intimate link between neuropathological processes and functional swallowing impairment will enable the clinician to be an actively contributing member of the specialist rehabilitation team. It is our hope that the approach of presenting biomechanical features of swallowing and their sensory and motor substrates at both a central and peripheral level will facilitate this clinical association between neuropathology and swallowing impairment.

Acknowledgments. We gratefully acknowledge Suzanne M. McAllister, who kindly created the figures included in this chapter. Sebastian Doeltgen is supported by a Postdoctoral Training Fellowship of the National Health and Medical Research Council of Australia.

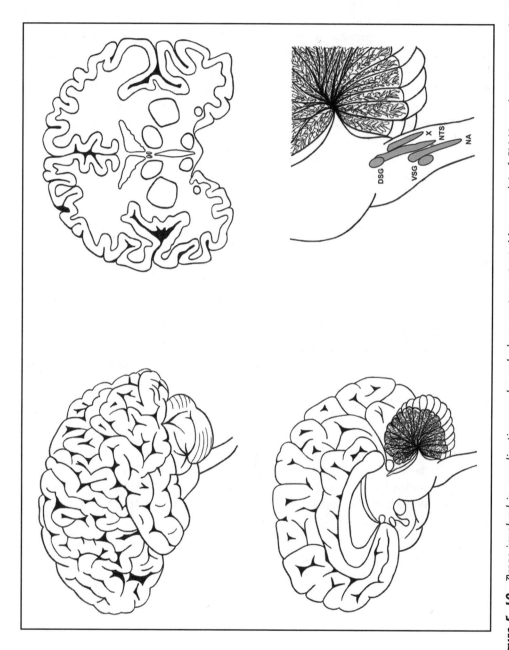

Figure 5–10. *Areas involved in coordinating esophageal phase motor output. Motor nuclei of CN X, nucleus tractus solitarius (NTS) and associated dorsal swallowing group (DSG), and nucleus ambiguus (NA) and associated ventral swallowing group (VSG).*

REFERENCES

Aziz, Q., & Thompson, D. G. (1998). Brain-gut axis in health and disease. *Gastroenterology, 114*(3), 559–578.

Babaei, A. Kern, M., Antonik, S., Mepani, R., Ward, D. B., Li, S. J., Hyde, J. & Shaker, R. (2010). Enhancing effects of flavored nutritive stimuli on cortical swallowing network activity. *American Journal of Physiology-Gastrointestinal and Liver Physiology, 299,* G422–G429.

Bear, M. F., Connors, B. W., & Paradiso, M. A. (2007). The chemical senses. In *Neuroscience* (3rd ed., pp. 251–275). Baltimore, MD: Lippincott, Williams & Wilkins.

Brodmann, K., & Garey, L. (2006). *Brodmann's localisation in the cerebral cortex: The principles of comparative localisation in the cerebral cortex based on the cytoarchitectonics.* New York, NY: Springer.

Carlson, N. R. (2001). *Physiology of behavior* (7th ed.). Boston, MA: Allyn and Bacon.

Cerf-Ducastel, B., & Murphy, C. (2003). FMRI brain activation in response to odors is reduced in primary olfactory areas of elderly subjects. *Brain Research, 986,* 39–53.

Chen, R., Corwell, B., Yaseen, Z., Hallett, M., & Cohen, L. G. (1998). Mechanisms of cortical reorganization in lower-limb amputees. *Journal of Neuroscience, 18*(9), 3443–3450.

Classen, J., Liepert, J.,Wise, S. P., Hallett, M. & Cohen, L. G. (1998). Rapid plasticity of human cortical movement representation induced by practice. *Journal of Neurophysiology, 79*(2), 1117–1123.

Daniels, S. K., & Foundas, A. L. (1999). Lesion localization in acute stroke patients with risk of aspiration. *Journal of Neuroimaging, 9*(2), 91–98.

Daniels, S. K., & Huckabee, M. L. (2008). *Dysphagia following stroke.* San Diego, CA: Plural.

Doeltgen, S. H., Dalrymple-Alford, C., Ridding, M. C., & Huckabee, ML. (2010). Differential effects of neuromuscular electrical stimulation parameters on submental motor evoked potentials. *Neurorehabilitation and Neural Repair, 24*(6), 519–527.

Doty, R. W., Richmond, W. H., & Storey, A. T. (1967). Effect of medullary lesions on coordination of deglutition. *Experimental Neurology, 17,* 91–106.

Fass, R. (2004). Sensory testing of the esophagus. *Journal of Clinical Gastroenterology, 38*(8), 628–641.

Fraser, C., Power, M., Hamdy, S., Rothwell, J., Hobday, D., Hollander, I., . . . Thompson, D. (2002). Driving plasticity in the human adult motor cortex is associated with improved motor function after brain injury. *Neuron, 34,* 831–840.

González-Fernández, M., Gardyn, M., Wyckoff, S., Ky, P. K. S., & Palmer, J. B. (2008). Validation of ICD-9 Code 787.2 for identification of individuals with dysphagia from administrative databases. *Dysphagia, 24*(4), 398–402.

Gow, D., Hobson, A. R., Furlong, P., & Hamdy, S. (2004). Characterising the central mechanisms of sensory modulation in human swallowing motor cortex. *Clinical Neurophysiology, 115,* 2382–2390.

Humbert, I. A., & Joel, S. (2012). Tactile, gustatory, and visual biofeedback stimuli modulate neural substrates of deglutition. *NeuroImage, 59,* 1485–1490

Jayasekeran, V., Singh, S., Tyrrell, P., Michou, E., Jefferson, S., Mistry, S., . . . Hamdy, S. (2010). Adjunctive functional pharyngeal electrical stimulation reverses swallowing disability after brain lesions. *Gastroenterology, 138,* 1737–1746.

Jean, A. (2001). Brainstem control of swallowing: Neuronal network and cellular mechanisms. *Physiological Reviews, 81*(2), 929–969.

Jean, A., & Dallaporta, M. (2006). Electrophysiologic characterization of the swallowing pattern generator in the brainstem. *GI Motility Online* (2006) doi:10.1038/gimo9. Retrieved January 23, 2012, from http://www.nature.com/gimo/contents/pt1/full/gimo9.html

Jefferson, S., Mistry, S., Michou, E., Singh, S., Rothwell, J. C., & Hamdy, S. (2009). Reversal of a virtual lesion in human pharyngeal motor cortex by high frequency contralesional brain stimulation. *Gastroenterology, 137,* 841–849.

Jenkins, W. M., Merzenich, M. M., Ochs, M. T., Allard, T., & Guic-Robles, E. (1990). Functional reorganization of primary somatosensory cortex in adult owl monkeys after behaviorally controlled tactile stimulation. *Journal of Neurophysiology, 63,* 82–104.

Kern, M. K, Birn, R. M., Jaradeh, S., Jesmanowicz, A., Cox, R. W., Hyde, J. S., & Shaker, R. (1998). Identification and characterization of cerebral cortical response to esophageal mucosal acid exposure and distention. *Gastroenterology, 115*(6), 1353–1362.

Kettenmann, B., Hummel, C., Stefan, H., & Kobal, G. (1997). Multiple olfactory activity in the human neocortex identified by magnetic source imaging. *Chemical Senses, 22*(5), 493–502.

Levine, M. W. (2000). *Levine and Shefner's fundamental of sensation and perception* (3rd ed.). Oxford, UK: Oxford University Press.

Mansson, I., & Sandberg, N. (1974). Effects of surface anesthesia on deglutition in man. *Laryngoscope, 84*(3), 427–437.

Martin, R. E., Goodyear, B. G., Gati, J. S., & Menon, R. S. (2001). Cerebral cortical representation of automatic and volitional swallowing in humans. *Journal of Neurophysiology, 85,* 938–950.

Neafsey, E.J., Hurley-Gius, K.M., & Arvanitis, D. (1986). The topographical organization of neurons in the rat medial frontal, insular and olfactory cortex projecting to the solitary nucleus, olfactory bulb, periaqueductal gray and superior colliculus. *Brain Research, 377*(2), 561–570.

Ridding, M. C., Brouwer, B., Miles, T. S., Pitcher, J. B., & Thompson, P. D. (2000). Changes in muscle responses to stimulation of the motor cortex induced by peripheral nerve stimulation in human subjects. *Experimental Brain Research, 131*(1), 135–143.

Roland, P., Larsen, B., Lassen, N., & Skinhof, E. (1980). Supplementary motor area and other cortical areas in organization of voluntary movements in man. *Journal of Neurophysiology, 43,* 118–136.

Teismann, I. K., Steinstraeter, O., Stoeckigt, K., Suntrup, S., Wollbrink. A., Pantev, C., & Dziewas R. (2007). Functional oropharyngeal sensory disruption interferes with the cortical control of swallowing. *BMC Neuroscience, 8,* 62.

Terreberry, R. R., & Neafsey, E. J. (1983). Rat medial frontal cortex: A visceral motor region with a direct projection to the solitary nucleus. *Brain Research, 278,* 245–249.

Wilson, D. A., Kadohisa, M., Fletcher, M. L. (2006). Cortical contributions to olfaction: Plasticity and perception. *Seminars in Cell and Developmental Biology, 17*(4), 462–470.

Chapter

6

BIOMECHANICAL ANALYSIS

James L. Coyle

INTRODUCTION

The transport of a bolus from the oral cavity to the esophagus through the pharynx results from a highly synchronized sequence of events lasting a very short duration. However, incoordination or abnormal obstruction of flow leads to varying degrees of dysphagia. Forces that generate and maintain intrabolus pressure, and those that produce hyolaryngeal excursion, are responsible for much of the efficient transfer of swallowed material to the digestive system as well as prevention of pulmonary aspiration. As videofluoroscopy is a dynamic assessment of function (versus an imaging modality designed to identify abnormal structure), an overly narrow diagnostic focus on the presence/absence of aspiration, and on patterns of residue, disables the examiner's ability to identify abnormal swallow biomechanics that may be amenable to intervention. This chapter describes the important biomechanical events of oropharyngeal swallowing, how they appear under videofluoroscopy, and how they may lead to bolus misdirection.

Purposes of Biomechanical Analysis: It's the Patient and Not the Barium

The presence or absence of abnormal airway penetration or of pharyngeal residue, are commonly reported without explanations of their causes. "Aspiration was observed" or "retention in the pyriform sinuses" often appears in examination reports without an assessment of the physiological disturbance that led to them. The videofluoroscopic swallowing study is not merely a screening tool for detecting these observations. If it were, we would not need trained radiologists, radiographers, and speech-language pathologists to perform these examinations; we could train anybody to see that barium had gone where it should not have gone. Aspiration, abnormal laryngeal penetration, and excessive pharyngeal residue are short-term outcomes of swallowing biomechanical errors. Efforts to eliminate them through tactics like texture modification or multiple swallows address the obviously abnormal movement of contrast but do not address the underlying abnormalities that caused abnormal flow in the first place. The dysphagia clinician cannot treat the barium, but he or she can treat the patient.

The radiology professional specializes in the diagnosis of disease through identification (via static and dynamic imaging) of anatomical or physiological aberrations from normal. The structure and function (normal and abnormal) of target organs can be observed and inferences regarding probable pathology produced. Traditionally, these professionals have not been involved in therapeutic efforts to remediate disease, though recent advances in interventional radiologic procedures have evolved. Modern interventional radiology was actually preceded by an interventional radiographic procedure more than three decades ago: the VFSS. The speech-language pathologist (SLP) can be trained to assess the structure and function of the upper aerodigestive tract, and then to propose and evaluate the effectiveness of interventions *during* the examination, using modern imaging technology. These therapeutic probes are essential components of the VFSS procedure, which is designed not just to observe and describe a disorder, but to assess effectiveness of interventions (Kahrilas, 1994; Logemann, 1993). The collaboration of the radiology and speech-language-swallowing professionals during the VFSS produces a unique diagnostic therapeutic trial that is unlike traditional radiographic procedures.

The VFSS, described in the early 1980s by Dr. Jeri Logemann (Logemann, 1983) and others, is both a diagnostic and interventional procedure. Without intervention, the VFSS merely documents impairments. Similarly, without characterizing the biomechanical causes of adverse short-term outcomes such as aspiration and post-swallow residue, the VFSS merely documents whether the patient aspirates what is swallowed or whether the bolus has been swallowed in its entirety, and does little to determine the cause or illuminate solutions for the problem. This chapter aims to review the biomechanical causes of the most common short-term outcomes of bolus

misdirection in an effort to remind us all of the goals of the instrumental swallowing study: diagnosis and treatment of dysphagia. The author summarizes the biomechanics of oropharyngeal swallowing with reference to the underlying physiology and links them to the radiographic findings commonly observed during the VFSS. The careful description of aberrant biomechanics will lead the clinician to effective interventions.

The Biomechanics of Swallowing

In Chapter 4, the anatomy and physiology of swallowing were discussed. Here we shall apply these principles to the movements of structures during swallowing and in the following sections, to the implications of abnormal movement patterns on short-term outcomes such as aspiration and post-swallow residue. Aspiration and post-swallow pharyngeal residue often receive more attention than necessary because the examiner does not instead focus on the more important biomechanical events causing aspiration and post-swallow residue.

Oropharyngeal Biomechanics and Swallowing

Although the oropharyngeal swallow is a continuum of temporally overlapping events, it is convenient to artificially divide this continuum into stages to describe what happens in the very short duration of the swallow. The mandible, soft palate, tongue, hyolaryngeal complex, and upper esophageal sphincter (UES) are active during the entire oropharyngeal swallow. However, activity of these structures may vary with bolus volume and viscosity, aging, and other factors described elsewhere in this book, and may actually shift from the performance of one action to another. Biomechanical analysis of oropharyngeal swallowing requires an understanding of normal swallow biomechanics.

The mandible, along with the hyoid bone and skull base, forms the anchoring attachment for the tongue. The mandible also anchors all of the anterior muscles responsible for hyolaryngeal excursion (HLE). During oral preparatory activity, stabilization of the mandible is necessary to ensure that forces generated within the lingual muscle fibers are transferred to their intended destinations. For example, the mandible is stabilized in a relatively "closed" or elevated position during oral bolus transit, enabling close contact of the tongue with the palate. This facilitates transfer of the tongue's propulsive forces to the bolus, which is progressively (from anterior to posterior) compressed between the tongue and hard palate (Tasko, Kent, & Westbury, 2002).

A common law of physics, Boyle's law, which indicates that decreasing the volume of a fluid within a closed cavity produces an increase in the fluid's pressure (or potential energy), illustrates how compression of the bolus generates potential energy in the form of intrabolus pressure (Nicosia & Robbins, 2001). Pressure generation is an "anterograde" or forward moving process with the propulsive forces transferred from the "beginning" of the oropharyngeal mechanism (i.e., anterior oral cavity) toward the "end" of the mechanism (the UES) as the bolus tail is progressively compressed. This pattern is stable during aging though the achievement of peak pressure generation takes longer in the elderly with liquid boluses (Nicosia et al., 2000). Generation of pressure between the tongue and palate is dependent on lingual force generation along with approximation of the tongue and palate to one another during oral transit. Were the mandible to be depressed during oral transit, (due to weakness in masseter and medial ptery-

goid or other condition reducing their ability to maintain mandible elevation), bolus compression would be compromised and oral residue after the initial swallow would be the result.

The tongue acts like a hydrostatic piston with its configuration almost constantly changing during bolus propulsion (Tasko et al., 2002). Only the extrinsic lingual muscles (except palatoglossus) have fixed bony origins causing the action of these muscles to always displace the entire tongue toward the site of these fixed attachments. For example, contraction of the genioglossus always displaces the tongue anteriorly (protrusion) toward the symphysis of the mandible. Intrinsic lingual muscles have no bony attachments, so their contractions only alter the shape of the tongue. Lingual movement during bolus propulsion can vary due to several conditions; however, there are relatively well-documented patterns of lingual motion producing bolus propulsion. The progressive (anterior to posterior) contact of the tongue to the palate produces a shrinking oral cavity volume propelling the bolus in the direction of the pharynx. When there is inadequate force of linguapalatal contact there is a reduction in intrabolus pressure generation which is a biomechanical error that will produce abnormal bolus flow or misdirection.

The palatoglossus muscles form the paired anterior faucial pillars that are described in Chapter 4 as the muscular-mucosal folds anterior to the palatine tonsils, and are considered to be the anatomical entrance to the pharynx. When each contract, its two unfixed, movable attachments (to the tongue base and soft palate) move toward each other. Linguavelar closure is the posterior barrier to passive flow of material from the oral cavity during oral preparatory activity. When either of its attachments is stabilized by other muscles (i.e., maintaining lingual depression or palatal elevation), the opposite, movable attachment is displaced toward the stabilized end. Thus, actions of the palatoglossus can contribute to elevation of the tongue base, depression of the soft palate or, as in the case of oral containment, approximation of the tongue base and soft palate to contain the bolus, as shown in Figures 6–1A and 6–1B.

Although most individuals tend to release the linguavelar valve at various times during oral preparation of soft and masticated solids, it remains relatively tightly shut during the preparation of liquid boluses (Hiiemae & Palmer, 1999; Saitoh et al., 2007). When oral transit and bolus propulsion begin, the linguavelar valve is initially closed and there may be a brief duration of time during which the bolus is compressed between the posteriorly-moving tongue and the stationary linguavelar valve, increasing intrabolus pressure (Sequence 6–1 in color insert). The linguavelar valve's release marks the release of oral containment and the bolus is ejected into the pharynx with a relatively high intrabolus pressure (Nicosia & Robbins, 2001). As pharyngeal pressure is near atmospheric pressure before the onset of oral transit (Cook, Dodds, Dantas, Kern, et al., 1989), the propelled bolus flows rapidly into an area of lower pressure. The soft palate shifts its position and rises to assume velopharyngeal closure while the tongue continues its progressively widening contact with the hard and soft palate, and lateral and posterior pharyngeal walls, literally injecting the bolus toward the floor of the pharynx in a fashion similar to what occurs when squeezing a tube of toothpaste.

The direction of lingual movements in the latter phases of its oral propulsive actions includes a short period of depression and retraction (Tasko et al., 2002). These movements not only propel the bolus through the pharyngeal cavity, they also act on the distal end of the epiglottis, literally pressing it down onto the rising laryngeal inlet. This contribution of the tongue to airway protection is often overlooked by examiners who attribute all airway protection events to non-oral structures and events. Additional protection of the airway is produced by the elevation and anterior displacement (out of the path of the oncoming bolus) of the larynx during hyolaryngeal excursion (HLE). The epiglottic petiole (attachment of the epiglottis to

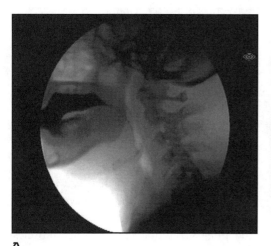
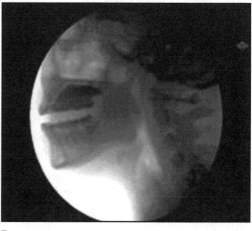

A   **B**

Figure 6–1. **A.** *Closure of the linguavelar is seen one frame prior to the onset of oral transit, in a healthy adult subject swallowing a large thin liquid bolus.* **B.** *Linguavelar closure prior to propulsion of a small thin liquid bolus in another healthy adult.*

the inner wall of the thyroid cartilage) is displaced superiorly and anteriorly which reorients it from its resting vertical position to a horizontal position. Combined with lingual propulsion which displaces the free end of the epiglottis inferiorly, epiglottic inversion and closure of the laryngeal inlet are completed, provided the remainder of the laryngeal inlet adequately rises to the level of the inverting epiglottis. This approximation of laryngeal inlet to epiglottis is produced by thyrohyoid muscles bilaterally and is seen radiographically as a shortening of the vertical distance between thyroid cartilage and hyoid bone.

Velopharyngeal closure is obviously a mechanism preventing nasopharyngeal regurgitation. This type of regurgitation is merely a reflection of the loss of intrabolus pressure (i.e., pressure leakage) to the nasopharynx when there is velopharyngeal incompetence. Two results occur from intrabolus pressure leaks here and elsewhere. First, the injection of pressurized material outside of the intended tube in which it is being propelled (i.e., through the site of the leak), and second, a loss of the propulsive forces generated by the propulsive organ (principally the tongue). The generating forces of the tongue decline as we age, thereby amplifying the effects of such leaks (Robbins, Levine, Wood, Roecker, & Luschei, 1995). Like velopharyngeal incompetence, incomplete laryngeal closure not only allows material to be injected into the airway, it reduces the net pressure within the bolus that enables it to completely pass into the esophagus.

Hyolaryngeal excursion (HLE) is an important and complex series of events that achieves several biomechanical outcomes in addition to the contribution to epiglottic inversion described above. Its motion is the net result of suprahyoid muscle actions that originate above and posterior (stylohyoid, posterior digastric), directly superior (hyoglossus) and anterior and superior (anterior digastric, mylohyoid, geniohyoid) to the hyoid bone. As all of these muscles originate above the hyoid, upward hyolaryngeal movement results from their combined contractions. As the force of contraction of the anteriorly originating muscles exceeds that of the posterior group, the net result of all of these muscular forces causes anterior hyoid displacement. The result is anterior and superior displacement of the hyolaryngeal complex. The hyoglossus is probably responsible for the small amount of counterclockwise rotation of the hyoid bone observed during swallowing (Dengel, Robbins, Coyle, & Sonies, 1996; Ekberg, 1986).

As the remainder of the entire hyolaryngeal complex is physically attached to the hyoid, it "follows along" in the hyoid's movement arc. As previously described, shortening of the distance between the hyoid and laryngeal inlet is produced by the thyrohyoid muscles. So the net result of HLE is upward and forward displacement of the entire hyolaryngeal complex which reorients the airway away from the oncoming bolus, and shortening of the larynx which brings the larynx under the inverting epiglottis (Sequence 6–2 in color insert). Due to the closure of the upper airway as described above and the adduction of the vocal folds that precedes HLE, transient apnea (cessation of respiration) is present during the pharyngeal stage of swallowing.

HLE is a contributor to opening of the upper UES. As the posterior wall of the larynx (i.e., the cricoid cartilage) is shared as the anterior wall of the UES, the muscular forces generated during HLE also produce traction on the anterior wall of the UES. The resting tone of the cricopharyngeal portion of the UES is inhibited moments before the delivery of these traction forces resulting in increased compliance of the UES at the moment HLE traction forces are delivered (Jean, 2001; McConnel, Cerenko, & Mendelsohn, 1988; Miller, 1986, 1997). The result of the combined "relaxation" of cricopharyngeal resting pressure and hyolaryngeal traction forces is distention of the UES which, in normal swallows of healthy young individuals, occurs before the arrival of the bolus head at the UES (Jacob, Kahrilas, Logemann, Shah, & Ha, 1989; McConnel et al., 1988). Applying Boyle's law in reverse order (increasing volume of a container produces a drop in intraluminal pressure), when UES opening precedes bolus head arrival, the increasing volume of the UES results in reduction of pressure within the UES in front of the bolus head, to a level below atmospheric pressure, which amplifies the effect of the generated intrabolus pressure on flow into and through the UES. McConnel and colleagues (1988) called this phenomenon an example of a "hypopharyngeal suction pump" to illustrate the pressure gradient produced by propulsive (pump) and anterograde "suction" (UES pressure decrease) forces in the UES.

Following the clearance of most of the bolus tail into the esophagus, the myoelectric activity of the muscles producing HLE returns to baseline. UES resting tone is restored and the tongue assumes its resting posture in the oral cavity. The hyolaryngeal complex descends to its resting position and the larynx reopens which enables restoration of breathing. Air typically is exhaled after the larynx reopens in healthy adults following single liquid swallows, although there is a greater tendency toward post-swallow inspiration during sequential swallows taken from a cup and in diseases such as stroke and chronic obstructive pulmonary disease (COPD) (Dozier, Brodsky, Michel, Walters, & Martin-Harris, 2006; Gross et al., 2008; Gross, Atwood, Ross, Olszewski, & Eichhorn, 2009; Leslie, Drinnan, Ford, & Wilson, 2002; Shaker et al., 1992).

The actions described above are clearly demonstrated in Sequence 6–3 (in color insert), of a single swallow of a large liquid bolus by a healthy elderly subject. It illustrates a complete swallow with a corresponding legend.

Biomechanical Analysis of Pharyngeal Onset Delay Versus Oral Containment Impairment

Abnormal penetration of swallowed material into the upper airway occurs during the oropharyngeal swallow event when one (or more) of three things happen: (1) when contrast arrives at the laryngeal inlet before the larynx is closed, (2) when laryngeal closure is incomplete or absent during the pharyngeal swallow, or (3) when the volume of material retained in the pharynx exceeds pharyngeal cavity volume and the pharyngeal residue overflows into the larynx.

The phrase "premature spillage" is often used when contrast is seen entering the pharynx before the pharyngeal stage has begun. For something to be premature, it must occur before it is supposed to happen. "Spillage" is not supposed to happen, making this term inappropriate. This term also does not differentiate between the two reasons that material might enter the pharynx before the pharyngeal stage: delayed onset of the pharyngeal response, and impaired oral containment. Delayed pharyngeal response is characterized by organized propulsion of the bolus to the pharynx with bolus head arrival at the laryngeal inlet before the onset of the neuromotor events we call the pharyngeal stage. Impaired oral containment is characterized by unorganized passive movement of bolus contents from the oral cavity toward the unprotected laryngeal inlet while the bolus is not being propelled. Both can lead to penetration of the airway before the pharyngeal stage onset. Delayed laryngeal closure and impaired posterior oral containment are very different, and it is important that these two are not made interchangeable by the examiner (Feinberg & Ekberg, 1991). If examiners expect to select appropriate interventions, they must first correctly identify the problem.

Delayed laryngeal closure is when the oral transit and pharyngeal stages of swallowing are separated by an abnormally long period of time, as defined by numerous studies of normal swallow physiology. The onset of pharyngeal swallow activity is marked by the onset of maximal HLE. This onset is defined as the moment at which the first movement of the body of the hyoid bone toward its eventual maximal superior and anterior pharyngeal-stage displacement that precedes a pharyngeal swallow. When a pharyngeal swallow is initiated, this hyoid movement is always preceded by active oral propulsion of the organized bolus. It should not be confused with the movement of the hyoid associated with lingual and mandibular movements during oral preparatory activity or speech. In healthy young individuals, typically there is no lapse of time between the entrance of the head of the organized liquid bolus head into the pharynx, and the onset of HLE, whereas in aging, there typically is an increasing pause (with HLE beginning later in relation to the entrance of the bolus head into the pharynx) between these two points in time (Ekberg & Feinberg, 1991).

Impaired posterior oral containment is an inadequacy in closure of the linguavelar valve (palatoglossus muscles) during prepharyngeal stage oral activity. Loss of oral contents results from the passive flow of material from the oral cavity when there has not been active oral propulsion. It is the result of incompetent barricading of oral contents in the mouth. Using VFSS, the examiner can observe how and why oral contents arrive at the laryngeal inlet before they are supposed to, and before the airway is closed, and whether it is due to impaired oral containment of pharyngeal onset delay. The duration of time between bolus propulsion and the pharyngeal reaction to bolus propulsion (i.e., the pharyngeal stage) can be measured by timing the flow

of the bolus head in comparison to the initiation of the pharyngeal stage movements of the hyolaryngeal complex. The onset of airway closure and subsequent apnea is an important component of the pharyngeal response along with HLE. In healthy young individuals, the onset of swallow-related apnea occurs primarily when the bolus head is either in the oral cavity or at the tongue base. However, for a small percentage, apnea begins while the bolus head is at the level of the valleculae (Perlman, He, Barkmeier, & Van Leer, 2005). As the vocal folds cannot be visualized radiographically, other standards for judging the timeliness of the pharyngeal onset have been devised using visually reliable anatomical landmarks.

The most widely used standard is the duration of stage transition (DST), also known as "pharyngeal delay time." DST, the biomechanical measure of pharyngeal onset delay, is the duration between the moment the bolus head crosses the mandibular ramus in the lateral view, and the onset of maximal HLE. Figures 6–2A, 6–2B, and 6–2C show the DST. Onset of hyoid movement is the beginning of DST and bolus entering pharynx is the end. If hyoid movement precedes bolus entry, the DST will be a negative duration, and if the bolus enters pharynx first, the DST will be a positive duration. In normal healthy young individuals, DST is zero or less than zero. It increases with age and in pathological conditions.

This duration generally has a "near-zero value" in young healthy individuals which means the examiner will observe the bolus head crossing the mandibular ramus at approximately the same time as the onset of HLE is observed (Leonard & McKenzie, 2006; McCullough, Rosenbek, Wertz, Suiter, & McCoy, 2007; Robbins, Hamilton, Lof, & Kempster, 1992). This duration increases with normal aging (HLE begins progressively later in relation to the entry of the bolus head

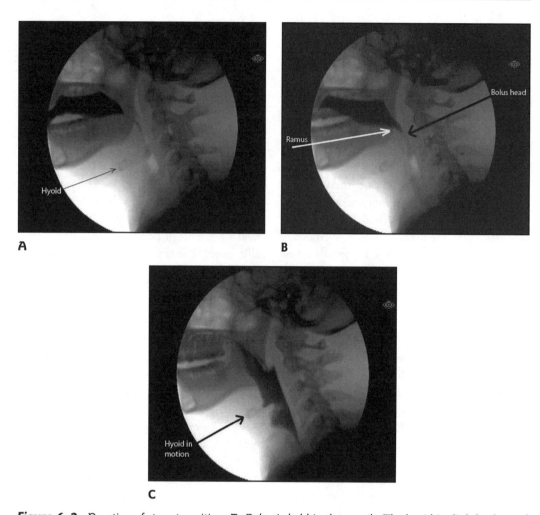

Figure 6–2. *Duration of stage transition.* **A.** *Bolus is held in the mouth. The hyoid is slightly elevated from rest due to oral activity. Oral transit began on this frame (time is zero).* **B.** *The first frame in which the head of the bolus (black arrow) is past the ramus of the mandible (white arrow). Time is 0.11 seconds after onset of oral transit.* **C.** *Time is 0.31 seconds after onset of oral transit. The onset of hyoid displacement associated with a pharyngeal swallow is detected using slow motion reviewing (arrow). It appears as the first blurring of the clearly outlined cortex of the resting hyoid body that leads is followed by a complete pharyngeal response. It should not be confused with hyoid movement associated with lingual or mandibular movement. As the onset of hyolaryngeal excursion is 0.31 seconds after the onset of oral transit, and the bolus entered the pharynx at 0.11 seconds after the onset of oral transit, the DST is Hyoid start (0.31) – bolus entering pharynx (0.11) = +0.2 seconds. Prolonged DST indicates that the bolus is inside the pharynx before the pharynx has reacted. If the events were reversed, the DST would have been Hyoid start (0.11) minus bolus entering pharynx (0.31) = −0.2 seconds DST.*

into the pharynx) and can become abnormally long or inconsistent with certain disease states such as stroke (Rosenbek, Roecker, Wood, & Robbins, 1996).

The examiner can easily measure DST with a digital timer or by simply counting frames during slow-motion playback and either characterize its contribution to airway penetration, or compare it to norms by correlating prolonged DST with other measures of airway compromise like the penetration-aspiration scale (Rosenbek, Robbins, Roecker, Coyle, & Wood, 1996). Depending on the video standard under which the recording is made, each frame of video constitutes 1/25th (the PAL format) or 1/30th (the NTSC format) of a second. So, a DST of 5 frames on a PAL formatted video sequence represents a 5/25ths or 0.20 second DST. The actual DST value is not necessary to make a diagnosis or form a treatment plan. The examiner can simply observe the position of the bolus head at the moment HLE begins. Regardless, it is essential that the biomechanical analysis determines whether an organized bolus was being propelled (in which case a DST issue might be the problem) or whether part of the as yet unpropelled bolus is passively flowing from the posterior oral cavity as described in the next section.

Posterior oral containment impairments will be observed as passive flow of disorganized oral contents into the pharynx from the oral cavity, typically filling the valleculae, which will eventually overflow caudally through the lateral channels into the pyriform sinuses. The passive flow of unorganized material to the mandibular ramus before the bolus head arrives at the same landmark is a clue indicating an oral containment impairment.

Either of these biomechanical causes of pre-pharyngeal flow into the pharynx can produce accumulating volumes in the pharyngeal recesses that are associated with an increased tendency for the material to enter the as yet unprotected airway. When contrast has filled the pyriform sinuses to 50% of their height, there is a significantly increased likelihood of swallow-related aspiration that can also be characterized with a pharyngeal retention scale (Eisenhuber et al., 2002; Perlman, Booth, & Grayhack, 1994).

In summary, the biomechanics of delayed pharyngeal onset and impaired oral contain-

ment are very different. If the examiner simply observes contrast and arbitrarily labels any contrast in the pharynx before the onset of HLE as "pharyngeal delay," an accurate diagnosis and any opportunities to alleviate the abnormality and its risks will be missed.

Biomechanical Analysis of Impaired Airway Closure

Failure of laryngeal closure can be caused by impairment or absence of a pharyngeal stage, mechanical obstruction, or complicated by vocal fold paralysis. Incomplete laryngeal vestibule closure facilitates penetration of the larynx during the high-pressure events of the pharyngeal phase. It can lead to aspiration during the pharyngeal swallow in the case of vocal fold paresis or paralysis (as material penetrates the larynx, but is allowed to enter the trachea), or post-swallow aspiration (as material that is held in the supraglottic area by the adducted vocal folds, is inhaled after the swallow). This latter pattern is seen in patients with COPD, and can be complicated by post-swallow inhalation. As post-swallow exhalation is the norm for healthy individuals, reversal of this pattern (i.e., inspiration after the swallow) raises the risk for aspiration when laryngeal penetration is present (Gross et al., 2009; Mokhlesi, Logemann, Rademaker, Stangl, & Corbridge, 2002; Shaker et al., 1992).

When completing the videofluoroscopic investigation, some subjects use the larynx as a pharyngeal reservoir without adverse consequence. Typically, the patient may exhibit poor vertical hyoid displacement, which causes impaired closure of the laryngeal vestibule, but is compensated for by adducting the vocal folds before swallowing, maintaining vocal fold adduction during the swallow, swallowing several times, and then exhaling after the swallow to clear the airway. Poor UES distension diameter and duration due to the HLE impairment may be apparent. Additionally, intrabolus pressure generation may also be observed as demonstrated by a gap between the tongue and posterior pharyngeal wall during oral propulsion. In cases like this, patients may be incorrectly prescribed thick liquids due to "deep laryngeal penetration." However, biomechanical analysis of the VFSS could potentially reveal the physiological causes of the laryngeal penetration as described here, and the simple interventions of "breath-hold before the swallow" combined with "multiple swallows" may alleviate the risk of aspiration, whereas active therapy would focus on attempting to restore impaired function.

The larynx closes from caudal to rostral with vocal fold adduction preceding the onset of HLE in healthy individuals (Shaker, Dodds, Dantas, Hogan, & Arndorfer, 1990). This is evident radiographically in cases of incomplete laryngeal closure without aspiration as described in the previous paragraph, where contrast enters the airway and penetrates to the level of the true vocal folds but not below. So, the depth of airway compromise is often mitigated by adducted vocal folds, even though the laryngeal vestibule may be open. A longer delay in the onset of vocal fold adduction or laryngeal closure naturally exposes the airway to more depth and volume of airway penetration.

The closure of the laryngeal vestibule is characterized by adduction of the arytenoid cartilages (which is not radiographically visible), shortening of the larynx through contraction of the thyrohyoid muscles which raise the laryngeal inlet toward the inverting epiglottis, and inversion of the epiglottis over the laryngeal inlet. This latter event is the combined result of the effects of HLE which pulls the petiole of the epiglottis anteriorly, and the combined retraction/depression of the tongue base along with the bolus. By displacing the epiglottic petiole, HLE changes epiglottic orientation from vertical to more horizontal, while the tongue base and bolus act on the

distal end of the epiglottis, literally pressing it down over the laryngeal inlet.

Failure of complete laryngeal vestibule closure is observed by the examiner when a portion of the bolus is injected into the space between the epiglottis and the shadow of the arytenoid cartilages during an otherwise timely pharyngeal stage. The laryngeal portion of the bolus will be seen descending to the level of the vocal folds (if they adduct in a timely manner), in the laryngeal ventricle (if the true vocal folds adduct after material has contacted them and before the false vocal folds adduct), or above the false vocal folds (if both true and false vocal folds have adducted before material penetrates the larynx).

Telltale (radiographic) signs of incomplete laryngeal closure include a visible space between the arytenoid cartilages and the epiglottis during a dry swallow, and a lack of approximation of the thyroid cartilage to the epiglottis. Incomplete HLE in either superior or anterior directions is the biomechanical cause of airway compromise in many cases by reducing approximation of the laryngeal inlet to the shadows of the hyoid and epiglottis. Inadequate lingual motion can reduce the inversion of the distal epiglottis over the laryngeal inlet. The biomechanics of these events are very easy to observe, yet are often overlooked or not differentiated by the examiner in favor of simple descriptions of whether or not material entered the airway. Laryngeal shortening from its baseline position (distance between hyoid bone and thyroid cartilage) causes approximation of the framework of the laryngeal inlet toward the hyoid bone (within which the epiglottis is situated) while the epiglottis becomes more horizontally oriented. The inversion of the distal epiglottis is very easy to observe. If HLE is impaired, the examiner will see little change in thyrohyoid distance, or a space between the lower mandibular shadow and hyoid body (or both) at the moment of maximal HLE. If the distal epiglottis is not inverted by the tongue base and bolus, the examiner may notice less than expected contact between the tongue base and posterior pharyngeal wall, or an actual air or contrast column between the two, and correctly identify the tongue as the impaired structure.

The biomechanics of laryngeal closure can also be impaired by cervical osteophytes (Strasser et al., 2000). If they are seen at the point of contact between the epiglottis and posterior pharyngeal wall, it is reasonable to conclude causation. If the epiglottis contacts the posterior pharyngeal wall but there is no mechanical obstruction preventing inversion, and there is no evidence of lingual propulsive impairment as just described, then the anterior displacement of the larynx is inadequate indicating weakness of the floor-of-mouth musculature. Osteophytes at more than one level are more likely to impede laryngeal closure and be associated with deglutitive aspiration (Strasser, et al., 2000). The examiner should observe the video frames at the moment of airway penetration to determine whether the epiglottis is in contact with the posterior wall of the pharynx. If it is, there may be evidence that the hyoid has been inadequately displaced, or that the epiglottis is either in contact with the posterior pharyngeal wall, or not being adequately contacted by the tongue base.

Pharyngeal edema as seen after radiation therapy to the head and neck, or other etiologies of thickening of the oropharyngeal mucosa such as candidiasis, can reduce the compliance and range of motion of structures like the epiglottis and contribute to incomplete closure of the airway.

Biomechanical Analysis of Pharyngeal Residue

As discussed earlier, material retained in the hypopharynx can be aspirated after the swallow. Excessive hypopharyngeal residue can be caused by more than one biomechanical error, each of which has its own etiology and rem-edy. This residue can passively overflow into the open larynx as respiration resumes, or during the subsequent swallow as it is injected into the larynx before the airway is completely closed (Eisenhuber et al., 2002). The examiner will observe the material entering the larynx from the pyriform sinuses instead of observing a portion of the oncoming bolus injected into the larynx. In some cases, however, a patient may exhibit airway penetration from both the pyriform sinuses before the arrival of the next bolus, and as a portion of the next bolus itself. Misidentification of this cause of aspiration can lead to erroneous selection of compensatory interventions. For example the chin-down posture has been shown to eliminate aspiration. However, in patients who aspirate from the pyriform sinuses, it is ineffective and may actually facilitate aspiration by biomechanically allowing gravity to direct residue into the airway (Shanahan, Logemann, Rademaker, Pauloski, & Kahrilas, 1993).

Opening of the UES is influenced by intrabolus pressure, hyolaryngeal traction forces, and timely inhibition of the resting closure pressure in the UES itself. Intrabolus pressure generation has been implicated as a significant source of complete clearance of swallowed material, due to its contribution to intrabolus radial forces pressing outwardly on the inner lumen of the UES (Cook, Dodds, Dantas, Massey, et al., 1989; Jacob et al., 1989). Impaired pressure generation in frail elderly subjects and stroke patients has been shown to be a cause of retained pharyngeal residue. The effects of a lingual exercise over a systematic 8-week program was shown to increase intrabolus pressure generation as well as reduce post-swallow pharyngeal residue in healthy and poststroke individuals (Kays & Robbins, 2006; Robbins et al., 2005; Robbins et al., 2007). Insufficient bolus propulsion can also contribute to reduced diameter of UES opening which, in turn, leads to separation and retention of the bolus tail in the pyriform sinuses and post-swallow airway penetration.

Propulsive forces can also be diminished due to incompetent valves (as in velopharyngeal incompetency with subsequent nasopharyngeal regurgitation). The additive contribution of valve incompetence to poor intrabolus pressure generation is twofold. Firstly, intrabolus pressure at the UES is partially lost to the leaky valve resulting in separation of a portion of the bolus and pharyngeal retention. Secondly, material is typically propelled through these incompetent and leaky valves (assuming pressure generation is adequate). In a case of velopharyngeal incompetency, this material then courses by gravity back into the pharynx increasing the volume of pharyngeal residue after the swallow and increasing aspiration tendency. The examiner will observe contrast that is injected rostrally, posterior to the soft palate, sometimes to the level of the hard palate. If the volume of this regurgitation is sufficient, gravity will cause the nasopharyngeal residue to return to the hypopharynx after the swallow (i.e., the pyriform sinuses will fill after the swallow has ended). Therefore, identifying the timing and origin of the hypopharyngeal residue through review of the videorecorded swallow events is essential to accurate diagnosis.

Impaired HLE can reduce the diameter or duration of UES distension and also cause bolus tail separation. HLE, described above as critical in the closure of the airway, is also critical to UES distension. As summarized in Chapter 4, traction forces applied to the hyolaryngeal framework by suprahyoid musculature displace the anterior wall of the UES anteriorly, moments after the resting tone of the UES is reduced via vagal inhibition (called UES "relaxation" by some, though the UES never fully relaxes). Impairments of HLE can be caused (as discussed above) by weakness of the anterior suprahyoid musculature, or by UES noncompliance itself. In either event, the examiner will observe reduced superior or anterior (or both) displacement of the

hyolaryngeal complex. There may be a gap between the hyoid body and the shadow of the mandible. The distance of expected displacement of the hyoid bone from its resting position has been described in several studies, and corresponds roughly to an anterior and superior displacement of approximately the vertical and horizontal dimensions of the vertebral body of one of the patient's cervical vertebrae (Cook, Dodds, Dantas, Massey, et al., 1989). It can be augmented in healthy individuals by increasing bolus volume and viscosity. Naturally, such manipulations should be employed judiciously during a VFSS examination.

UES noncompliance can result from absent or reduced inhibition of UES resting tone, fibrosis of the cricopharyngeal musculature or its surrounding mucosal envelope following radiotherapy, or by denervation. Any of these phenomena can increase UES inertia such that HLE traction forces cannot overcome them, and hence, reduced UES opening diameter and duration may be observed (Franzmann, Lundy, Abitbol, & Goodwin, 2006). The mistiming of UES "relaxation" can affect transsphincteric flow of material and produce hypopharyngeal retention as described earlier. The examiner might see a similarly reduced HLE because the hyolaryngeal complex is tethered to the noncompliant UES. Thus, in some cases it can be difficult to assign the biomechanical cause to either weakness of HLE traction forces or cricopharyngeal noncompliance.

The cricopharyngeal bar (CPB) is another example of UES noncompliance that can cause bolus tail separation and subsequent pharyngeal residue. It is characterized by a fingerlike muscular projection appearing to protrude from the posterior wall of the UES into its lumen. In healthy individuals, a CPB affects UES opening diameter without concomitant changes in the duration of other swallowing-related biomechanical events; so additional pathology is necessary to produce clinically adverse sequelae (Dantas et al., 1990). The addition of neuromuscular weakness or other sources of impaired intrabolus pressure generation can interact with a CPB to produce hypopharyngeal retention and subsequent aspiration. The cricopharyngeal bar is a probable precursor to the Zenker's diverticulum because intrabolus pressure proximal to the CPB is excessively high, contributing to distortion of the mucosal envelope of the UES through the posterolateral inferior constrictor wall (Coyle, 2009; McConnel, Hood, Jackson, & O'Connor, 1994).

Hypopharyngeal retention must be assessed through the biomechanical analysis. The biomechanical events characterizing each are radiographically observable to the examiner, but they need to be sought in the data analysis. Hypopharyngeal residue can be aspirated. The residue itself is not to blame, but moreover results from one or more of the biomechanical errors described in this section.

SUMMARY

Abnormal penetration of swallowed material into the airway and post-swallow retention of bolus components are commonly identified abnormalities in dysphagic patients. It is important to remember that each of these outcomes is the result of one or more specific biomechanical error(s) that must be identified by the examiner in order to be remediated effectively by the treating clinician. Efforts to manage dysphagia that focus on reducing residue or eliminating aspiration by means that do not address the underlying biomechanical errors causing bolus misdirection may inefficiently achieve the goal of improved function, or completely fail to do so. Improving patient function is a process that focuses on restoration of impaired structures and systems, or physical compensation for impairments either permanently, or during a period of restoration, not on alteration of the environment as is the case with diet modification. Alteration of food and liquid viscosity may buy time while the patient is properly rehabilitated, but it is not a viable long-term option in patients with impairments that are amenable to aggressive restorative interventions. The VFSS is a therapeutic trial; the x-ray contrast is the visual aid/tool. Accurate biomechanical analysis is essential not only to detection and listing of impairments, but toward the endpoint of accurately focused interventions.

REFERENCES

Cook, I. J., Dodds, W. J., Dantas, R. O., Kern, M. K., Massey, B. T., Shaker, R., & Hogan, W. J. (1989). Timing of videofluoroscopic, manometric events, and bolus transit during the oral and pharyngeal phases of swallowing. *Dysphagia*, *4*(1), 8–15.

Cook, I. J., Dodds, W. J., Dantas, R. O., Massey, B., Kern, M. K., Lang, I. M., . . . Hogan, W. J. (1989). Opening mechanisms of the human upper esophageal sphincter. *American Journal of Physiology*, *257*(5 Pt. 1), G748–G759.

Coyle, J. L. (2009). Zenker's Diverticulum. In H. Jones & J. C. Rosenbek. (Eds.), *Dysphagia in rare conditions*. San Diego, CA: Plural.

Dantas, R. O., Cook, I. J., Dodds, W. J., Kern, M. K., Lang, I. M., & Brasseur, J. G. (1990). Biomechanics of cricopharyngeal bars. *Gastroenterology*, *99*(5), 1269–1274.

Dengel, G. A., Robbins, J. A., Coyle, J. L., & Sonies, B. C. (1996, 1996). Hyoid rotation during swallowing, *Proceedings of Fifth Scientific Meeting*, Dysphagia Research Society; Aspen, CO.

Dodds, W. J., Taylor, A. J., Stewart, E. T., Kern, M. K., Logemann, J. A., & Cook, I. J. (1989). Tipper and dipper types of oral swallows. *American Journal of Roentgenology*, *153*(6), 1197–1199.

Dozier, T. S., Brodsky, M. B., Michel, Y., Walters, B. C., & Martin-Harris, B. (2006). Coordination of swallowing and respiration in normal sequential cup swallows. *Laryngoscope, 116*(8), 1489–1493.

Eisenhuber, E., Schima, W., Schober, E., Pokieser, P., Stadler, A., Scharitzer, M., & Oschatz, E. (2002). Videofluoroscopic assessment of patients with dysphagia: Pharyngeal retention is a predictive factor for aspiration. *American Journal of Roentgenology, 178*(2), 393–398.

Ekberg, O. (1986). The normal movements of the hyoid bone during swallow. *Investigative Radiology, 21*(5), 408–410.

Ekberg, O., & Feinberg, M. J. (1991). Altered swallowing function in elderly patients without dysphagia: Radiologic findings in 56 cases. *American Journal of Roentgenology, 156*(6), 1181–1184.

Feinberg, M. J., & Ekberg, O. (1991). Videofluoroscopy in elderly patients with aspiration: Importance of evaluating both oral and pharyngeal stages of deglutition. *AJR American Journal of Roentgenology, 156*(2), 293–296.

Franzmann, E. J., Lundy, D. S., Abitbol, A. A., & Goodwin, W. J. (2006). Complete hypopharyngeal obstruction by mucosal adhesions: A complication of intensive chemoradiation for advanced head and neck cancer. *Head and Neck, 28*(8), 663–670.

Gross, R. D., Atwood, C. W., Ross, S. B., Eichhorn, K. A., Olszewski, J. W., & Doyle, P. J. (2008). The coordination of breathing and swallowing in Parkinson's disease. *Dysphagia, 23*(2), 136–145.

Gross, R. D., Atwood, C. W., Ross, S. B., Olszewski, J. W., & Eichhorn, K. A. (2009). The coordination of breathing and swallowing in chronic obstructive pulmonary disease. *American Journal of Respirotary Critical Care Medicine, 179*(7), 559–565.

Hiiemae, K. M., & Palmer, J. B. (1999). Food transport and bolus formation during complete feeding sequences on foods of different initial consistency. *Dysphagia, 14*(1), 31–42.

Jacob, P., Kahrilas, P. J., Logemann, J. A., Shah, V., & Ha, V. (1989). Upper esophageal sphincter opening and modulation during swallowing. *Gastroenterology, 97*(6), 1469–1478.

Jean, A. (2001). Brain stem control of swallowing: Neuronal network and cellular mechanisms *Physiologic Reviews, 81*(2), 929–969.

Kahrilas, P. J. (1994). Anatomy, physiology and pathophysiology of dysphagia. *Acta Oto-Rhino-Laryngologica Belgica, 48*(2), 97–117.

Kays, S., & Robbins, J. A. (2006). Effects of sensorimotor exercise on swallowing outcomes relative to age and age-related disease. *Seminars in Speech and Language, 27*(4), 245–259.

Leonard, R., & McKenzie, S. (2006). Hyoid-bolus transit latencies in normal swallow. *Dysphagia, 21*(3), 183–190.

Leslie, P., Drinnan, M. J., Ford, G. A., & Wilson, J. A. (2002). Swallow respiration patterns in dysphagic patients following acute stroke. *Dysphagia, 17*(3), 202–207.

Logemann, J. A. (1983). *Evaluation and treatment of swallowing disorders*. San Diego, CA: College-Hill Press.

Logemann, J. A. (1993). The dysphagia diagnostic procedure as a treatment efficacy trial. *Clinics in Communication Disorders, 3*(4), 1–10.

McConnel, F. M., Cerenko, D., & Mendelsohn, M. S. (1988). Manofluorographic analysis of swallowing. *Otolaryngologic Clinics of North America, 21*(4), 625–635.

McConnel, F. M., Hood, D., Jackson, K., & O'Connor, A. (1994). Analysis of intrabolus forces in patients with Zenker's diverticulum. *Laryngoscope, 104*(5, Pt. 1), 571–581.

McCullough, G. H., Rosenbek, J. C., Wertz, R. T., Suiter, D., & McCoy, S. C. (2007). Defining swallowing function by age: Promises and pitfalls of pigeonholing. *Topics in Geriatric Rehabilitation, 23*(4), 290–307.

Miller, A. J. (1986). Neurophysiological basis of swallowing. *Dysphagia, 1*(2), 91–100.

Miller, A. J. (1997). *Neuroscientific bases of swallowing and dysphagia*. San Diego, CA: Singular.

Mokhlesi, B., Logemann, J. A., Rademaker, A. W., Stangl, C. A., & Corbridge, T. C. (2002). Oropharyngeal deglutition in stable COPD. *Chest, 121*(2), 361–369.

Nicosia, M. A., Hind, J. A., Roecker, E. B., Carnes, M., Doyle, J., Dengel, G. A., & Robbins, J. A. (2000). Age effects on the temporal evolution of isometric and swallowing pressure. *Journals of Gerontology Series A: Biological Sciences and Medical Sciences, 55*(11), M634–M640.

Nicosia, M. A., & Robbins, J. A. (2001). The fluid mechanics of bolus ejection from the oral cavity. *Journal of Biomechanics, 34*(12), 1537–1544.

Perlman, A. L., Booth, B. M., & Grayhack, J. P. (1994). Videofluoroscopic predictors of aspiration in patients with oropharyngeal dysphagia. *Dysphagia, 9*(2), 90–95.

Perlman, A. L., He, X., Barkmeier, J., & Van Leer, E. (2005). Bolus location associated with videofluoroscopic and respirodeglutometric events. *Journal of Speech, Language, and Hearing Research, 48*(1), 21–33.

Robbins, J., Gangnon, R. E., Theis, S. M., Kays, S. A., Hewitt, A. L., & Hind, J. A. (2005). The effects of lingual exercise on swallowing in older adults. *Journal of the American Geriatrics Society, 53*(9), 1483–1489.

Robbins, J., Hamilton, J. W., Lof, G. L., & Kempster, G. B. (1992). Oropharyngeal swallowing in normal adults of different ages. *Gastroenterology, 103*(3), 823–829.

Robbins, J., Kays, S. A., Gangnon, R. E., Hind, J. A., Hewitt, A. L., Gentry, L. R., & Taylor, A.J.(2007). The effects of lingual exercise in stroke patients with dysphagia. *Archives of Physical Medicine and Rehabilitation, 88*(2), 150.

Robbins, J., Levine, R., Wood, J., Roecker, E. B., & Luschei, E. (1995). Age effects on lingual pressure generation as a risk factor for dysphagia. *Journals of Gerontology Series A: Biological Sciences and Medical Sciences, 50*(5), M257–M262.

Rosenbek, J. C., Robbins, J. A., Roecker, E. B., Coyle, J. L., & Wood, J. L. (1996). A penetration-aspiration scale. *Dysphagia, 11*(2), 93–98.

Rosenbek, J. C., Roecker, E. B., Wood, J. L., & Robbins, J. A. (1996). Thermal application reduces the duration of stage transition in dysphagia after stroke. *Dysphagia, 11*(4), 225–233.

Saitoh, E., Shibata, S., Matsuo, K., Baba, M., Fujii, W., & Palmer, J. B. (2007). Chewing and food consistency: Effects on bolus transport and swallow initiation. *Dysphagia, 22*(2), 100–107.

Shaker, R., Dodds, W. J., Dantas, R. O., Hogan, W. J., & Arndorfer, R. C. (1990). Coordination of deglutitive glottic closure with oropharyngeal swallowing. *Gastroenterology, 98*(6), 1478–1484.

Shaker, R., Li, Q., Ren, J., Townsend, W. F., Dodds, W. J., Martin, B. J., . . . Rynders, A. (1992). Coordination of deglutition and phases of respiration: Effect of aging, tachypnea, bolus volume, and chronic obstructive pulmonary disease. *American Journal of Physiology, 263*(5 Pt. 1), G750–G755.

Shanahan, T. K., Logemann, J. A., Rademaker, A. W., Pauloski, B. R., & Kahrilas, P. J. (1993). Chin-down posture effect on aspiration in dysphagic patients. *Archives of Physical Medicine and Rehabilitation, 74*(4), 736–739.

Strasser, G., Schima, W., Schober, E., Pokieser, P., Kaider, A., & Denk, D. M. (2000). Cervical osteophytes impinging on the pharynx: Importance of size and concurrent disorders for development of aspiration. *American Journal of Roentgenology, 174*(2), 449–453.

Tasko, S. M., Kent, R. D., & Westbury, J. R. (2002). Variability in tongue movement kinematics during normal liquid swallowing. *Dysphagia, 17*(2), 126–138.

Chapter

7

THE NORMAL AGING SWALLOW

Margaret Coffey

INTRODUCTION

An understanding of the normal swallow and the changes that are experienced with age is a vital underpinning to the interpretation of instrumental swallow examinations for the clinical team managing dysphagia. Population aging is widespread across the world and most advanced in highly developed countries due to a decrease in birth rates together with an increase in the average life span in the second half of the 20th century (United Nations, 2002). From 2000 to 2030 the worldwide population aged over 65 years is projected to increase by approximately 550 million to 973 million (United Nations, 2002). Although swallowing difficulties can affect all age groups, the majority of patients requiring dysphagia evaluations are drawn from those over 60 years.

Disease processes are not always responsible for the changes in swallowing that occur with age. Healthy individuals as young as 45 years may experience changes to their swallow (Robbins, Hamilton, Lof, & Kempster, 1992) but the progression of change in the normal swallow becomes most noticeable over the age of 60 years. The term *presbyphagia* refers to the age-related changes in the oropharyngeal

and esophageal swallowing of healthy adults (Robbins, Bridges, & Taylor, 2006). Knowledge of how the normal swallow changes with time equips clinicians with the skills to interpret videofluoroscopy or other instrumental evaluations appropriately in the older individual. Without this knowledge, there is a risk of over-managing swallowing in the elderly by unnecessarily modifying diets, introducing compensatory techniques (McCullough, Rosenbek, Wertz, Suiter, & McCoy, 2007) or introducing enteral feeding, all of which can limit quality of life. Equally, the under-management of swallowing in this group can lead to medical complications including dehydration, malnutrition, pneumonia, and, in extreme cases, death (Holas, Halvorson, & Reding, 1990). An important consideration in managing older individuals with swallowing difficulty is the notion of functional reserve, a concept defined as the ability to adapt to stress (Prendergast, Fisher, & Calkins, 1993). The older adult experiences an age-related diminishment in functional reserve and when faced with challenges such as an acute illness, fracture, or a change in medication, they have a greater risk of developing dysphagia than a younger individual. The ability of the team to differentiate between *presbyphagia* and *dysphagia* is vital in the management of those healthy older patients whose vulnerability with illness may precipitate a transition from a functional swallow into swallowing difficulty.

The normal age-related changes associated with swallowing encompass physiological, anatomical and sensory aspects. In addition, there is emerging evidence that the cortical processing of swallowing (Martin et al., 2007; Teisman et al., 2010) and the function of respiration related to swallowing is altered with age (Martin-Harris, 2006; Martin-Harris, Brodsky, Michel, Lee, & Walters, 2007; Teisman et al., 2010). These changes have the potential to affect oral, pharyngeal, and esophageal stages of swallowing and will be discussed in this chapter. Readers are encouraged to familiarize themselves with the anatomy and physiology of normal swallowing as explained in Chapter 4, and the biomechanical analysis of swallowing explained in Chapter 6.

CHANGES ASSOCIATED WITH AGE

The Oral Stage of Swallowing

Changes in Physiology with Age

Physiological aging can be distinguished between *primary aging* which involves the deterioration in structure and function of the body and *secondary aging* which causes changes to physiology arising from such factors as disease, radiation exposure, diet, alcohol, and physical inactivity (Easterling, 2008). *Sarcopenia* is the specific age-related process that describes the degree of loss of skeletal muscle mass, organization, and strength (Rosenberg, 1997). Sarcopenia has the potential to cause 30 to 40% loss of muscle strength by 80 years of age (Easterling, 2008). Recent research has found that tongue strength, particularly tongue lat-

eralization and protrusion, is affected by sarcopenia with a significant diminishment in function with age (Clark & Solomon, 2011). It has been suggested that generalized age-related changes in skeletal muscle strength may affect labial and buccal strength, compromising aspects of the oral swallow such as cup drinking (Schindler & Kelly, 2002). However, it appears that the effects of sarcopenia have a greater impact on the muscles of the tongue than on labial or buccal musculature. The concept of functional reserve previously discussed is relevant in discussing oral stage swallowing in the older individual. Although swallow pressures remain similar across the lifespan overall, lingual pressure reserve appears to particularly decline with age (Robbins et al., 2005). The consequence of reduced lingual pressure reserve is that older people may need to take more time and may work lingual muscles harder to produce adequate pressure to propel a bolus from the anterior to posterior oral cavity (Robbins, Levine, Wood, Roecker, & Luschei, 1995). This extra time taken may actually benefit older individuals as it allows an increase in the number of motor units to be recruited, enabling a critical buildup of lingual pressure (Robbins et al., 2006). Although it may be tempting to provide therapy to attempt to speed up the swallow in an older individual, there can be potential detrimental effects to this approach. Speeding up the swallow may prevent the buildup of sufficient lingual pressure (Robbins et al., 2006) and may result in less efficient oral stage bolus transit.

Changes in Transit Time with Age

Healthy swallowing in the elderly generally occurs more slowly (Robbins et al., 2006). Oral transit time has been shown to be significantly delayed in older adults as compared to younger adults (Shaw et al., 1995). It is important to note that oral transit times may be influenced by the pattern of oral swallow technique used.

Studies (Cook et al., 1989; Dodds et al., 1989) have distinguished between a "tipper" swallow (tongue tip elevated with bolus on the posterior surface of the tongue) or "dipper" swallow (initial forward movement of the tongue to pick up the bolus from under the tongue position and transport it to the posterior surface of the tongue). Those over age 60 were more likely to present with a "dipper" type swallow, which increased oral transit time by 0.5 seconds (Dodds et al., 1989). The clinician should avoid the temptation to misconstrue the "dipper" pattern as an abnormal or lazy swallow when it is in fact a variant of a normal swallow with increased prevalence in those over the age of 60.

Changes in Dentition with Age

Age-related reduction in the efficiency and timeliness of the oral stage swallow may also be related to anatomical changes in dentition. It is not simply the number of teeth present but the functional arrangement and type of teeth in the oral cavity which influences the ability to masticate food adequately (Hildebrandt, Dominguez, Schork, & Loesche, 1997). While a full set of dentures appears to facilitate the oral stage swallow (Leidberg, Stoltze, & Owall, 2005) (Furaya, 1999), they may also have a negative effect on taste perception (Hermel, Schonwetter, & Samueloff, 1970), although the latter remains poorly understood and researched. Poorly fitting or an incomplete set of dentures can compromise mastication and prolong oral stage transit in the absence of any other disease process. As a consequence, those with poor or no dentition (Figure 7–1) may have difficulty chewing and may avoid stringy food (such as meat), crunchy food (such as vegetables) or dry solid foods (such as bread or toast). It has been found that older adults often accommodate to deficits such as tooth loss (Arcury et al., 2009). Some of these compensations include avoiding foods that are difficult to chew or that

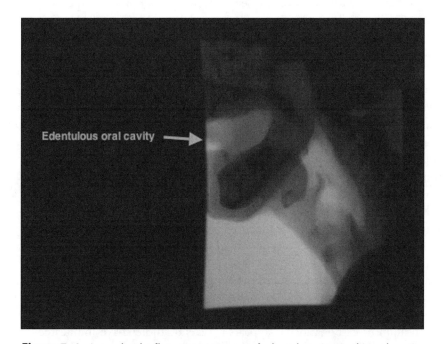

Figure 7–1. *Lateral videofluoroscopic image of edentulous (no teeth) oral cavity.*

interfere with removable prostheses. Further compensations involve modifying size, shape, and consistency of food to make it more comfortable to eat (Quandt et al., 2010). These compensations do not necessarily indicate an abnormality of the oral stage swallow but a dietetic evaluation may be advisable to ensure an adequate caloric intake is maintained on a modified diet.

Changes in Taste, Smell, and Chemesthesis with Age

Changes in taste and smell affect the sensory aspects of swallowing. Changes in taste with normal aging have been well documented (Mojet, Christ Hazelhof, & Heidema, 2001; Schiffman 1997; Weiffenbach, Baum, & Burghauser, 1982). Aging itself does not appear to reduce the number of taste buds despite early research suggesting this as a phenomenon (Frank, 1994; Mistretta, 1984). Changes occur primarily in how taste bud receptors process different flavors. This leads to alterations in the perception of taste intensity with taste essentially fading with age (Pelletier, 2007). Similar physiological factors may be responsible for the changes in the sense of smell documented with age, though this may be less prevalent than previously thought (Mackay-Sim, Johnston, Owen, & Burne, 2006).

Clearly, more research is required in this area. Extrinsic factors such as medications, infection and smoking may also exacerbate the changes in sensations of both taste and smell that occur with age. Chemesthesis is another aspect that requires considerastion when examining oral sensation in the older individual. Chemesthesis happens when certain sensory receptors are stimulated by the chemical compounds in some foods. This results in the awareness of sensations such as the "hotness" of chili, the "coolness" of menthol, and the tingling sensation of carbonation. It appears as though chemesthesis does not decline with aging to the same extent as taste (Fukunaga, Uematsu, & Sugimoto, 2005). It is likely that changes in taste and smell may influence food choices and the use of extra flavor enhancers can potentially improve nutrition in the older individual.

Xerostomia

Xerostomia, defined as the subjective sensation of oral dryness (Smidt, Torpet, Nauntofte, Heegaard, & Pedersen, 2011), is a common complaint in adults above the age of 65 and appears to be more prevalent in women (Narhi, 1994; Neville, Damm, Allen, & Bouquot, 2002). Xerostomia may be caused by physiological age-related changes in salivary gland function. However, the use of prescription medications may also increase the likelihood of an older adult experiencing xersotomia (Thomson, Chalmers, Spencer, & Slade, 2000; Turner & Ship, 2007). Cardiac, respiratory, and neurological agents and antineoplastic drugs have been found to be associated with oral dryness (Smidt, Torpet, Nauntoffe, Heegard, & Pedersen, 2011). Dry mouth may lead to an increased intake of liquids and may result in modifications to the diet to avoid dry and more solid foods that may be more challenging to swallow. In other populations with xerostomia, such as those with a diagnosis of head and neck cancer, xerostomia appears not to delay oral transit but rather disrupts the perception and comfort of eating (Logemann et al., 2001; Logemann et al., 2003). As a consequence, diet choices may be altered.

Pharyngeal Stage

Changes in Initiation of Swallowing with Age

Several studies have implicated age as causing a delay in triggering the pharyngeal swallow (Robbins et al., 1992; Tracy et al., 1989). Although there is conflict in the literature as to which specific bolus positions or anatomical markers should be used to define pharyngeal swallow initiation, onset of hyoid movement has often been selected because it is frequently identified as indicating swallow initiation (Leonard & McKenzie, 2006). The transition between the oral and pharyngeal stages of swallowing has been defined as starting when the bolus head reaches the point where the lower edge of the mandible crosses the tongue base and ends when laryngeal elevation begins (Logemann, 1998). Delayed pharyngeal swallow initiation has been defined as the temporal difference between the bolus head arrival at the posterior angle of the mandible and the onset of hyoid motion (Martin-Harris et al., 2007). It has been found that healthy adults over 50 years were delayed in initiating the pharyngeal swallow compared with more youthful individuals (Martin-Harris et al., 2007). In a further study, normal subjects over 60 years old had delay times of 0.4 to 0.5 seconds whereas those under 60 years old had delay times of 0.02 seconds (Tracy et al., 1989). Delayed initiation of the pharyngeal swallow may be indicative of the normal slowing down of swallowing seen with age and another factor in presbyphagia. However, if the swallow delay is significant and related to an underlying disease process causing dysphagia, the risk of aspiration may increase (Kim, McCullough, & Asp, 2005).

Changes in Movement of the Hyoid and Suprahyoid Muscles with Age

Once pharyngeal swallow initiation is completed, the bolus passes into the pharynx, the tongue base retracts, and the hyoid bone and larynx are pulled superiorly and anteriorly. This movement of the hyolaryngeal complex is a critical biomechanical component of normal swallowing function (Kim

& McCullough, 2008). The movement of the hyoid superiorly and anteriorly protects the airway during swallow and facilitates safe passage of the bolus from the pharynx to the esophagus. It has been shown that the range of anterior hyoid movement diminishes with age although superior displacement appears to be maintained (Kim & McCullough, 2008). The suprahyoid muscles play a significant role in the superior and anterior movement of the hyoid. It appears that because more muscles are involved in the superior movement of the hyoid, they may be less susceptible to fatigue (Kim & McCullough, 2008). The reduction in anterior displacement may similarly be due to progressive weakness of the suprahyoid muscles associated with age. Decreased anterior displacement of the hyoid may also result in reduced opening of the upper esophageal sphincter and increase the propensity of pharyngeal residue buildup in older individuals (Kim & McCullough, 2008).

Changes in Bolus Transit and Residue with Age

Several earlier studies have suggested that bolus transit from the pharynx to the esophagus slows with age (Cook et al., 1994; Rademaker, Pauloski & Colangelo 1998; Robbins et al., 1992; Tracy et al., 1989). This delay in bolus transit through the pharynx can result in increased pharyngeal residue. One study compared young adults between 20 and 40 years with older adults between 66 and 84 years and found that the older adults had increased pharyngeal residue (Butler, Stuart, & Kemp, 2009). However, this study examined only 2 types of consistencies: water and milk, with greater residue occurring on milk. A more recent study (Kelly, Macfarlane, Ghufoor, Drinnan, & Lew-Gor, 2008) looked at post-swallow residue in a group of subjects under 40 years and a group over 65 years on a range of consistencies, including different volumes of liquid, yogurt, chopped banana, and cheese sandwich. In contrast to previous studies, this research found that young and older subjects had equally efficient clearance of pharyngeal residue, with older participants having marginally less residue than young participants. It is notable that this study excluded subjects with medical conditions such as diabetes, cancer, cardiovascular, or neurological disease or surgery to the upper digestive tract and those taking medications at the time of recruitment. In a study that differentiated between adults over 65 years old with no medical problems and those with well-controlled medical problems (including hypertension, osteoarthritis, diabetes, hypercholesterolemia) it was found that the overall time of pharyngeal transit was significantly prolonged in the group of subjects with medical problems (Kendall, Leonard, & McKenzie, 2004a). The subjects with a diagnosis of hypertension had the most significant delays in pharyngeal bolus transit.

Changes to the Mechanism of Airway Protection with Age

Timely hyolaryngeal elevation is important to facilitate epiglottic tilt and protection of the airway during swallowing (Kim et al., 2005). Successful swallowing involves closing the supraglottis and protecting the airway through the elevation of the arytenoids, forward movement of the epiglottis (Kendall, Leonard, & McKenzie, 2004b), and closure of vocal folds. Closure of the supraglottic structures should be completed no later than 0.1 seconds after the head of the bolus arrives at the upper esophageal sphincter (UES) irrespective of age in those with a normal swallow (Kendall et al., 2004b). It appears as though older individuals close the supraglottic airway earlier than younger subjects. However, the interval between onset of vocal fold closure and other swallow events appear similar in young and older individuals. The interval between the onset of vocal fold closure and UES relaxation is reported to be shorter in older participants compared with younger individuals (Mendell & Logeman, 2007). Maintaining vocal fold closure is one of the primary airway protective mechanisms against aspiration.

Reduction in airway protection increases the risk of laryngeal penetration and aspiration. Laryngeal penetration has been described as entry of material into the airway with aspiration defined as entry of material into the larynx (Daniels et al., 2004). Laryngeal penetration is often considered a *normal* phenomenon with research suggesting that 53.1% of subjects without dysphagia demonstrate some degree of laryngeal penetration (Daggett, Logemann, Rademaker, & Pauloski, 2006) (Figure 7–2). However, the same research found a notable decline in airway protection in adults over the age of 70. Laryngeal penetration has been reported to be present in 9.3% of the normal population over 65 years of age and is six times more likely to occur in older adults compared with younger ones (Daniels et al., 2004). Additionally, the frequency of laryngeal penetration on liquid boluses in normal subjects above the age of 50 is almost twice the frequency of that seen below the age of 50 (Daggett et al., 2006). Laryngeal penetration of other consistencies such as pudding, cookie, and apple also appear to occur more frequently after age 50 whereas penetration on these consistencies did not occur at all before the age of 50 in one study (Daggett et al., 2006). Care therefore should be taken not to interpret all episodes of laryngeal penetration as abnormal. It is also worthwhile considering that although laryngeal penetration does appear to increase in normal subjects with age, aspiration is never considered a normal finding (Allen, White, Leonard, & Belafsky, 2010). Aspiration should always warrant further investigation.

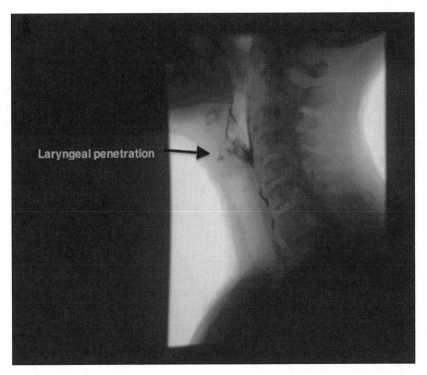

Figure 7–2. *Lateral videofluoroscopic image of laryngeal penetration in an 85-year-old female.*

Esophageal Stage

Upper Esophageal Sphincter

A complete videofluoroscopic evaluation will involve lateral, oblique, and anterior-posterior views and will involve the review of the esophageal stage of swallowing, often in consultation with a radiologist who will decide whether a more detailed investigation is required. An understanding of some of the changes expected with age in the esophageal stage of swallowing is therefore beneficial.

As the bolus is propelled from the pharynx to the esophagus, it needs to pass through the upper esophageal sphincter and then be propelled by peristaltic forces through the esophagus to the lower esophageal sphincter, which relaxes to allow food to pass into the stomach. Movement of the hyolaryngeal structure and, specifically, anterior displacement of the hyoid is not only crucial to airway protection (as previously discussed) but also assists in opening the upper esophageal sphincter to allow the bolus to pass from the pharynx to the esophagus. It appears that age (Bardan, Kern, & Arndorfer, 2006) not only brings a delay in the opening of the upper esophageal sphincter but also a physiological reduction in the range of opening of the sphincter. The phenomenon of delayed and/or reduced upper esophageal sphincter opening may not always be pathological and may act as protection for the increased risk of gastroesophageal reflux with age (Kim & McCullough, 2008). Although acid reflux occurs with equal frequency in younger and older individuals, crucially, the duration of the reflux may be longer in those who are older (Lee et al., 2007) and therefore prolonged protection may be required. Structural changes to the upper esophageal sphincter, such as the presence of a *cricopharyngeal bar* may further reduce its ability to open and impede bolus transit from pharynx to esophagus. A cricopharyngeal bar is a structural abnormality of the UES that can be a common finding on videofluoroscopy swallow examinations, the radiographic appearance of which is due to fibrosis rather than spasm or failed UES relaxation (Cook, 2006). It is thought that one-third of older individuals have a cricopharyngeal bar that may reduce the width of the upper esophageal sphincter (Leonard, Kendall, & McKenzie, 2004). Cricopharyngeal bars are often visible on instrumental swallowing evaluation tools including videofluoroscopy (Figure 7–3; see Chapter 15 for further information).

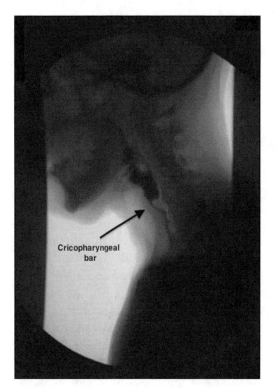

Figure 7–3. *Lateral videofluoroscopic image of cricopharyngeal bar in a 71-year-old male.*

Peristalsis

Transit of liquid and food through the esophagus is achieved through peristalsis. There is a distinction made between *primary peristalsis* which is induced by swallowing and *secondary peristalsis* which is caused by local distension of esophageal muscles (Patterson, Hildreth, & Wilson, 2007; Ren et al., 1995) and which helps clear residual bolus or refluxate (Robbins et al., 2006). Primary peristalsis occurs in a sequential, coordinated contraction wave to propel food to the stomach. Bolus transit through the esophagus may be reduced in efficiency as a consequence of the changes in peristalsis that occur with age (Grande et al., 1999; Ren et al., 2000). It has been suggested that significant peristaltic changes with esophageal swallowing occur primarily in individuals over 80 years of age (Bhutto & Morley, 2008). A failure of peristaltic contractions and incomplete esophageal emptying has been found in some older individuals (Ferioli, Dantas, Oliveira, & Braga, 1996) (Figure 7–4).

Lower Esophageal Sphincter

There is limited research in this area in normal older subjects. However, a recent study by (Besanko et al., 2011) found that basal lower esophageal pressure was reduced in older subjects compared to younger and episodes of incomplete lower esophageal sphincter relaxation were higher in older subjects, particularly with liquid.

RESPIRATION AND SWALLOWING

The respiratory system is intricately linked with swallowing. The predominant respiratory pattern in adults is *expiration* before and after the swallow (Martin-Harris et al., 2005). It duration (Leslie, Drinnan, Ford, & Wilson, 2005). This means that older people may need larger, more flavorsome boluses, not smaller amounts of bland food as conventionally thought in the past (Leslie et al., 2005). It has been found that swallowing affects additional areas of respiration other than post-swallow inspiration and increased duration of apnea. These include increased respiratory rate and higher levels of oxygen desaturation over the age of 60 (Hirst, Ford, Gibson, & Wilson, 2002).

CORTICAL PROCESSING OF SWALLOWING AND AGE

Neuroimaging studies have suggested that cortical processing of swallowing happens in multiple regions of the cerebral cortex (Hamdy et al., 1999; Martin, Goodyear, Gati, & Menon, 2001; Martin et al., 2004). The most prominent swallow-related cortical activation areas appear in the lateral pericentral and perisylvian cortices, anterior cingulated gyrus cortex, adjacent supplementary motor area, right insula/operculum, and precuneus (Martin et al., 2004; Martin et al., 2007). Just as physiological changes occur with swallowing with age, it appears as though neural processing for swallowing may also be susceptible to change. Although much information has yet to emerge from the field of neural plasticity in relation to age-related changes to swallowing, there is some evidence to suggest that older adults demonstrate greater activation in right motor, pre-motor, and pre-frontal regions than younger subjects (Robbins et al., 2008). It has been posited that the increased cortical activation seen when older subjects swallow may represent a neural compensation for the changes that happen in oral sensory motor function with age (Martin et al., 2004). A study undertaken with a small group of female subjects over 60 years found that brain

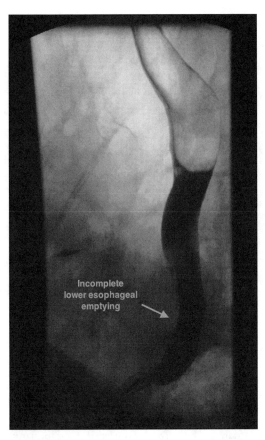

Figure 7–4. *A/P videofluoroscopic image of incomplete lower esophageal emptying in a 74-year-old male.*

has been found that healthy individuals older than 65 years tend to demonstrate a pattern of *inhaling* before and after swallowing rather than exhaling. *Apnea* refers to the period during swallowing when respiration ceases temporarily. It occurs at the initiation of the pharyngeal swallow and is typically between 1.0 seconds and 1.5 seconds in healthy adults (Martin-Harris, 2006). The duration of apnea increases with age. It is possible that apnea is a protective mechanism allowing compensation for other age-related changes such as longer oropharyngeal and hypopharyngeal transit times and delayed initiation of maximum hyolaryngeal excursion. Increasing the volume of a bolus appears critical in increasing apnea activation on a water swallow was substantially greater to that activated by a saliva swallow (Martin et al., 2007). A later study used magneto encephalography (MEG) to map brain activity in nine healthy older subjects between 60 and 85 years compared with nine healthy younger subjects between 22 and 26 years (Teisman et al., 2010). This study found increased somatosensory cortical activation during swallowing of water in the older age group. The somatosensory system receives and interprets information from joints, ligaments, muscles, and skin (Anderson, Keith, Novak, & Eliot, 2002). The primary postcentral gyrus of the parietal lobe is the location for the primary somatosensory area of the human cortex. The conclusions of this study suggest that this finding may indicate a compensation for the relative impreciseness that occurs in swallowing with age.

CONCLUSION

Some research into the normal changes that occur with swallowing as an individual ages require increased scrutiny. Many studies have not examined the "oldest old," those above 80 years (McCullough et al., 2007). Some studies have focused on a single consistency only. Bolus viscosity and size are often inconsistent among studies, reducing the generalizability of findings. Many studies have not controlled for diseases that may have an impact on swallowing with the result that some of the changes seen may not be due to age alone.

Nonetheless, knowledge of presbyphagia and the appreciation of the differences between presbyphagia and dysphagia are becoming more commonplace. Care should be taken not to pigeonhole those with normal changes in swallowing as being dysphagic simply because they are older. Videofluoroscopic studies should be as comprehensive as those with younger patients. As reported by McCullough et al. (2007), it is helpful to remember that overmanaging older patients with postural adjustments, strategies, or thickened liquids may compromise their quality of life.

REFERENCES

Allen, J., White, C., Leonard, R., & Belafsky, P. (2010). Prevalence of penetration and aspiration on videofluoroscopy in normal individuals without dysphagia. *Otolaryngology-Head and Neck Surgery, 142*(2), 208–213.

Aly, Y., & Abdel-Aty, H. (1999). Normal oesophageal transit time on digital radiography. *Clinical Radiology, 54*(8) 545–549.

Anderson, D., Keith, J., Novak, P., & Eliot, M. (2002). *Mosby's medical, nursing and allied health dictionary* (6th ed.). London, UK: Mosby.

Arcury, T., Bell, R., Anderson, A., Chen, H., Kohrman, T., & Quandt, S. (2009). Oral health self-care behaviors of rural older adults. *Journal of Public Health Dentistry, 69*(3), 182–189.

Bardan, E., Kern M, Arndorfer, R. C., Hofmann, C., & Shaker R. (2006). Effect of aging on bolus kinematics during the pharyngeal stage of swallowing. *American Journal of Physiology. Gastrointestinal and Liver Physiology, 290*(3), G458–G465.

Besanko, L., Burgstad, C., Mountfield, R., Andrews, J., Heddle, R., Checklin, H., & Fraser R. (2011). Lower oesophageal sphincter relaxation is impaired in older patients with dysphagia. *World Journal of Gastroenterology, 17*(10), 1326–1331.

Bhutto, A., & Morley, J. (2008). The clinical significance of gastrointestinal changes with aging. *Current Opinion in Clinical Nutrition and Metabolic Care, 11*(5) 651–660.

Butler, S., Stuart, A., & Kemp, S. (2009). Flexible endoscopic evaluation of swallowing in healthy young and older adults. *Annals of Otology, Rhinology and Laryngology, 118*(2), 99–106.

Clark, H., & Solomon, N. (2011). Age and sex differences in orofacial strength. *Dysphagia*. epub ahead of print. Springer online. doi: 10.1007/s00455-011-9328-2

Cook, I. (2006). Clinical disorders of the upper esophageal sphincter. *GI Motility Online*. doi: 10.1038/gimo37

Cook, I., Dodds, W., Dantas, R., Kern, M., Massey, B., Shaker, R., & Hogan WJ. (1989). Timing of videofluoroscopic, manometric events, and bolus transit during the oral and pharyngeal phases of swallowing. *Dysphagia, 4*(1), 8–15.

Cook, I., Weitman, M., Wallace, K., Shaw, D., McKay, E., Smart, R., & Butler S. (1994). Influence of aging on oral pharyngeal bolus transit and clearance during swallowing: Scintigraphic study. *American Journal of Physiology, 26*(6), G972–G977.

Daggett, A., Logemann, J., Rademaker, A., & Pauloski, B. (2006). Laryngeal penetration during deglutition in normal subjects of various ages. *Dysphagia, 21*(4), 270–274.

Daniels, S., Corey, D., Hadskey, L., Legendre, C., Priestly, D., Rosenbek, J., & Foundas A., (2004). Mechanism of sequential swallowing during straw drinking in healthy young and older adults. *Journal of Speech, Language, and Hearing Research, 47*(1), 33–45.

Dodds, W., Taylor, A., Stewart, E., Kern, M., Logemann, J., & Cook, I. (1989). Tipper and dipper types of oral swallows. *American Journal of Roentgenology, 153*(6) 1197–1199.

Easterling, C. (2008). Does exercise aimed at improving swallow function have an effect on vocal function in the healthy elderly. *Dysphagia, 23*(3), 317–326.

Ferioli, E., Dantas, R., Oliveira, R., & Braga, F. (1996). The influence of aging on oesophageal motility after ingestion of liquids with different viscosities. *European Journal of Gastroenterology and Hepatology, 8*(8), 793–798.

Frank, M. (1994). *Effects of aging on structure and function of taste buds.* Boca Raton, FL: CRC Press.

Fukunaga, A., Uematsu, H., & Sugimoto, K. (2005). Influences of aging on taste perception and oral somatic sensation. *Journals of Gerontology-Series A Biological and Medical Science, 60*(1), 109–113.

Furaya, J. (1999). Effects of wearing complete dentures on swallowing in the elderly. *Journal of the Japanese Stomatology Society, 66*(4), 361–369.

Grande, L., Lacima, G., Ros, E., Pera, M., Ascaso, C., & Visa, J. (1999). Deterioration of oesophageal motility with age: A manometric study of 79 healthy subjects. *American Journal of Gastroenterology, 94*(7), 1795–1801.

Hamdy, S., Mikulis, D., Crawley, A., Xue, S., Law, H., Henry, S., & Diamant N. (1999). Cortical Activation during human volitional swallowing: an event related fMRI study. *American Journal of Physiology-Gastrointestinal and Liver Physiology, 277*(1 Pt. 1), G219–G225.

Hermel, J., Schonwetter, S., & Samueloff, S. (1970). Taste sensation and age in man. *Journal of Oral Medicine, 25*(2) 39–42.

Hildebrandt, G., Dominguez, B., Schork, M., & Loesche, W. (1997). Functional units, chewing, swallowing and food avoidance among the elderly. *Journal of Prosthetic Dentistry, 77*(6), 588–595.

Holas, M., Halvorson, K., & Reding, M. (1990). Videofluoroscopic evidence of aspiration and relative risk of pneumonia or death following stroke. *Clinical Research, 11*, 93–98.

Hurst, L., Ford, G., Gibson, G., & Wilson, J. (2002). Swallow induced alterations in breathing in normal older people. *Dysphagia, 17*(2), 152–161.

Kelly, A., Macfarlane, K., Ghufoor, K., Drinnan, M., & Lew-Gor, S. (2008). Pharyngeal residue across the lifespan: A first look at what's normal. *Clinical Otolaryngology, 33*(4), 348–351.

Kendall, K., Leonard, R., & McKenzie, S. (2004a). Common medical conditions in the elderly: Impact on pharyngeal bolus transit. *Dysphagia, 19*(2), 71–77.

Kendall, K. A., Leonard, R. J., & McKenzie, S. (2004b). Airway protection: Evaluation with videofluoroscopy. *Dysphagia, 19*, 65–70.

Kim, Y., & McCullough, G. (2008). Maximum hyoid displacement in normal swallowing. *Dysphagia, 23*(3), 274–279.

Kim, Y., McCullough, G., & Asp, C. (2005). Temporal measurements of pharyngeal swallowing in normal populations. *Dysphagia, 20(4)*, 290–296.

Lee, J., Anggiansah, A., Anggiansah, R., Young, A., Wong, T., & Fox, M. (2007). Effects of age on gastroesophageal junction, esophageal motility and reflux disease. *Clinical Gastroenterology and Hepatology, 5*(12), 1392–1398.

Leidberg, B., Stoltze, K., & Owall, B. (2005). The masticatory handicap of wearing removable dentures in elderly men. *Gerodontology, 22*(1), 10–16.

Leonard, R., Kendall, K., & McKenzie, S. (2004). UES opening and cricopharyngeal bar in non-dysphagic elderly and nonelderly adults. *Dysphagia, 19*(3), 182–191.

Leonard, R., & McKenzie, S. (2006). Hyoid-bolus transit latencies in normal swallow. *Dysphagia, 21*(3), 183–190.

Leslie, P., Drinnan, M., Ford, G., & Wilson, J. (2005). Swallow respiratory patterns and aging: Presbyphagia or dysphagia. *Journal of Gerontology, 60A*(3), 391–395.

Logemann, J. (1998). *Evaluation and treatment of swallowing disorders* (2nd ed.). Austin, TX: Pro-Ed.

Logemann, J., Pauloski, B., Rademaker, A., Lazurus, C., Mittal, B., Gaziano, J., . . . Newman, L. (2003). Xerostomia: 12-month changes in saliva production and its relationship to perception and performance of swallow function, oral intake, and diet after chemoradiation. *Head and Neck, 25*(6), 432–437.

Logemann, J., Smith, C., Pauloski, B., Rademaker, A., Lazurus, C., Colangelo, L., . . . Newman, L. (2001). Effects of xerostomia on perception and perception and performance of swallow function. *Head and Neck, 23*(4), 317–321.

Mackay-Sim, A., Johnston, A., Owen, C., & Burne, T. (2006). Olfactory ability in the healthy population: Reassessing presbyosmia. *Chemical Senses, 31*(8), 763–771.

Martin, R., Barr, A., MacIntosh, B., Smith, R., Stevens, T., Taves, D., . . . Hachinski V. (2007). Cerebral cortical processing of swallowing in older adults. *Experimental Brain Research, 176*(1) 12–22.

Martin, R., Goodyear, B., Gati, J., & Menon, R. (2001). Cerebral cortical representation of automatic and volitional swallowing in humans. *Journal of Neurophysiology, 85*(2), 938–950.

Martin, R., Macintosh, B., Smith, R., Barr, A., Stevens, T., Gati, J., & Menon R. S. (2004). Cerebral areas processing swallowing and tongue movement are overlapping but distinct: A functional magnetic resonance imaging study. *Journal of Neurophysiology, 92*(4), 2428–2493.

Martin-Harris, B. (2006). Co-ordination of respiration and swallowing. *GI Motility Online*. doi:10.1038/gimo10

Martin-Harris, B., Brodsky, M., Michel, Y., Ford, C., Walters, B., & Heffner, J. (2005). Breathing and swallowing dynamics across the adult life-span. *Archives of Otolaryngology-Head and Neck Surgery, 131*(9), 762–770.

Martin-Harris, B., Brodsky, M., Michel, Y., Lee, F., & Walters, B. (2007). Delayed initiation of the pharyngeal swallow: Normal variability in adult swallows. *Journal of Speech, Language and Hearing Research, 50*(3), 585–594.

McCullough, G., Rosenbek J. C., Wertz, R., Suiter, D., & McCoy, S. (2007). Defining swallowing function by age. promises and pitfalls of pigeonholing. *Topics in Geriatric Rehabilitation, 23*(4), 290–307.

Mendell, D., & Logeman JA (2007). Temporal sequence of swallow events during the oropharyngeal swallow. *Journal of Speech, Language, and Hearing Research, 50*(5), 1256–1271.

Mistretta, C. (1984). Aging effects on anatomy and neurophysiology of taste and smell. *Gerontology, 3*(2), 131–136.

Mojet, J., Christ Hazelhof, E., & Heidema, J. (2001). Taste perception with age: Generic or specific losses in threshold sensitivity to the five basic tastes. *Chemical Senses, 26*(7), 845–860.

Narhi, T. (1994). Prevalence of subjective feelings of dry mouth in the elderly. *Journal of Dental Research, 73*(1), 20–25.

Neville, B., Damm, D., Allen, C., & Bouquot, J. (2002). *Oral and maxillofacial pathology*. Philadelphia, PA: W. B. Saunders.

Patterson, J., Hildreth, A., & Wilson, J. (2007). Measuring edema in irradiated head and neck cancer patients. *Annals of Otology, Rhinology, and Laryngology, 116*(8), 559–564.

Pelletier, C. (2007). Chemosenses, aging and oropharyngeal dysphagia. *Topics in Geriatric Rehabilitation, 23*(3), 249–268.

Prendergast, D., Fisher, N., & Calkins, E. (1993). Cardiovascular, neuromuscular and metabolic alterations with age leading to frailty. *Journal of Gerontology, 48* (Spec No), 61–67.

Quandt, S., Chen, H., Bell, R., Savoca, M., Anderson, A., Leng, X., . . . Arcury, T. (2010). Food avoidance and food modification practices of older rural adults: Association with oral health status and implications for service provision. *Gerontologist, 50*(1), 100–111.

Rademaker, A., Pauloski, B., & Colangelo, L. (1998). Age and volume effects on liquid swallowing function in normal women. *Journal of Speech, Language, and Hearing Research, 41,* 275–284.

Ren, J., Shaker, R., Kusano, M., Podvrsan, B., Metwally, N., Dua, K., & Sui Z. (1995). Effect of aging on the secondary esophageal peristalsis: Presbyesophagus revisited. *American Journal of Physiology, 268*(5 Pt. 1), G772–G779.

Ren, J., Xie, P., Lang, I., Bardan, E., Sui, Z., & Shaker, R. (2000). Deterioration of the pharyngo-UES contractile reflex in the elderly. *Laryngoscope, 110*(9), 1563–1566.

Robbins, J., Bridges, A. D., & Taylor, A. (2006). Oral, pharyngeal and esophageal motor function in aging. *GI Motility Online.* doi:10.1038/gimo39

Robbins, J., Butler, S., Daniels, S., Diez-Gross, R., Langmore, S., Lazarus, C., Martin-Harris B., . . . Rosenbek, J. (2008). Swallowing and dysphagia rehabilitation: Translating principles of neuroplasticity into clinically oriented evidence. *Journal of Speech, Language, and Hearing Research, 51,* S276–S300.

Robbins, J., Gangnon, R., Theis, S., Kays, S., Hewitt, A., & Hind, J. (2005). The effects of lingual exercise on swallowing in older adults. *Journal of the American Geriatrics Society, 53*(9), 1483–1489.

Robbins, J., Hamilton, J., Lof, G., & Kempster, G. (1992). Oropharyngeal swallowing in normal adults of different ages. *Gastroenterology, 103*(9), 823–829.

Robbins, J., Levine, R., Wood, J., Roecker, E., & Luschei, E. (1995). Age effects on lingual pressure generation as a risk factor for dysphagia. *Journal of Gerontology A: Biological Sciences and Medical Sciences, 50A*(5), M257–M262.

Rosenberg, R. (1997). Sarcopenia: Origins and clinical relevance. *Journal of Nutrition, 27*(3), 990S–991S.

Schiffman, S. (1997). Taste and smell losses in normal aging and disease. *Journal of the American Medical Association, 278*(16), 1357–1362.

Schindler, J., & Kelly, J. (2002). Swallowing disorders in the elderly. *Laryngoscope, 112*(4), 589–602.

Shaw, D., Cook, I., Gabb, M., Holloway, R., Simula, M., Panagopoulos, V., & Dent, J. (1995). Influence of normal aging on oropharyngeal and upper esophageal sphincter function during swallowing. *American Journal of Physiology, 268*(3 Pt. 1), G389–G396.

Smidt, D., Torpet, L., Nauntoffe, B., Heegard, K., & Pedersen, A. (2011). Associations between oral and ocular dryness, labial and whole salivary flow rates, systemic diseases and medications in a sample of older people. *Community Dentistry and Oral Epidemiology, 39*(3), 276–288.

Teisman, I., Steinstraeter, O., Schmidt, W., Ringelstein, E., Pantev, C., & Dziewas, R. (2010). Age-related changes in cortical swallowing processing. *Neurobiology of Aging, 31*(6), 1044–1050.

Thomson, W., Chalmers, J., Spencer, A., & Slade, G. (2000). Medication and dry mouth: Findings from a cohort study of older people. *Journal of Public Health Dentistry, 60*(1), 12–20.

Tracy, J., Logeman J. A., Kahrilas, P., Jacob, P., Kobara, M., & Krugler, C. (1989). Preliminary observations on the effects of age on oropharyngeal deglutition. *Dysphagia, 4*(2), 90–94.

Turner, M., & Ship, J. (2007). Dry mouth and its effects on the oral health of elderly people. *Journal of American Dental Association, 138*(Suppl.), 15S–20S.

United Nations 2002 Population Division. Retrieved April 14, 2011, from http://www.un.org

Weiffenbach, J., Baum, B., & Burghauser, R. (1982). Taste thresholds: quality specific variation with human aging. *Journal of Gerontology, 37*(3), 372–377.

Chapter

EFFECTIVE USE OF IMAGING TECHNOLOGY

Elizabeth Judson and Julie M. Nightingale

INTRODUCTION

The radiographer has a vital role within videofluoroscopy; therefore, this chapter explains the range of fluoroscopy and ancillary equipment used, plus the associated health and safety and radiation safety requirements for the patient, carers, and staff. The chapter also builds on the extensive knowledge of specialist fluoroscopic radiographers by discussing best practice in image acquisition and radiation safety, and introduces the concept of fluoroscopy to those professionals involved in the procedure who do not have a background in radiation science.

The videofluoroscopy clinic is a multiprofessional clinic with consultant radiologists, radiographers, and speech-language pathologists (SLP) working together. In many centers, particularly within the United Kingdom, the radiographer may have advanced

their role to include image acquisition traditionally undertaken by the radiologist. They may be working as an advanced or consultant practitioner, supported in the smooth running of the procedure by a radiographer, nurse, or radiographic assistant. The advanced practitioner radiographer will assume the role of the radiologist, providing an opinion on the imaging and performing the fluoroscopy element of the procedure. This chapter outlines the role of the radiographer who is responsible for the technical aspects of the examination, and focuses in particular on safety aspects, ensuring that the environment is safe, and that radiation safety principles are adhered to.

The essential equipment is described together with some basic radiation physics and radiation safety principles, which serve as a reminder and reference tool for radiographers and experienced SLPs, or as an introduction to SLPs new to the videofluoroscopy environment.

INTRODUCTION TO RADIATION SCIENCE

The Emergence of the Radiography and Radiology Professions

X-rays were first discovered in 1895 by Wilhelm Roentgen, a German physicist who was experimenting with passing electrical currents through vacuum tubes. He noticed that photographic plates stored in his laboratory were become inexplicably blackened, which he deduced were as a result of some unknown rays or particles emitted from the vacuum tubes—these he termed "x-rays." For the first few years this new technology was used indiscriminately for "pleasure" photographs, with little or no awareness of the inherent dangers of radiation. However, the advent of the First World War saw the medical applications of x-rays come to the forefront; battlefield photographers and engineers effectively became the first radiographers.

It was some time later that the medical fraternity saw the value of x-ray technologies, and sought to ensure that although "laymen" could produce x-ray images, the interpretation of those images required a medical background. It was in the mid-1920s that the new profession of radiographers within the U.K. was legally barred from reporting images (Price, 2005), and medically trained radiologists placed reporting firmly within their domain. This is the way it remained for many years, until the 1970s and 1980s when laws were relaxed to enable radiographers to contribute to a report.

At the present time, in the U.K. radiographers are able to provide a definitive report provided they have been appropriately trained, work within agreed protocols, are subject to regular audit and engage in continuing professional development (see Chapter 3). Although there is still some resistance to radiographer-reporting from some sections of the radiologist community, there is no reason why a radiographer should not take on the management of the videofluoroscopy procedure, to include image acquisition as well as contributing to the written report (usually in conjunction with an SLP).

The Production of the X-Ray Beam

The generation of x-rays requires, in simplified terms, a cathode and filament that emits electrons when a current (mA) is applied. This lies opposite an anode with a target made of tungsten. The cathode and anode are placed within an evacuated glass cylinder (Figure 8–1). When a large potential difference (kV) is applied to the cylinder, the electrons are fired rapidly at the target. Interaction of the target molecules with the high-speed electrons causes energy to be released in the form of x-rays. Manipulation of the current in milliampere seconds (mAs) controls the "quantity" of electrons, while manipulation of the kilovoltage (kV) affects the speed and energy of the electrons. Therefore, the manipulation of kV and mAs are the two primary exposure factors at the radiographer's disposal to influence the quantity (density) and the quality (penetration) of the x-ray beam.

X-rays are emitted from the target in all directions, and so require shielding in the form of a lead casing with the exception of the port of the x-ray tube, which can be varied in size by the operator by the use of rectangular or circular lead collimators (see Figure 8–1). Before exiting the collimators the x-ray beam passes through copper or aluminum filtration to remove the low energy x-rays; these are insufficiently penetrating to pass through tissue, but will still potentially damage skin and other tissues.

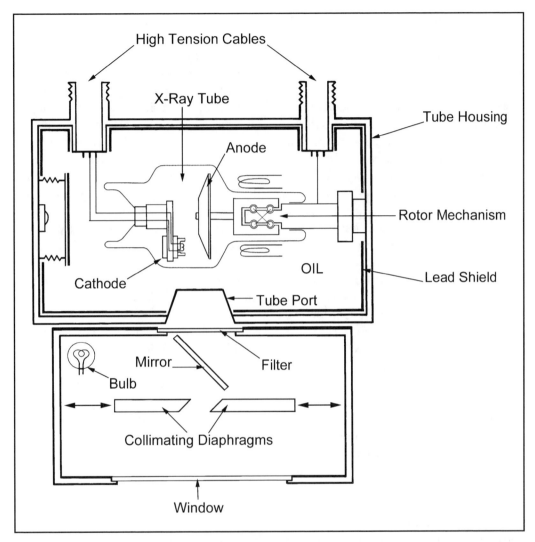

Figure 8–1. *Schematic diagram demonstrating a rotating anode x-ray tube within the tube housing and lead shield. The diaphragm mechanism is attached, which includes the light beam diaphragm and collimator mechanism. (Diagram created by Graham Nightingale).*

The side effect of the production of x-rays is the generation of a massive amount of heat, approximately 1% of any exposure results in x-rays, with 99% of the energy given out as heat. Therefore, much of modern x-ray tube technology is devoted to dissipating heat. For example, the glass tube is encased in oil that allows heat to be removed by convection (see Figure 8–1). This means that the x-ray tube housing is bulky. The anode rotates at high speed during the exposure to distribute the electron beam around a wider surface area to prevent the target from melting. It takes a short time to get up to speed, which accounts for the brief prep time (with accompanying increasing noise) before an exposure can be made.

The Production of the X-Ray Image

The radiographer is able to adjust the x-ray beam to suit the clinical situation, by manipulating kVp, mAs, image size (collimation), and source-image distance (previously known as focus-film distance). In some cases they are also able to manipulate the focus/target size: smaller targets provide sharper images, but at the expense of generation of increased heat.

In a conventional x-ray examination, the radiographer positions the patient appropriately, and then centers (positions) the x-ray beam at a predetermined centering point on the patient's body, and collimates the beam to include only the relevant anatomy. Centering and collimation are aided by a light-beam diaphragm and targeted laser lights. Movement unsharpness is a particular problem, so the patient is immobilized or asked to arrest respiration during the exposure. The x-ray beam passes through the patient, with some x-rays being absorbed by the tissue, some being transmitted through the patient unchanged, and some being scattered in different paths. Scattered radiation is a particular problem as it reduces image quality and increases dose to the patient and staff, so a number of steps are taken to reduce the amount of scatter a) being produced (e.g., tissue compression, collimation) and b) reaching the image receptor (e.g., grids).

An imaging receptor is placed beneath the patient's anatomy; traditionally, this would have been an x-ray film placed within a cassette containing light-emitting screens. The light is important to greatly amplify the effect of the x-rays: for each x-ray penetrating the screen, many light photons are emitted, thus enabling the amount of radiation required to be reduced. Modern radiology departments will now be using either computed radiography (CR) using cassettes that require further "processing" to create a digital image, or acquiring digital images directly without the use of a cassette (direct digital radiography or DDR).

Principles of Fluoroscopy

The x-ray equipment used for videofluoroscopy is a fluoroscopy unit of which there are two types, the traditional fluoroscopy unit and the C-arm, both using an x-ray tube coupled with an image intensifier and image display system to provide real-time moving images. After the x-rays pass through the patient, instead of using traditional cassettes to acquire the image, the x-ray beam is captured by the image intensifier and converted into light. The light is then captured by a TV camera and displayed on a monitor (MedicineNet .com, 2011).

An image intensifier is a device that converts x-rays emitted through the patient into a visible light output, which is then converted into a digital image viewed on a monitor. Unlike conventional x-rays, which have a single millisecond exposure, the fluoroscopy x-ray tube is capable of emitting low dose x-ray beams either in pulses (pulsed fluoroscopy) or in a continuous stream (continuous fluoroscopy). The pulse rate can be varied by the operator. The system is also able to acquire conventional images (single or multiple exposures, higher dose but higher quality) at several frames per second, and to "grab" images from the monitor (at no extra dose to the patient, but lower quality).

The traditional fluoroscopy unit may have the x-ray tube positioned permanently below the fluoroscopy couch (hidden from view), with the image receptor (known as an *explorator*) above the patient. This configuration is known as an under-couch fluoroscopy tube, and has some limitations in terms of lack of space for larger patients, poor access to the patient, and additional dose for staff (as the operator must be close to the patient during exposures).

In comparison, an over-couch fluoroscopy configuration (with the x-ray tube above the patient) gives some advantages as it is less restrictive for the patient and has the potential to be operated remotely.

The C-arm units have the image intensifier coupled to the x-ray tube in a C-shaped configuration, using either a fixed or a mobile unit that can rotate around the patient couch (Figure 8–2). This has advantages for more immobile patients, as the equipment can move

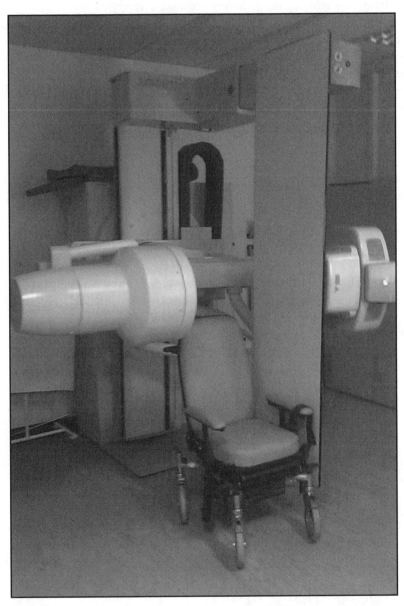

Figure 8–2. *A modern fluoroscopy unit (Toshiba Ultimax from Toshiba Medical Systems), with the image intensifier seen closest to the camera, and the x-ray tube behind the fluoroscopy table. A specialist videofluoroscopy chair is positioned ready to receive the patient ("The Mangar Porter" chair from Mangar Aids Ltd). A full-color version of the figure can be seen in the color insert.*

around them more easily. Modern C-arm units are generally digital, thereby giving higher quality, but often at lower doses.

As the aim of a videofluoroscopy examination is to study the swallowing dynamics, it is essential to have real-time imaging. Although the equipment has the ability to acquire detailed images, it is usually sufficient for VFSS to store the fluoroscopy-acquired (captured) images and video clips, thus limiting radiation dose. By storing images produced during an examination, and in particular using the last image hold function on the monitor where available, it enables review of images during the examination and may reduce the need for additional exposures. It will also aid report writing after the examination. VFSS images can be stored in several ways: images can be captured by acquiring images (a high resolution "still") in a single exposure or at a few frames per second; "grabbing" fluoroscopy images (low resolution); or storing fluoroscopy images to a hard drive. In modern radiology departments these images are also stored to PACS (Picture Archiving and Communication System) creating a permanent digital storage of images, which can be viewed throughout a department or hospital-wide network. The images can also be stored to a DVD or CD that the SLP can take away; this can be useful for home visits for patient and carer education.

The additional benefit of image storage is that if during the examination either the SLP or radiologist/radiographer is uncertain of the findings (e.g., whether they saw aspiration), the stored imaging can be reviewed immediately, with the potential of reducing the radiation dose as the swallow may not need repeating.

RADIOBIOLOGY AND THE RISKS OF RADIATION

The use of radiation for medical investigation carries with it tremendous benefits, but also

a risk of potential harm. It is incumbent on the referrer and the radiographer/radiologist to ascertain that the potential benefits of the procedure outweigh the potential harm: this is known as the risk-benefit analysis, or justification. However, in order to justify a procedure, it is essential to have an understanding of the type and level of potential risks.

X-rays were first discovered in 1895, with natural radioactivity identified a year later. Both x-rays and gamma rays are classified as ionizing radiation and are part of the electromagnetic spectrum, which also includes nonionizing radiation (microwaves, visible light, and radiowaves). Nonionizing radiation has sufficient energy to "move" atoms, but not alter them chemically. Ionizing radiation, however, is capable of removing electrons from atoms, which can potentially damage the DNA within living cells.

Exposure of the population to ionizing radiation is not restricted to man-made radiations (medical or nuclear power). It is estimated that 80% of the dose to the public comes from natural radiation sources, such as cosmic radiation when flying at altitude, and radiation emanating from radon gas and rocks such as granite (USEPA, 2007). In order to reassure the public, medical exposures are often compared for simplicity to natural background radiation; for example, one chest x-ray equals approximately 3 days of natural background radiation, or one flight across the Atlantic Ocean. As a chest x-ray is seen to be a typical "low dose" investigation, it is often used as a comparison for other radiographic procedures. For example, VFSS in one center was calculated for risk explanations to be equivalent to 10 chest x-rays (Zammit-Maempel, Chapple, & Leslie, 2007).

Practical radiation protection in health care is based on the assumption that radiation is carcinogenic, and may have other less likely adverse effects including genetic defects of children born to exposed parents, and physical or mental defects in a fetus exposed in utero. The scientific basis for these conclusions comes from epidemiological studies following populations exposed to large doses of radiation, including large medical exposures (mainly high-dose radiotherapy). However the vast majority of our knowledge has been gained from the Lifespan Study following over 100,000 survivors of the Nagasaki and Hiroshima nuclear bombs. From this, several important facts have been established (USEPA, 2007):

- At extremely high doses, there is a threshold dose below which certain effects are not seen (for example, radiation burns, gastrointestinal damage, or neurological damage). These threshold-based effects are known as deterministic effects.
- The greater the dose, the greater the chance of developing cancer. However, different individuals will have different risk from the same exposure.
- There is thought to be no lower threshold for developing cancer (this is known as a stochastic (chance) effect)
- Radiation-induced cancers appear many years after initial exposure.

These findings are based on individuals receiving extremely high exposures, which are then extrapolated down mathematically to be made to "fit" with low dose exposures (those characteristically below 20 mSv). However, surprisingly, the risk of developing cancer following either acute or cumulative doses below 100 mSv cannot be directly proved (Harbron, 2012). One of the confounding factors is that all the known radiation-induced effects, including cancer, may occur naturally, or as a result of lifestyle factors such as smoking. A definite link between low dose radiation and cancer is almost impossible to prove. From an epidemiological research perspective, another serious barrier is presented. As radiation dose decreases, the required sample size to "prove" cancer links dramatically increases. Harbron (2012) estimates that the numbers required to demonstrate cancer risk following a common radiographic procedure such as a chest x-ray would be billions. Thus, it is not possible to statistically prove whether diagnostic radiography exposures are harmful or not; the risk is either too small to detect or does not exist at all (Harbron, 2012).

The lack of evidence of the risk of inducing cancer at low doses seen in diagnostic imaging exposures poses a problem for radiographers and radiologists. Although they may have no proof of risk, equally they have no evidence that categorically states that risk is absent. On this basis, radiation protection assumes that there is a *potential* risk, even at small doses (i.e., no threshold dose), and that a single radiation track has the ability to initiate significant damage to the DNA of an individual cell, which theoretically, could induce the development of cancer.

Evidence suggests that not all human tissues are equally radiosensitive. Tissues which are rapidly dividing are at greater risk of radiation damage; these include the skin and gastrointestinal tract, known to be adversely affected by very high therapy doses (skin burns, alopecia, and vomiting and diarrhea). The testes and ovaries are also thought to be more radiosensitive, with potential risks to offspring, so where possible they are shielded in clinical practice. However, there is little convincing evidence for carcinogenic effects crossing the generation gap, and evidence for hereditary effects is unreliable.

Nevertheless, greater attention is paid to the risks related to the rapidly dividing and differentiating tissues of the fetus. The risks of high doses of radiation are not the same at all stages of pregnancy, with the pre-implantation phase (0–3 weeks gestation) being thought to be most susceptible to lethal effects, and the embryonic period (3–8 weeks) being the most susceptible for teratogenic (abnormality forming) effects. However, the potential frequency of cancer and leukemia induction is not thought to be influenced by the stage of pregnancy (Krovak & Nightingale, 2005).

All radiology departments should have a policy regarding the imaging of female patients of reproductive capacity (12–55 years). This should encompass two key protocols: avoiding inadvertent irradiation of the early embryo in an unknown pregnancy, and ensuring a dose reduction strategy once a pregnancy is known (Krovak & Nightingale, 2005). International (ICRP 84, 2000) and European (ECRP 100, 1998) legislation has helped to shape these policies, including the introduction of two frameworks for protection of the unborn child. The first of these is the application of the "10 day rule" for high dose procedures (e.g., CT abdominal scans), which ensures that the patient is scanned within the first 10 days of the start of menstruation, when a pregnancy is not possible. However, this rule has been relaxed for many procedures because of the exceptionally low risk of damage to an embryo within the first two weeks of pregnancy. The second framework, known as the "28 day rule," is more universally applied within diagnostic radiology for procedures that may involve exposure to the abdomen and pelvis. The woman is questioned about the date of her last menstrual period, and for the examination to proceed this should have occurred within the last 28 days. Where pregnancy is suspected, a pregnancy test may be requested, and an alternative nonionizing procedure may be considered. Alternatively the examination may go ahead if essential, but with additional shielding for the patient's abdomen. The VFSS procedure is highly unlikely to yield a significant dose to the abdomen, so there is questionable cause for ascertaining pregnancy status. However, where imaging is used to explore the lower esophagus or stomach, uterine doses could be higher.

ENSURING RADIATION SAFETY FOR PATIENTS

Radiation safety should be considered in relation to patients, operators, other staff, and carers, the aim being to protect these personnel from both the primary beam and secondary (scattered) radiation (Ball & Moore, 1997).

The primary beam is the radiation that exits the x-ray tube through the collimators. When this beam passes through the body it interacts with the patient. Much of it will be absorbed by the tissues, or will pass through to the image receptor. However, some x-rays will be scattered when they interact with tissue; this scattered radiation can exit the patient in any direction. Scattered radiation can degrade image quality (blackens the image without adding any anatomical information) and it can also reach other parts of the patient, staff, and carers.

Radiation safety in the U.K. is guided by both the Ionising Radiation (Medical Exposure) Regulations 2000 (IRMER, 2000) which has a focus on reducing radiation dose to the patient, and the Ionising Radiation Regulations (1999) which mainly considers radiation doses to staff. The Health and Safety Executive (HSE) in the U.K. enforces the legal requirements and these are detailed in approved codes of practice (IRR, 1999). In the United States, The Nuclear Regulatory Commission (NRC), the Food and Drug Administration (FDA), and other federal and state agencies regulate medical procedures that use radiation (USEPA, 2007). These agencies also issue guidance designed to reduce unnecessary use of radiation and ensure that technicians, equipment, and techniques meet standards for minimizing radiation exposure. The Environmental Protection Agency (EPA) also issues standards and guidance to limit human exposure to radiation (USEPA, 2007).

Although legislation will differ between nations, three basic principles of radiation protection of patients should be followed by all, regardless of nationality or professional group. These are the principles of justification, optimization, and limitation.

Justification

The SLP and radiologist/radiographer should consider whether the benefit of the procedure will outweigh the risk of the procedure, or the risk of not doing the procedure. Sometimes these benefits can be difficult to quantify, but if the management of the patient will not be altered by the videofluoroscopy, the examination should not go ahead (Ball & Moore, 1997).

Optimization

The minimum amount of radiation should be used to produce images that provide sufficient information for the clinician. The ALARP (As Low As Reasonably Practicable) principle should be adhered to and the responsibility for this lies with the radiographer and the radiologist. Using this principle keeps the radiation dose to the patient and therefore any risk from harm to a minimum. It will also reduce the radiation received by other personnel in the room. Optimization involves ensuring the best functionality of equipment, and the appropriate selection and manipulation of exposure factors commensurate with an optimized dose with a satisfactory image quality. Fluoroscopy rooms are regularly checked for safety and accuracy by medical physics departments and internally by the radiology quality assurance team so that there is early warning of problems such as overexposure, deteriorating image quality, or inaccurate collimation. Any faults detected during routine use should also be notified to the manager or supervisor, equipment manufacturer, and if necessary the room should be taken out of use. Orga-

nizations such as the United States Food and Drug Administration's Center for Devices and Radiological Health establishes standards for x-ray machines and other electronic products to ensure that human health is protected through safe operation (USEPA, 2000).

Limitation

The dose received shall not exceed the recommended dose for that procedure (see Radiation Dosimetry section). The radiographer and radiologist will choose and set up the equipment and technical factors to reduce the dose to the patient. The equipment used should be suitable for purpose and used judiciously to ensure doses are minimized. Various dose reduction strategies are outlined in Table 8–1.

ENSURING RADIATION SAFETY FOR PERSONNEL

The managers and clinical leads in the radiology department will work with the Radiation Protection Advisor (RPA) (an independent radiation expert) to ensure that the regulations are adhered to, and that protocols and risk assessments are written and reviewed. Most radiology departments will have in place Radiation Protection Supervisors (RPS) or Radiation Safety Officers (RPO) who are responsible for radiation safety within a particular specialist area, including fluoroscopy. All staff (including anyone accessing the fluoroscopy suite, such as cleaners) should be aware of the local rules (radiation safety protocols) and employer's procedures (IRMER, 2000). The local rules should be clearly visible within the fluoroscopy room. The radiographer is responsible for ensuring that everyone in the room adheres to these rules and procedures. In addition, radiation safety guidance

Table 8–1. Dose Reduction Strategies

Strategy	Purpose
Use high output x-ray tube	Can generate higher energy beam with less heating over longer periods
Select high kVp	Ensures a high energy beam with less low energy photons (damaging but add no value)
Use automatic exposure devices (AEDs)	Have the potential to maintain an appropriate image brightness with minimal lag when movement is apparent
Use pulsed fluoroscopy at a low frame rate where possible	Preferable to continuous radiation—will reduce overall radiation dose without significantly affecting image quality
Collimate the beam	Reduces the area of tissue exposed to primary radiation and also reduces the amount of scattered radiation, consequently improving image quality
Use last image hold	The unit retains the last image on the monitor screen and allows review of the image without exposing the patient to unnecessary radiation
Maintain the image intensifier as close to the patient as possible	Reduces the distance between the patient and image detector, with the x-ray tube as far away from the patient as possible. This reduces unsharpness and reduces the skin dose to the patient.
Do not overuse the magnification mode	The aim to use the largest field size possible, particularly if the equipment has the option to magnify images in postprocessing, i.e., acquisition. Magnification tends to improve image quality but at the expense of patient dose.
Set fluoroscopy timers	An audible alarm is activated when a predetermined fluoroscopy time is reached (e.g., 5 minutes) to remind the operator that a reasonable time has expired. Although it may be clinically appropriate to continue, it is worthwhile considering whether the examination can be brought to a conclusion. If this time is frequently reached the team may wish to consider reviewing practice or techniques in the future.

is also issued in professional documents such as the ASHA Guidelines for Speech-Language Pathologists Performing Videofluoroscopic Swallowing Studies (2004).

The technical measures described in the previous section will endeavor to reduce the dose to patients, which in turn will also reduce the dose received by staff and carers. There are, however, some additional measures that will further reduce dose to staff and carers. These include the use of distance and location, and personal protective equipment (PPE), and minimizing the radiation dose generated.

Distance and Staff Location

The use of distance is explained by the *inverse square* law. Radiation spreads out as it travels away from the source, and in doing so the intensity reduces. The inverse square relationship indicates that doubling the distance from a radiation source decreases the radiation level by a factor of four. Conversely, halving the distance increases the radiation level by a factor of four. Intelligent application of this principle can yield significant reductions in operator and staff radiation exposures. Therefore, if staff and carers are required to stay in the room, they are advised to keep as much distance between the x-ray tube and themselves as is practicable.

The radiographer and radiologist will advise on the correct place for the speech-language pathologist and other professionals and relatives to stand during fluoroscopy. In a traditional under-couch tube configuration, when the patient is stood or seated with their back to the fluoroscopy table, the majority of the scattered radiation will pass backward toward the x-ray tube (back-scatter). Similarly, a lot of scattered radiation will be emitted to the side of the patient, with less being scattered in a forward direction (Figure 8–3). The

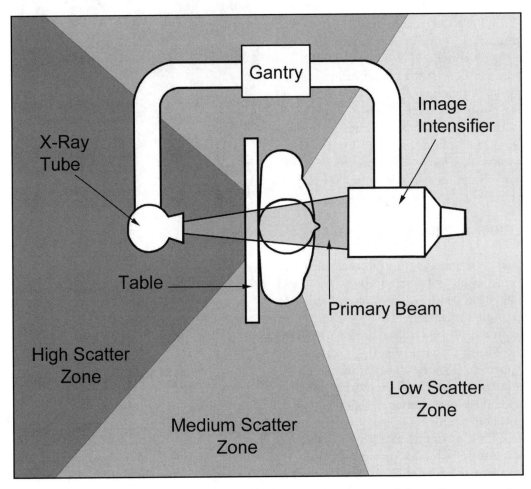

Figure 8–3. *Schematic diagram to demonstrate the scatter patterns created during fluoroscopy using a traditional undercouch x-ray configuration (overhead view). The high scatter zone is toward the x-ray tube, with the low scatter zone toward the image intensifier. Staff should attempt to remain in the low scatter zone during fluoroscopy, and as far away from the patient as is feasible. (Diagram created by Graham Nightingale).*

most appropriate place to stand is therefore facing the patient, but at an angle where the equipment (and the operator) will shield the staff from the main scatter. Similarly, where a C-arm fluoroscopy unit is in operation, staff should be aware of the relative position of the x-ray tube and image intensifier, standing towards the intensifier side of the C-arm where possible. The operator (radiologist or radiographer) should be alert to staff and carer position at all times and should not initiate fluoroscopic exposure until everyone is in as safe a place as possible. Only those essential to the examination (e.g., the radiographer, radiologist and SLP) should remain within the controlled area, which is the area around the source of radiation (Farr & Allisy-Roberts, 1998). The other personnel, such as students or relatives, should be outside the controlled area, behind the protective screen or outside the room. Placing the operator's hands in the primary beam should be avoided at all times; this is particularly relevant to this procedure if it is a requirement for someone to feed the patient.

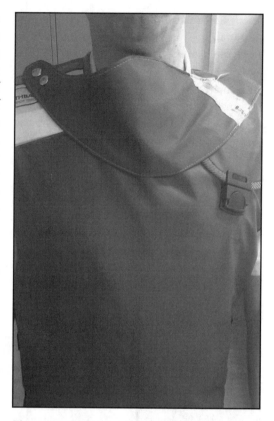

Figure 8–4. Lead rubber protective apron and thyroid shield.

Personal Protective Equipment (PPE)

Staff or relatives within the controlled area should wear a lead rubber apron, 0.35mm lead equivalent, which reduces scattered radiation exposure to the torso. They are also advised to wear a thyroid collar, as the thyroid is more sensitive to radiation (Figure 8–4). This equipment is not designed for use within the primary beam. There should be sufficient lead rubber garments for all staff that need to remain in the room outside of the controlled area. If the patient requires help with feeding, it is usually better if a known carer does this as it is may be more likely to be successful for some patient groups (e.g., pediatrics, or patients with learning disabilities; see Chapters 11 and 12). In turn, the SLP receives fewer cumulative doses of radiation if present

at many clinics. Leaded gloves designed to be used within the primary beam can be worn if hand placement within the x-ray beam is briefly necessary or if the hands are positioned nearby for extended periods of time.

Personnel Monitoring

The radiology department will generally use a dosimetry service to monitor doses received by staff working with radiation. There are various types of monitoring: environmental monitoring within the x-ray room, Thermoluminescent dosimeters (TLDs), film badges and personal digital monitors. TLDs and film badges can also be used to monitor doses received by carers, where a communal badge is worn and the details of the individual recorded. If any high readings are highlighted, an investigation is carried out. The dosimeter is either worn at lapel level, or worn inside the lead rubber apron. Some centers require two dosimeters to be worn, one located outside the apron and one underneath. In a study of the doses received by SLPs during VFSS procedures, Hayes et al. (2007) estimated that the mean radiation dose recorded on a dosimeter worn on the front of the lead apron at chest level was 0.15 mR (0.0015 mGy).

RADIATION DOSIMETRY

The radiology department will also be likely to use a dosimetry service to monitor doses received by patients. The dose to the patient may be measured via a Dose Area Product (DAP) meter (attached to the x-ray tube collimator port), having first taken the height and weight of the patient, or dose may be measured directly using thermoluminescent dosimeters attached to the patient. The DAP reading in grays per square centimeter (Gy/cm^2) can be converted mathematically to take into account the sensitivities of different tis-

sues to radiation, giving a measurement of what is known as effective dose, measured in millisieverts (mSv) (Chau & Kung, 2009).

DAP data and fluoroscopy screening times can be audited to ensure that doses are kept within national and regional limits, known as diagnostic reference levels (DRLs). Dose reference levels should be visible to operators to refer to so that they are aware of regional and national limits. These limits can be overridden, but routinely the operator should be working within these limits.

Hart, Hillier, and Wall (2009) recommended the national DRLs based on 2005 U.K. data for Barium Swallow should be 9 Gy/cm^2 DAP with a fluoroscopy time of 2.3 minutes. There currently are no national DRLs for VFSS in the U.K. or in the United States. However, VFSS DAPs would be expected to be lower, with fluoroscopy time possibly higher. With sound fluoroscopic technique, effective doses from VFSS can be as low as 0.2 mSv: the equivalent of approximately 10 chest x-rays, and considerably less than the dose from a lumbar spine x-ray (Zammit-Maemple et al., 2007). Published research has identified variable VFSS dose data as demonstrated in Table 8–2. However, caution should be applied when directly comparing figures from

Table 8–2. *Comparison of DAP and Fluoroscopy Times Across Several Studies*

Research Study	Patient Group	Mean Dose Area Product (Gy/cm²)	Mean Fluoroscopy Time (minutes)
Wright et al. (1998)	Adult	4	4.8
Crawley et al. (2004)	Adult	3.5	3.7
Zammit-Maempel et al. (2007)	Adult	1.4	3
Chau et al. (2009)	Adult	2.4	4.2
Weir et al. (2007)	Child	0.3	2.5

Source: Adapted from Chau et al., 2009.

different studies, because they are influenced not only by patient demographics (e.g., size), but by the skills of the operator and the equipment configuration. Under-couch x-ray tube configurations may give considerably higher doses than over-couch or C-arm units (Wright, Boyd, & Workman, 1998), with digital units potentially giving additional dose savings.

In the absence of national VFSS DRLs, local and regional DRLs may be available when doses from various institutions are measured and submitted to a dosimetry service. The analyzed DRL data are issued to the department and can be used to ensure best practice is adhered to. If the doses are outside the norm for the region, then a local investigation should take place. Medical physics experts together with the radiology team will consider the following:

- Are higher doses seen across all examinations, or related to certain sessions where a particular radiologist/radiographer is present?
- Is it a particular SLP session?
- Has the equipment been serviced regularly?
- Have medical physics checks been undertaken and any recommendations applied?

Medical physicists may also attend a session, as part of an investigation, to observe practices, and will submit a report with their observations and any recommendations. The report should be shared with the speech-language pathologists.

HEALTH AND SAFETY MEASURES

An initial risk assessment will have been carried out on a newly installed fluoroscopy room and any risks identified together with recommendations and safety measures to avoid incidents. A separate radiation risk assessment is carried out to identify particular risks associated with radiation.

For each session and for individual patients the potential health and safety risks should be assessed, including whether there are any moving and handling issues, the health of the patient and whether there is significant risk of aspiration. Any necessary strategies should be discussed and put in place. Table 8–3 outlines the roles and responsibilities of the radiographer managing the VFSS procedure from a health and safety viewpoint. Radiation protection of staff and dose reduction for patients is clearly a primary responsibility of the radiographer, but they are also required to ensure ancillary equipment is used safely and effectively. The imaging room essentials required for a swallowing clinic include a specialist or adapted chair, suction, and feeding accessories. These include cups; straws; food; barium sulfate preparation; food thickener; spoons; and mouth wipes.

VFSS Chair

Commercially available chairs suitable for VFSS are often used (Figure 8–5), enabling the examination to be performed with the patient in a seated position, the normal position for eating and drinking. In able-bodied patients the procedure can be undertaken standing, but it is important where possible that swallowing is assessed in a normal, natural position so that the patient feels comfortable and it demonstrates normal feeding/swallowing. The chair, ideally, should have armrests for support, footrests and wheels. The wheels allow easier positioning particularly with the less mobile patients or patients who are unable to keep still for long periods.

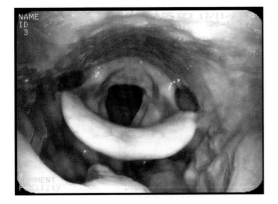

Figure 2–1. *Image showing the scope in the high position.*

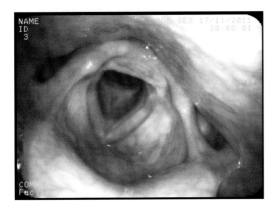

Figure 2–2. *Image showing the scope in the low position.*

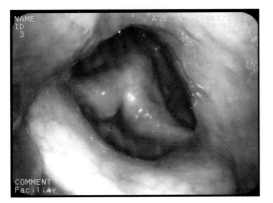

Figure 2–3. *Image showing a voluntary breath-hold used in the supraglottic swallowing maneuver.*

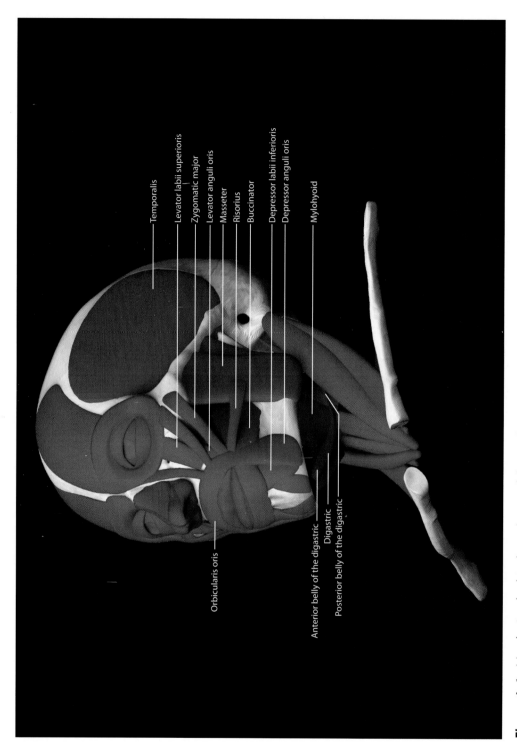

Temporalis

Levator labii superioris

Zygomatic major

Levator anguli oris

Masseter

Risorius

Buccinator

Depressor labii inferioris

Depressor anguli oris

Mylohyoid

Orbicularis oris

Anterior belly of the digastric

Digastric

Posterior belly of the digastric

Figure 4–1. Muscles involved in the oral stage of the swallow.

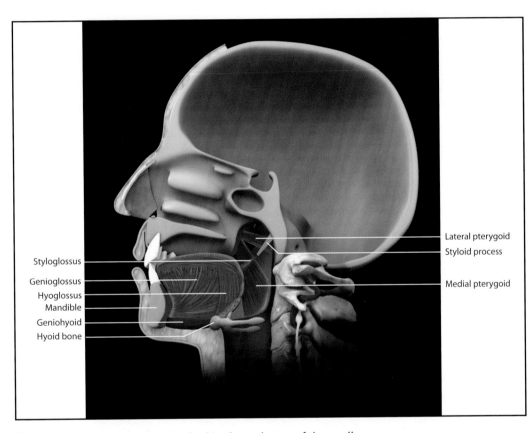

Figure 4–2. Further muscles involved in the oral stage of the swallow.

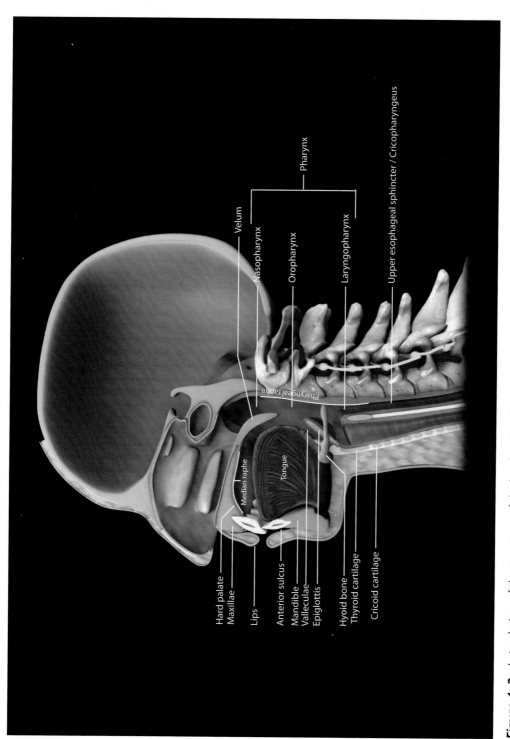

Figure 4–3. Lateral view of the structures of the head and neck.

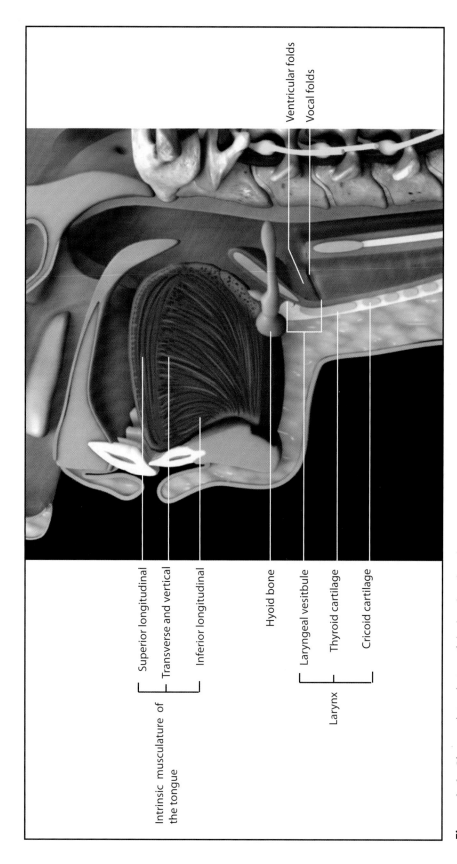

Figure 4-4. *Close-up lateral view of the head and neck.*

Intrinsic musculature of the tongue
- Superior longitudinal
- Transverse and vertical
- Inferior longitudinal

Hyoid bone

Larynx
- Laryngeal vesitbule
- Thyroid cartilage
- Cricoid cartilage

Ventricular folds

Vocal folds

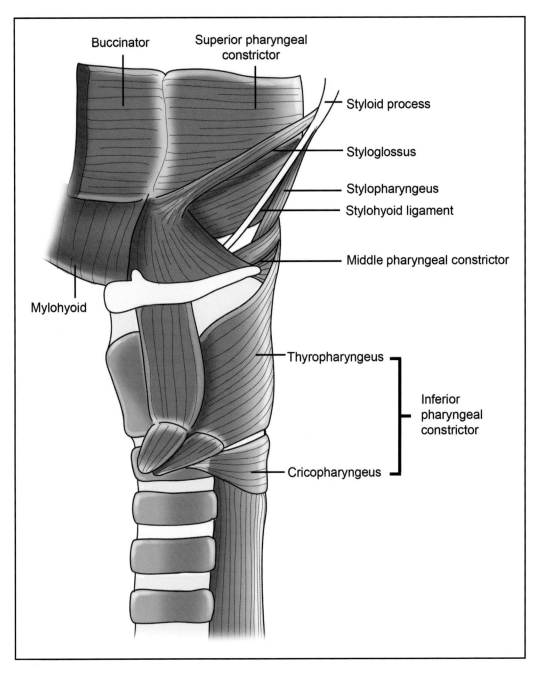

Figure 4–5. *Muscles involved in the pharyngeal stage of the swallow.*

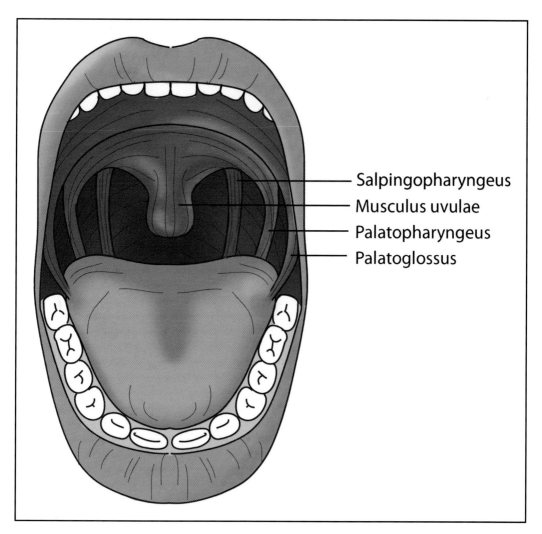

Figure 4–6. *Anterior-posterior view of the oral cavity showing further muscles involved in the pharyngeal stage of the swallow.*

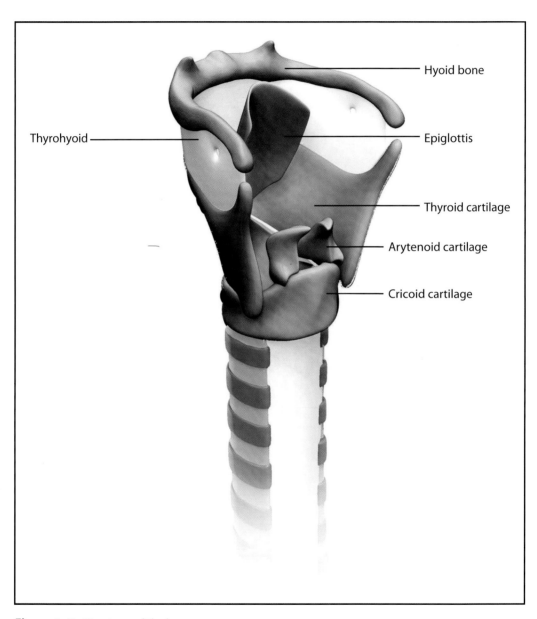

Figure 4–7. *Structures of the larynx.*

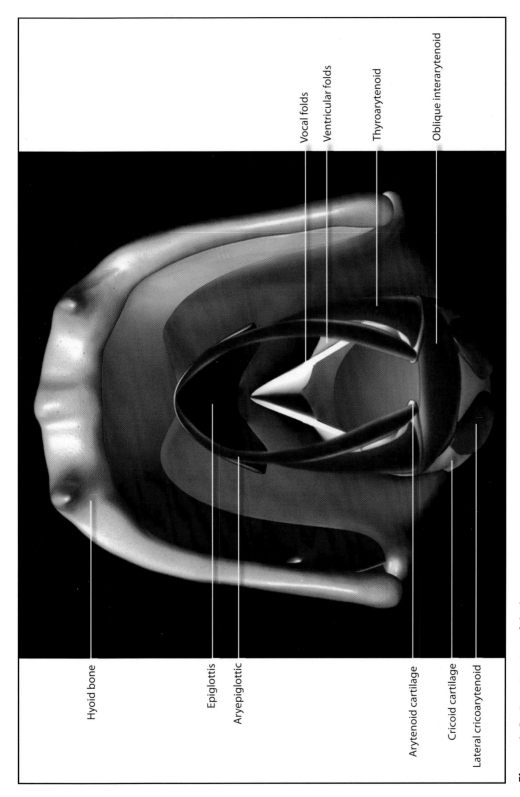

Hyoid bone

Epiglottis

Aryepiglottic

Arytenoid cartilage

Cricoid cartilage

Lateral cricoarytenoid

Vocal folds

Ventricular folds

Thyroarytenoid

Oblique interarytenoid

Figure 4–8. Superior view of the larynx.

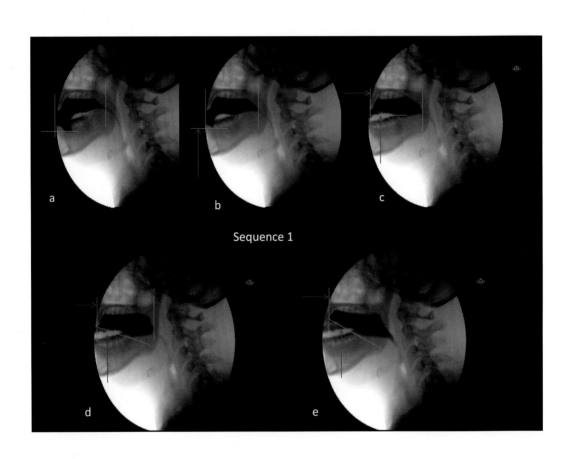

Sequence 1

Sequence 6–1. Frame a. *The large liquid bolus is held in the oral cavity with the linguavelar valve closed. The bolus tail is seen in the floor of mouth. This subject uses a "tipper" pattern of oral transit (Dodds et al., 1989). The blue vertical lines indicate the anterior and posterior margins of the bolus. The horizontal blue line indicates the position of the bolus tail which is held by the tongue tip.* Frame b. *The tongue tip has risen (red arrow) from its baseline position in Frame a, yet the position of the bolus head is the same as in Frame a. Bolus compression is beginning as the bolus is being compressed into a smaller volume while the linguavelar valve remains closed.* Frame c. *Continued posterior movement of the tongue tip displacing the bolus tail is seen. The tail is moved posteriorly while the linguavelar valve remains closed. The tongue base has lowered to accommodate the compressed bolus.* Frame d. *The anterior tongue is not tilted with the bolus tail further compressed. The tip of the bolus head is positioned more posteriorly as the linguavelar valve remains closed.* Frame e. *The linguavelar valve is released and the bolus head crosses the ramus of the mandible, the radiographic landmark denoting the entrance of the pharynx. Continued posterior movement of the anterior tongue propels the bolus. The potential energy created by bolus compression is converted to kinetic energy as intrabolus pressure is transferred to the pharynx.*

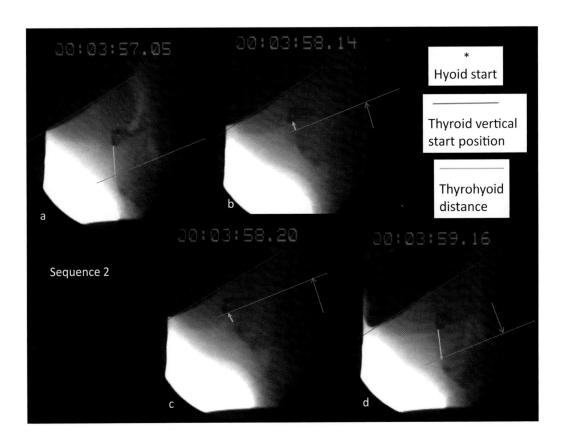

00:03:57.05   00:03:58.14

*
Hyoid start

_____
Thyroid vertical
start position

_____
Thyrohyoid
distance

a   b

00:03:58.20   00:03:59.16

Sequence 2

c   d

Sequence 6-2. *Hyolaryngeal excursion biomechanics during a dry swallow (no contrast). Dry swallows are useful in isolating biomechanics without the distraction of contrast. The red diagonal line indicates the inferior border of the mandible which is used as a landmark against which hyoid position is compared to assess vertical hyoid motion. The blue line indicates the plane of the superior margin of the thyroid cartilage. The green line indicates the distance between the anterior superior thyroid cartilage and the hyoid body. It changes to an arrow to indicate direction of motion. This timer indicates elapsed time in minutes, seconds and then in frames (after the decimal). NTSC video scans at 30 frames per second so each tic after the decimal point indicates one frame elapsed. One frame is the equivalent of 1/30 (0.033) of a second. So a timer value of 02:45.27 on a frame indicates that 2 minutes, 45 seconds plus 27 frames (27/30 = 0.9 seconds), or 2:45.90 seconds, have elapsed. This timer uses frames after the decimal because the video images of timer values of less than 1/30 of a second can be hard to decipher when the fields generating the frame (each frame is the product of two interlaced video fields) contain two different timer values (of less than 1/30 of a second). Frame a. Hyoid at rest at frame zero (timer = 03:57.05). The red dot will follow the hyoid body as it moves. The blue line indicates the superior margin of the thyroid cartilage. The distance between the thyroid cartilage and hyoid is marked by the green line at rest. All structures are at rest. Frame b. Thirty-nine frames after frame a, at timer value 3:58.14 (1 second plus 9 frames = 39 frames = 1.3 seconds). The hyoid has risen from its resting position (distance between red dot and plane of mandible) because of contraction of suprahyoid muscles. The thyrohyoid has not only risen along with the hyoid due to its connection to the hyoid (elevation of the blue line), the distance between the thyroid and the hyoid has shortened due to contraction of the thryrohyoid muscle (shortening of the green line). Frame c. Six frames (0.2 seconds) later at timer value 3:58.20. Further approximation of hyoid to mandible, and of thyroid to hyoid, are seen. Both hyoid and thyroid are also now displaced both toward the plane of the mandible and anteriorly as well. Frame d. Twenty-six frames (0.86 seconds) later at timer value 3:59.16. Hyoid and thyroid cartilage are descending toward their resting positions as the pharyngeal stage comes to an end and suprahyoid muscles resume their resting activity. Distance between the hyoid and thyroid increases as thyrohyoid muscle contraction ceases. Elapsed time from Frames a to d: 2.33 seconds.*

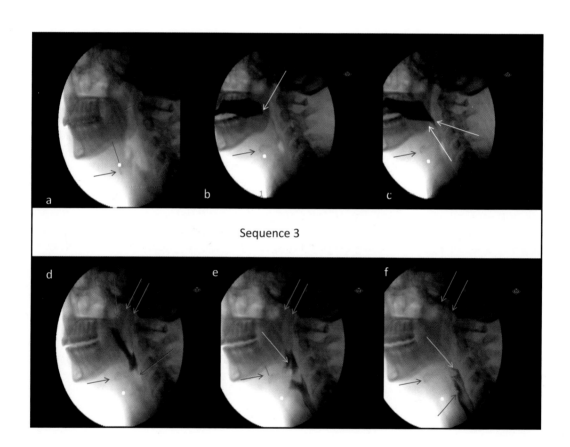

Sequence 3

Sequence 6–3. *One swallow biomechanics. Throughout this sequence the white dot is placed at the starting position of the body of the hyoid bone. The lower red arrow points to the body of the hyoid bone and the vertical line drawn to its right indicates the vertical distance between the hyoid and mandible at rest. The upper red arrow indicates the width of the open nasopharyngeal port and the horizontal line below it shows the anterior-posterior dimension available for nasal breathing at rest. Note that this area disappears in Frame 2. Frame a. We see the subject at rest without a bolus in the mouth. The two mandibular rami are not aligned in this frame though they are perfectly aligned in Frames b and c. Frame b. A bolus is seen in the oral cavity with slightly elevated hyoid due to oral activity. The subject has just initiated oral transit. The air space in the oropharynx has disappeared. The bolus head is shown by the yellow arrow. The nasopharyngeal port has been occluded by some anterior movement of the posterior pharyngeal wall. Already, we can see some upward movement of the hyoid has occurred. Frame c. The bolus head (yellow arrow) is seen crossing the plane formed by the ramus of the mandible (white arrow), the anatomical landmark that indicates the entrance to the pharynx. The hyoid remains in the same position as in Frame b. In Frame c and then more so in Frame d, the soft palate (or velum) has ascended to its typical position forming the valve separating the nasal from oral cavities. Frame d. Further hyoid elevation and now some anterior or forward movement. Here we can also see the onset of UES opening as the air space in the pyriform sinus elongates inferiorly. This increase in UES volume increases the pressure gradient ahead of the bolus increasing its speed toward the esophagus. Frame e. A small red line has been drawn to demonstrate the vertical distance that the hyoid has been displaced. Compare this line to the same marker in Frame 1. The green arrow in Frame e is pointing to the free end of the epiglottis. Frame f. The green arrow is pointing to the now inverted epiglottis. Here the hyoid's further movement is seen and the bolus tail is now seen well into the UES. The soft palate has returned to near its resting position. In Frames d through f, we can see that the subject is rotating her head while swallowing as indicated by the presence of two mandibular shadows that seem to be increasing in distance from one another by Frame 6. Note the overall distance traveled by the hyoid from its resting position which is indicated by the white dot in all frames.*

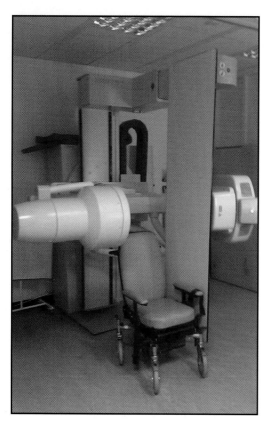

Figure 8–2. *A modern fluoroscopy unit (Toshiba Ultimax from Toshiba Medical Systems), with the image intensifier seen closest to the camera, and the x-ray tube behind the fluoroscopy table. A specialist videofluoroscopy chair is positioned ready to receive the patient ("The Mangar Porter" chair from Mangar Aids Ltd).*

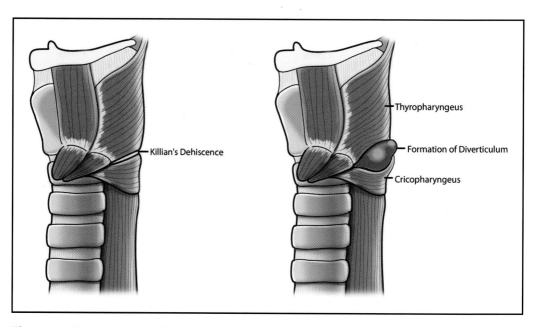

Figure 15–4. *Lateral view of the thyropharyngeus and cricopharyngeus muscles, with the triangular space between the two known as Killian's dehiscence. A Zenker's diverticulum can be seen forming via compression of the posterior pharyngeal wall through the dehiscence, creating the outpouching seen with such diverticula.*

Table 8–3. *Radiographer Role Within VFSS*

Phase of Procedure	Activity	Explanation
Preparation	Fluoroscopy equipment	The equipment is placed in appropriate position (e.g., table erect) and seating secured. Check equipment is clean and tidy. Patient identification entered into computer, recording devices switched on and ready to record.
	Ancillary equipment and contrast materials	Ensure adequate materials and ease of access.
	Justification	The radiographer will ensure there is a correctly completed requisition (a request for an x-ray exposure) by either a medical practitioner or speech pathologist
	VFSS aims	The radiographer should liaise with the speech pathologist to understand the patient history, VFSS aims and the strategies to be trialed during the test
Introduction to Patient	Identification and pregnancy status	The radiographer will make sure the patient identification policy has been followed, and will check pregnancy status where relevant.
	Consent	The radiographer should seek consent following department policy (usually verbal informed consent). Where appropriate carers will be present during the explanation of the procedure.
	Role of carer	The role the carer may play should be explained, including where to stand, and whether to assist in feeding.
Prior to exposure	Patient positioning	The radiographer or speech pathologist will seat the patient, ensuring they are safe and comfortable, so that the patient feels secure and is able to follow and comply with instructions.
	Staff protection	The radiographer will ensure that everyone is wearing the required protective wear and radiation monitoring badges where relevant. Check they are in the safest position in the room, ideally behind the x-ray tube and more than 6 feet away from the x-ray source.
	Monitor positioning	The monitor should be situated so that the speech pathologist, radiologist, and radiographer can readily view the imaging without twisting.
	Selection of materials and positioning	The speech pathologist will normally determine the sequence of food textures and trials of position and techniques to improve swallowing or prevent aspiration.

continues

Table 8–3. continued

Phase of Procedure	Activity	Explanation
During procedure	Initial imaging (control positioning)	The radiographer or radiologist will image the patient (usually lateral position) to determine if the patient is in the correct position and will collimate the beam to reduce the dose to the patient and staff. The area of interest is the lips anteriorly, the upper esophagus inferiorly, the soft palate superiorly, and the cervical spine posteriorly.
	Further collimation	Once the oral phase has been assessed the radiographer can collimate further to only show the pharynx.
	Repositioning	The patient often remains in the lateral position but anterior-posterior imaging is possible either by moving the patient through 90 degrees if mobile, moving the chair or the x-ray tube (C-arm units).
	Coordination of imaging	Good communication between SLP and radiographer/radiologist is vital so that the radiation dose is reduced. The SLP can indicate when he/she is ready for imaging to commence, or the radiographer can commence screening once the patient has taken a mouthful of food.
	Fluoroscopy use during procedure	Fluoroscopy should only continue for the minimum time required to make a decision for treatment or a diagnosis. It is, however, important not to stop too soon and miss second or third clearing swallows; therefore, the procedure needs to be undertaken by experienced practitioners who understand swallowing. If imaging is prematurely stopped to reduce dose, this may be false economy if the swallow needs to be repeated.
	Swallows without imaging	If fatigue is thought to contribute to the patients swallowing difficulties, the patient can swallow further boluses without imaging (to reduce dose), then image a further swallow.
	Termination of procedure	Good communication is required between the speech pathologist and radiographer so that the imaging can be terminated when sufficient information has been acquired. Similarly, a decision to stop prematurely due to significant aspiration or deteriorating patient condition should be made promptly. The radiographer should initiate appropriate referral if required (e.g., to physiotherapist). The radiographer should ensure that images have been appropriately captured, labeled, and stored.

Table 8–3. *continued*

Phase of Procedure	Activity	Explanation
Aftercare	Patient comfort	The patient should be offered a drink of water or a mouthwash if required and mouth wipes should be made available for the patient before they leave the room. They should be warned that stools may be white for a few days.
	Results	The patient should be informed where and when they are likely to receive their results.
	Room preparation	The radiographer should prepare the room for the next patient and should clean surfaces and utensils.

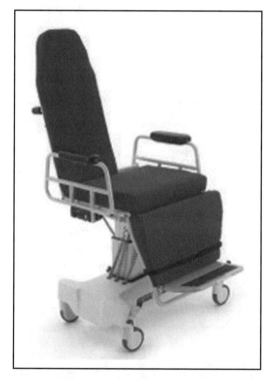

Figure 8–5. *An example of an adapted chair suitable for videofluoroscopy. Photo courtesy of TransMotion Medical Inc., USA.*

Some commercially available chairs have radiolucent backrests, which allow the passage of the x-ray beam without degrading the image, giving an additional benefit of being able to perform an anteroposterior view without moving the patient, but by moving the chair or the fluoroscopy equipment.

It is possible to use an ordinary chair but this will limit the session to the more able-bodied patients, and could exclude some patients with neurological deficits.

Suction Apparatus

As many patients referred for videofluoroscopy are being assessed for aspiration, suction should always be available, and staff should be trained and deemed competent to use it. In some clinics a physiotherapist or nurse is always present, in others they may attend on request when at risk patients are scheduled.

Feeding Accessories

Feeding accessories such as cups, spoons, straws and other accessories for feeding should be readily available. In certain circumstances (for example learning disability), patients and carers will be encouraged to bring their own feeding utensils and favorite foods with them. Cleanliness of feeding utensils is essential, with many centers using disposable products.

SUMMARY

The VFSS examination, undertaken by a skilled operator using modern well-functioning fluoroscopy equipment, is a relatively low dose procedure. Nevertheless, there are inherent risks associated with this procedure, with the potential risks of radiation being of primary concern. Although there is little evidence of the risk of cancer related to low doses of radiation, the principle of radiation protection is based on an assumption that there is a potential risk even from a single radiation track within a low dose procedure.

It is the radiographer's responsibility to ensure that the VFSS procedure is properly justified, and that protocols are followed to ensure that inadvertent exposure does not occur (e.g., incorrect patient, or irradiation of a fetus). It is incumbent on the operator (radiographer or radiologist) to employ practices to ensure that the dose delivered to the patient is as low as reasonably practicable (ALARP), by applying the principles of dose optimization and dose limitation. Careful application of dose minimizing procedures will reduce the dose to the patient, but will also potentially reduce staff doses. The radiographer has ultimate responsibility for ensuring the safety of staff, students, and carers who may be required to be present within the fluoroscopy room during exposures. The judicious application of fluoroscopy, recognizing the important principles of distance and location, application of protective equipment, and personnel monitoring, will all keep staff doses to negligible levels.

The speech-language pathologist working within the fluoroscopy environment is obliged to familiarize themselves with local radiation protection rules and practices, and observe these on all occasions. Prior to the commencement of fluoroscopy screening, the SLP should carefully assess the patient's needs and formulate appropriate aims for the VFSS procedure. Effective communication of these aims to the radiographer or radiologist is likely to yield a more efficient procedure, with a reduction in fluoroscopy screening time, and ultimately a lower radiation dose to the patient and the attending staff.

REFERENCES

American Speech-Language-Hearing Association. (2004). Guidelines for speech-language pathologists performing videofluoroscopic swallowing studies. *ASHA Supplement, 24,* 77–92.

Ball, A. D., & Moore, J. (1997). *Essential physics for radiographers* (3rd Ed.). Oxford, UK: Blackwell Science.

Chau, K. H. T., & Kung, C. M. A. (2009). Patient dose during videofluoroscopy swallowing studies in a Hong Kong public hospital. *Dysphagia, 24,* 387–390.

Crawley, M. T., Savage, P., & Oakley, F. (2004). Patient and operator dose during fluoroscopic examination of swallow mechanism. *British Journal of Radiology, 77,* 654–656.

Department of Health. (2000). *Ionising Radiation (Medical Exposure) Regulations. Statutory Instrument 2000 No. 1059.* The Stationary Office, London. Retrieved January 12, 2012, from http://www.hse.gov.uk/radiation/ionising/

European Commission. (1998). *Guidance for protection of unborn children and infants irradiated due to parental medical exposures.* Radiation Protection 100.

Farr, R. F., & Allisy-Roberts, P. J. (1998). *Physics for medical imaging.* London, UK: Saunders.

Harbron, R. W. (2012). Cancer risks from low dose exposure to ionizing radiation—Is the liner no-threshold model still relevant? *Radiography, 18,* 28–33.

Hart, D., Hillier, M. C., & Wall, B. F. (2009). National reference doses for common radiographic, fluoroscopic and dental x-ray examinations in the UK. *British Journal of Radiology*, *82*, 1–12.

Hayes, A., Alspaugh, J. M., Bartelt, D., Campion, M. B., Eng, J., Gayler, B. W., . . . Haynos, J. (2009). Radiation safety for the speech-language pathologist. *Dysphagia*, *24*, 274–279.

ICRP International Commission on Radiation Protection. (2000). *Pregnancy and medical radiation*. ICRP 84.

Ionising Radiation Regulations. (1999). The Stationary Office, London, UK.

Krovak, B., & Nightingale, J. (2005) Radiation protection of female patients of reproductive capacity: A survey of policy and practice in Norway. *Radiography*, *13*, 35–43.

MedicineNet.com. (2011). *Definition of fluoroscopy*. Retrieved February 22, 2012, from http://www.medterms.com/script/main/art.asp?articlekey=3488

Price, R. (2005, June). Critical factors influencing the changing scope of practice: The defining periods. *Imaging and Oncology*, pp. 6–11.

USEPA United States Environmental Protection Agency. (2007). Radiation: Risks and realities. Retrieved February 20, 2012, from http://epa.gov/radiation/docs/402-k-07-006.pdf

Weir, K. A., McMahon, S. M., Long, G., Bunch, J. A., Pandeya, N., Coakley, K. S., & Chang, A. B. (2007). Radiation doses to children during modified barium swallow studies. *Pediatric Radiology*, *37*, 283–290.

Wright, R. E. R., Boyd, C. S., & Workman, A. (1998). Radiation doses to patients during pharyngeal videofluoroscopy. *Dysphagia*, *13*, 113–116.

Zammit-Maempel, I., Chapple, C. L., & Leslie, P. (2007). Radiation dose in fluoroscopic swallow studies, *Dysphagia*, *22*, 13–15.

Part

II

CLINICAL INDICATIONS

Chapter

9

STROKE

Stephanie K. Daniels and Joseph Murray

INTRODUCTION

Dysphagia is a major source of disability following stroke affecting quality of life, nutrition, hydration, pulmonary status, and increasing healthcare costs. Half of patients presenting with stroke and dysphagia are more likely to be malnourished than stroke patients with intact swallowing (Davalos et al., 1996) and are three times more likely to develop pneumonia regardless of severity of swallowing impairment or presence of aspiration (Martino et al., 2005). Length of hospitalization is increased for stroke patients with dysphagia, and these patients are more likely to be discharged to nursing homes in contrast to patients without dysphagia (Odderson, Keaton, & McKenna, 1995). The videofluoroscopic swallowing study (VFSS) is a critical component in the precise identification of abnormal bolus flow (pooling, residue, airway invasion) as well as the underlying physiologic impairment resulting in abnormal bolus flow. A detailed evaluation protocol and thorough interpretation of the VFSS are required to effectively recommend and implement nutritional intake and management of swallowing dysfunction.

INCIDENCE

Stroke is a major medical problem affecting 2000 people per million worldwide each year (Thorvaldsen, Asplund, Kuulasmaa, Rajakangas, & Schroll, 1995), occurring in approximately 700,000 individuals annually in the United States (Broderick et al., 1998) and 100,000 individuals annually in the United Kingdom (Wolfe, 2000). In both countries, it is the third leading cause of death (Broderick et al., 1998). The specific incidence of dysphagia in stroke is unclear due, in part, to variable patient selection methods (i.e., referrals to speech pathology versus consecutive stroke patients), evaluation methods (i.e., questionnaire, clinical swallowing evaluation [CSE], instrumental assessment), and how one defines dysphagia. That is, is identification of dysphagia determined by occurrence of aspiration or specific swallowing impairment which may or may not result in aspiration? For instance, patients may have clinically significant dysphagia (e.g., severe pharyngeal residue) but no airway invasion. Moreover, recent research indicates that healthy adults, particularly those with advancing age, may demonstrate incidental aspiration (Butler, Stuart, Markley,

& Rees, 2009; McCullough, Rosenbek, Wertz, Suiter, & McCoy, 2007; see Chapter 7, The Normal Aging Swallow). This suggests that the determination of dysphagia should be based on specific swallowing impairment, yet we must understand normal deglutitive variations to prevent over-identification. Is dysphagia based on the result of a single swallow? Again, research suggests that determining dysphagia based on a single swallow does not distinguish between healthy adults and individuals following stroke with and without dysphagia (Daniels et al., 2006; Daniels et al., 2009). Abnormality across multiple swallows appears to be a more robust method in defining dysphagia. An exception to this rule would be an individual whose swallowing on a single trial is deemed so severely disabling that the patient's safety would be compromised should the evaluation be continued.

Knowing the limitations in defining dysphagia, it appears that when dysphagia is identified via VFSS, it occurs in approximately 65% of acute stroke patients (Daniels et al., 1998; Mann, Hankey, & Cameron, 1999) with the incidence of aspiration occurring in about half (Daniels, McAdam, Brailey, & Foundas, 1997; Mann et al., 1999). Of acute stroke patients who aspirate, 40 to 70% do so silently (Daniels et al., 1998; Splaingard, Hutchins, Sulton, & Chaudhuri, 1988). That is, there is no overt sign of aspiration such as cough or voice change when material contacts the true vocal folds or enters the trachea.

PATHOPHYSIOLOGY

The central pattern generator for swallowing is located in the medulla, and damage to this region can result in profound dysphagia. A lateral medullary (Wallenberg) stroke is associated with a fairly circumscribed swallowing pattern in the acute phase of stroke.

Frequently, the initial presenting swallowing impairment following this type of stroke is an absent pharyngeal swallow in which the patient cannot even swallow their own saliva resulting in continual expectoration. As the patient recovers, common dysphagia features are weak pharyngeal swallow, reduced hyolaryngeal excursion, unilateral pharyngeal hemiparesis, and reduced pressure to drive the bolus through the pharynx into the upper esophageal sphincter. The oral stage of swallowing is generally intact following this type of stroke.

Acute and chronic dysphagia, however, can occur following a single unilateral cortical or subcortical stroke to either hemisphere. Similar regions important in swallowing have been identified with functional imaging studies in healthy adults and lesion studies in stroke patients. These regions include the primary motor, supplementary motor, and primary somatosensory cortices, insula, anterior cingulate, basal ganglia, as well as white matter pathways that connect these regions (Daniels & Huckabee, 2008; Figure 9–1). It was previously suggested that swallowing impairments were dependent upon which hemisphere sustained the infarct (Robbins & Levine, 1988; Robbins, Levine, Maser, Rosenbek, & Kempster, 1993). Individuals with right hemispheric stroke were identified with pharyngeal stage dysfunction and a greater occurrence of aspiration than individuals with left hemispheric stroke who demonstrate oral stage dysfunction and infrequent aspiration. More current research, however, contradicts this notion as oral and pharyngeal stage dysfunction and occurrences of airway invasion have been identified equally in individuals with right or left hemispheric stroke (Daniels, Brailey, & Foundas, 1999; Daniels & Foundas, 1999; Theurer, et al., 2008). Differences in functional swallowing, perhaps, may appear worse in individuals with right hemispheric damage due to cognitive deficits and lack of

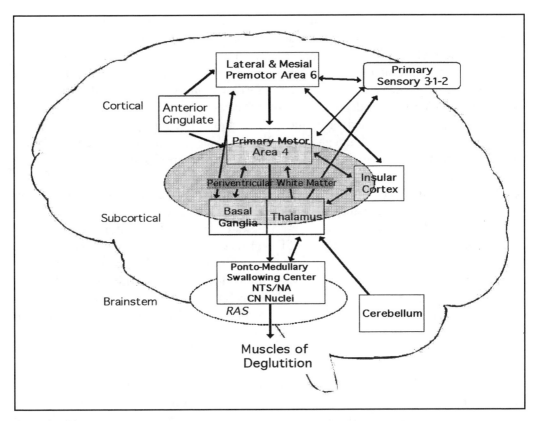

Figure 9–1. *Proposed model of the neural networks of swallowing. CN = cranial nerve nuclei, NA = nucleus ambiguus, NTS = nucleus tractus solitarius, RAS = reticular activating system. Source: From Dysphagia Following Stroke by S. K. Daniels and M. L. Huckabee, 2008, p. 20. Copyright © 2008 by Plural Publishing. Used with permission.*

awareness of swallowing problems. Supramedullary stroke is not characterized by a particular swallowing pattern; almost any type of specific swallowing impairment involving the oral and/or pharyngeal stages of swallowing may be evident.

CLINICAL PRESENTATION

Clinically, individuals with stroke may have their swallowing screened at the bedside as a frontline measure to identify the risk of dysphagia and aspiration and, where appropriate, to expedite referral for more in-depth swallowing assessment. For individuals with stroke, given the fact that swallowing should be screened prior to provision of oral intake, including medication (Adams et al., 2007), it is likely that nursing staff and/or physicians will complete the screening, thus screening tools must be valid and reliable as well as feasible to administer.

If risk of dysphagia is identified by the screening, the individual is generally referred to a speech-language pathologist (SLP) for completion of a CSE. The CSE allows the SLP to determine if an instrumental evaluation of swallowing is warranted, develop a hypothesis of the specific swallowing impairment, and develop strategies concerning management. The CSE is generally composed of patient history and interview, basic gross motor observation, observation of cognition and communication (and in-depth examination at a later point if warranted), assessment of oral structure integrity, a thorough cranial nerve assessment, and evaluation of actual swallowing. Completion and interpretation of these components will ensure that the CSE is not relegated to screening status (Rosenbek, McCullough, & Wertz, 2004).

When completing a screening or CSE on individuals with stroke, it is important to remember that they may not present with obvious clinical signs of dysphagia. Prandial features of dysphagia may include drooling, reduced mastication, throat clearing, coughing and choking, nasal regurgitation, and complaints of residue in the oral cavity and pharynx. Coughing, choking, and voice change after swallow will not be present in individuals who aspirate silently. Moreover, reduced sensation or cognition, which can result from stroke, may impair an individual's awareness of the symptoms. Individuals may continue to ingest liquid even when coughing or choking (Parker et al., 2004), which indicates anosognosia (unawareness of deficits) or anosodiaphoria (unconcern or indifferent to deficits). Therefore, clinicians must not equate the absence of complaints of dysphagia with intact swallowing. Although it is important to ask individuals with stroke about their swallowing problem, the astute SLP will also look for clinical signs that may not be directly related to swallowing. Various clinicians have developed clusters of features evident on the CSE that are associated with dysphagia or aspiration (for example, Daniels et al., 1997, 1998; Logemann, Veis, & Colangelo, 1999; McCullough, Wertz, & Rosenbek, 2001; McCullough et al., 2005), but these must be viewed in the context of

the entire CSE and presentation of the individual patient. For example, dysphonia, dysarthria, weak volitional cough, abnormal gag reflex, cough or throat clear after trial water swallows, and voice change after trial water swallows were each identified to be predictive of risk of aspiration (penetration with laryngeal residue) in acute stroke patients (Daniels et al., 1998). Specificity for each item, however, was reduced indicating that each feature had the potential to over-identify risk of aspiration when used independently. Continued research revealed that identification of any two of these six clinical features identified above provided the best yield of correctly identifying individuals with and without risk of aspiration (Daniels et al., 1997), whereas another study found that identification of any four of the six features provided the best validity (McCullough et al., 2001). Further research in this area has revealed other features such as response to a 3-oz water swallow test (i.e., cough, wet voice), dysphonia, and jaw weakness to be the best predictors of aspiration in stroke patients (McCullough et al., 2005).

Even the most perceptive clinician completing the most in-depth CSE can only infer so much from this assessment. Hyolaryngeal elevation may be determined by manual palpation, but the timing of hyolaryngeal movement in relationship to the location of the bolus is unknown. Thus, on the CSE whereas pooling of material in the pharynx may be suspected, it is unclear if the bolus is in the valleculae or pyriform sinus. Likewise, residue can be posited but location and underlying cause cannot be discerned on the CSE. A cough may or may not indicate that aspiration has occurred, and cessation of a cough may not indicate that aspiration has resolved; therefore, implementation of compensatory strategies, such as thickened liquid, would appear unwise until evaluated with VFSS.

Findings from the CSE can facilitate conduction of the VFSS as well as recommendations. The VFSS is ideally completed in a precise environment in which the patient is seated at 90 degrees, distraction is minimal, and the evaluation time is unlimited. Obviously, this is not the real world, especially on a hospital ward. Thus, data from the CSE on posture in the bed or chair, attention, neglect, memory, fatigue, and so forth will inform the SLP on possible influences on swallowing and the potential for successful implementation of compensatory strategies.

ROLE OF VFSS IN THE MANAGEMENT OF THIS PATIENT GROUP

The VFSS is critical in determining dysphagia in individuals with stroke as it allows identification of the specific swallowing impairment that can be targeted by the clinician for rehabilitation or compensation. As stroke frequently affects both the oral and pharyngeal stages of swallowing, VFSS is the optimal instrumental tool to assess swallowing in this patient population as it allows the examiner to view the actual swallowing biomechanics of both stages in a single viewing. If esophageal dysfunction or structural issues are believed to contribute the complex of presenting problems, the esophageal stage can be examined fluoroscopically during the examination. The VFSS is generally completed with a SLP and radiologist/radiographer present. In the United Kingdom (and various other countries) a radiographer is a highly specialized clinician trained in radiographic imaging and subsequent interpretation and reporting of the findings. The radiology staff, like the SLP, has an interest in performing a complete evaluation of the structure and function that identifies specific swallowing impairment(s) while attempting all compensatory strategies that may enhance swallowing safety or efficiency.

It is important for SLPs to develop a standard protocol that can be initially implemented in all individuals with stroke but then individualized after the first or second swallow depending on the patient findings. The idea is to develop a protocol that can effectively detail swallowing and allow time for implementation of compensatory strategies yet be efficient to limit the amount of radiation exposure (Lemen, 2004; Zammit-Maempel, Chappel, & Leslie, 2007). Every consistency that can be swallowed cannot be tested in VFSS. The astute clinician must evaluate a limited number of consistencies, generally three (thin liquid, semi-solid, solid), and then infer function across consistencies. Additional consistencies that are required for testing specific swallowing complaints (e.g., rice) or for use as a compensatory strategy of course should be introduced on an individualized basis.

The VFSS should be initiated with the patient in the lateral view. An anterior-posterior view can be obtained to distinguish between unilateral and bilateral pyriform sinus residue or to evaluate proximal esophageal dysfunction. Whenever possible, the patient should self-administer the trials as this is the most natural and will provide the best representation of typical feeding behaviors. Ideally two trials of each volume and consistency should be presented (Lazarus et al., 1993) to allow for the observation of variability in the manipulation and advancement of the bolus and variation in the timing of onset of the pharyngeal swallow.

As aspiration is frequently suspected in patients with stroke who are referred for VFSS, starting the examination with a small calibrated bolus of thin liquid facilitates safety. Five milliliters (ml), is a good initial volume that generally can be administered to most, if not all, patients. It is small enough, approximately one teaspoon, to prevent complications if aspirated but large enough for a person to comfortably swallow from a cup or other method of delivery. Limiting the amount to be presented is good practice at the start of the VFSS as individuals with frontal lobe or right hemisphere lesions may exhibit disinhibition, poor judgment, and impaired impulse control. If provided with a larger amount, they may not appropriately regulate the volume with subsequent harmful effect prompting the termination of the procedure before the salient components are tested. Verbally cuing a patient to swallow has been shown to affect the timing of oral and pharyngeal transfer in healthy older adults and individuals with mild dementia (Daniels, Corey, Schulz, Foundas, & Rosenbek, 2007; Daniels, Schroeder, DeGeorge, Corey, & Rosenbek, 2007) and should be omitted if possible. Even if aspiration is evident with the first 5ml swallow, unless there are significant concerns for the patient's safety, a second liquid trial should be administered. Some individuals, particularly those who have not had any recent oral intake, may need this initial swallow to prime the swallowing system. If significant aspiration or post-swallow residue is not identified with both 5ml trials, continue with a self-regulated cup sip followed by 5ml of a puree/semi-solid texture. Finally, present the solid texture consisting of half a cookie or cracker topped with barium, or foods with barium impregnated in the product to replicate familiar "real-world" food materials. Depending on the result of the liquid trials and if significant aspiration is not evident, the patient should sequentially swallow a large volume (e.g., 100ml) of thin liquid barium as the biomechanics of sequential swallowing has been proven to be different than discrete swallows (Chi-Fishman & Sonies, 2000; Daniels & Foundas, 2001; Daniels et al., 2004; Murguia, Corey, & Daniels, 2009). If the patient demonstrates consistent airway invasion or post-swallow residue, then evaluate the effects of compensatory strategies.

Although it has been suggested that viscosity and volume should be presented in an order that is individualized for each assessment based on suspected dysfunction (Kuhlemeier, Palmer, & Rosenberg, 2001), the authors rarely consider starting with a thick consistency. Even though a person may not aspirate the thicker consistency, if retained, the thicker consistencies can fill the spaces in the pharynx and potentially alter the bolus flow of subsequent liquids. For example, if a clinician initially administers barium pudding, or even nectar or honey consistency barium, and severe vallecular residue is evident, a subsequent swallow of thin liquid may be aspirated more readily as it could not "pool," or rest in the valleculae until the pharyngeal swallow was evoked. Further, the retained thick liquid may obscure the structures and the head and/or tail of any new bolus that is presented making a fair assessment of subsequent liquid presentations difficult or impossible.

When viewing the VFSS, it is important that clinicians: (1) identify any anatomic abnormalities, (2) judge bolus flow in terms of pharyngeal pooling (material entering the pharynx before onset of the pharyngeal swallow), airway invasion, and residue, and (3) determine the underlying swallowing impairment that is resulting in the abnormal bolus flow. When assessing bolus flow, it is important to understand normal swallowing and to attempt to be as objective as possible. From research of healthy young and older adults, it is known that the bolus head may proceed past the angle of the mandible prior to onset of the pharyngeal swallow (Martin-Harris, Brodsky, Michel, Lee, & Walters, 2007; Stephen, Taves, Smith, & Martin, 2005). In fact, during sequential swallowing, individuals may initiate the swallow with the bolus head in the pyriform sinuses (Daniels et al., 2004). These findings suggest that normal variations in swallow timing onset, which do not impact safety (airway invasion) or efficiency (post-swallow residue), may not represent a clinically significant impairment and should be viewed in terms of the individual's overall deglutitive function.

The penetration-aspiration scale (Rosenbek, Robbins, Roecker, Coyle, & Wood, 1996) is an objective way to score airway invasion by delineating the depth of bolus travel, clearance of material that is penetrated or aspirated into the airway, and response to the airway invasion as factors in scoring. These components add critical vital information to the clinician and is far more useful that the binary "present or absent" that is frequently used to score airway invasion. Likewise, using a semi-objective means to quantify the amount of residue (Eisenhuber et al., 2002; Hind, Nicosia, Roecker, Carnes, & Robbins, 2001; Perlman, Booth, & Grayhack, 1994) can provide more information and be used to document improvement or decline in a more precise way than employing binary scoring methods. As discussed earlier, however, one must identify dysphagia based on more than a single swallow (Daniels et al., 2009).

Interpretation of the VFSS is not limited to evaluation of bolus flow. It is imperative that the SLP identify the specific swallowing impairment(s). It is the specific swallowing impairment that is at the heart of the oropharyngeal dysphagia and what clinicians treat with rehabilitative approaches. The knowledgeable clinician can use findings of pooling, residue, and airway invasion to help determine the specific swallowing impairment. Table 9–1 provides a sample of a score sheet used to identify underlying swallowing impairment. While this scoring system helps the SLP evaluate various aspects of swallowing, it only uses a binary scoring method, and as noted earlier, identifying levels of severity is preferred. The MBSImp uses a semi-quantitative method to evaluate severity of impairment (Martin-Harris, et al., 2008); however, use of this tool requires formal training before implementation.

Another important element of the VFSS is the evaluation of the effects of any compensatory strategy that may be considered for use during oral intake. Compensatory strategies should not be applied randomly but should be based on the specific symptoms observed during the VFSS, for example, pyriform sinus residue yielding aspiration (Table 9–2). During the examination the clinician may believe that the physiologic basis of an observed symptom (e.g., an event of aspiration) can be ameliorated with a direct intervention (e.g., chin tuck). If this occurs, the intervention should be attempted on the next swallow using the same volume, consistency, and manner of bolus delivery to determine if the compensation is effective. If it does prove effective, that intervention should be employed for successively larger boluses or more challenging bolus types. Moreover, one should incorporate findings from the CSE, such as poor attention, when choosing a compensation for a specific patient. Research has identified both chin tuck and thickened liquids to reduce liquid aspiration in individuals with aspiration before the swallow (Logemann et al., 2008; Shanahan, Logemann, Rademaker, Pauloski, & Kahrilas, 1993) due either to a delayed pharyngeal swallow or reduced oral control. Evaluating both in VFSS is ideal, but the final recommendation to use one or the other may be based, in part, on the cognitive status of the patient. Use of a chin tuck, even if it reduces aspiration, is not feasible in a client with poor memory, unless family or staff can be present for all meals to assist in cuing the patient to use the intervention. Certain compensatory strategies such as sour bolus have been identified as facilitating swallowing (Logemann et al., 1995; Pelletier & Lawless, 2003); however, the patient may not find this type of bolus palatable and will likely reject it if offered. Some interventions, while demonstrably effective, may not be practical for implementation during meals. Given this, the clinician should carefully consider the practical applicability of the intervention before attempting these in the fluoroscopy suite.

Table 9–1. *An Example of a Videofluoroscopic Swallowing Study Score Sheet*

VIDEOFLUOROSCOPIC SWALLOWING STUDY					

Name: _____ ID#: _____

Study Conditions:

View: _____ Lateral _____ A-P   **Delivery Method:** _____ Cup _____ Straw _____ Syringe

Code: L1 = liquid trial 1; L2 = liquid trial 2; P1 = pudding trial 1; P2 = pudding trial 2;
S1 = solid trial 1; cont = continuous drinking 100ml

Circle appropriate consistency/sequence	5ml	cup sip	pudding	solid	cont
Oral Stage: _____ Normal					
A. Anterior loss	L1 L2	L1 L2	P1 P2	S1	L1
B. Premature spillage	L1 L2	L1 L2	P1 P2	S1	L1
Pooling to: valleculae	L1 L2	L1 L2	P1 P2	S1	L1
pyriform sinus	L1 L2	L1 L2	P1 P2	S1	L1
C. Delayed initiation	L1 L2	L1 L2	P1 P2	S1	L1
D. Uncoordinated initiation	L1 L2	L1 L2	P1 P2	S1	L1
E. Multiple lingual gestures	L1 L2	L1 L2	P1 P2	S1	L1
F. Piecemeal deglutition	L1 L2	L1 L2	P1 P2	S1	L1
G. Residue	L1 L2	L1 L2	P1 P2	S1	L1
Pharyngeal Stage: _____ Normal					
A. Delayed swallow	L1 L2	L1 L2	P1 P2	S1	L1
Pooling: valleculae	L1 L2	L1 L2	P1 P2	S1	L1
pyriform sinus	L1 L2	L1 L2	P1 P2	S1	L1
B. ↓ velopharyngeal closure	L1 L2	L1 L2	P1 P2	S1	L1
C. ↓ tongue base retraction	L1 L2	L1 L2	P1 P2	S1	L1
D. ↓ vocal fold closure	L1 L2	L1 L2	P1 P2	S1	L1
E. ↓ laryngeal movement	L1 L2	L1 L2	P1 P2	S1	L1
F. ↓ epiglottic inversion	L1 L2	L1 L2	P1 P2	S1	L1
G. ↓ supraglottic closure	L1 L2	L1 L2	P1 P2	S1	L1
H. Mistimed laryngeal closure	L1 L2	L1 L2	P1 P2	S1	L1
I. ↓ pharyngeal contraction	L1 L2	L1 L2	P1 P2	S1	L1
J. ↓ UES opening	L1 L2	L1 L2	P1 P2	S1	L1

Table 9–1. *continued*

K. Penetration (P-A 2-5)*	LI L2	LI L2	PI P2	SI	LI
L. Aspiration (P-A 6-8)*	LI L2	LI L2	PI P2	SI	LI
M. Residue: valleculae**	LI L2	LI L2	PI P2	SI	LI
pyriform sinus**	LI L2	LI L2	PI P2	SI	LI
aryepiglottic folds	LI L2	LI L2	PI P2	SI	LI
pharyngeal wall	LI L2	LI L2	PI P2	SI	LI

*Penetration-Aspiration Scale

**Rate severity   I—Mild (> coating but < 25% filling of space); 2—Moderate (25–50% filling); 3—Severe (> 50% filling)

Cognitive status during testing (circle all that apply):

Alert   Cooperative   Drowsy   Inattentive   Neglect   Agitated   Confused   Anosognosia

Comments/Recommendations: _____

_____

THERAPEUTIC TECHNIQUES

_____ Chin Tuck	_____ Head turn (Right/Left)	_____ Cyclic ingestion
_____ Thick liquids (nectar/honey)	_____ Effortful swallow	_____ Breath hold
_____ Mendelsohn maneuver	_____ Other (List)	_____ Combination (list)

Study Conditions:

View: _____ Lateral _____ A-P   **Delivery Method:** _____ Cup _____ Straw _____ Syringe

Circle appropriate consistency/sequence   5ml   cup sip   pudding   solid   cont

Oral Stage: _____ Normal

A. Anterior loss	LI L2	LI L2	PI P2	SI	LI
B. Premature spillage	LI L2	LI L2	PI P2	SI	LI
Pooling to: valleculae	LI L2	LI L2	PI P2	SI	LI
pyriform sinus	LI L2	LI L2	PI P2	SI	LI
C. Delayed initiation	LI L2	LI L2	PI P2	SI	LI
D. Uncoordinated initiation	LI L2	LI L2	PI P2	SI	LI
E. Multiple lingual gestures	LI L2	LI L2	PI P2	SI	LI
F. Piecemeal deglutition	LI L2	LI L2	PI P2	SI	LI
G. Residue	LI L2	LI L2	PI P2	SI	LI

continues

Table 9–1. *continued*

Pharyngeal Stage:	_____ Normal							
A. Delayed swallow	LI	L2	LI	L2	PI	P2	SI	LI
Pooling: valleculae	LI	L2	LI	L2	PI	P2	SI	LI
pyriform sinus	LI	L2	LI	L2	PI	P2	SI	LI
B. ↓ velopharyngeal closure	LI	L2	LI	L2	PI	P2	SI	LI
C. ↓ tongue base retraction	LI	L2	LI	L2	PI	P2	SI	LI
D. ↓ vocal fold closure	LI	L2	LI	L2	PI	P2	SI	LI
E. ↓ laryngeal movement	LI	L2	LI	L2	PI	P2	SI	LI
F. ↓ epiglottic inversion	LI	L2	LI	L2	PI	P2	SI	LI
G. ↓ supraglottic closure	LI	L2	LI	L2	PI	P2	SI	LI
H. Mistimed laryngeal closure	LI	L2	LI	L2	PI	P2	SI	LI
I. ↓ pharyngeal contraction	LI	L2	LI	L2	PI	P2	SI	LI
J. ↓ UES opening	LI	L2	LI	L2	PI	P2	SI	LI
K. Penetration (P-A 2-5)*	LI	L2	LI	L2	PI	P2	SI	LI
L. Aspiration (P-A 6-8)*	LI	L2	LI	L2	PI	P2	SI	LI
M. Residue: valleculae**	LI	L2	LI	L2	PI	P2	SI	LI
pyriform sinus**	LI	L2	LI	L2	PI	P2	SI	LI
aryepiglottic folds	LI	L2	LI	L2	PI	P2	SI	LI
pharyngeal wall	LI	L2	LI	L2	PI	P2	SI	LI

*Penetration-Aspiration Scale

**Rate severity   1—Mild (> coating but < 25% filling of space); 2—Moderate (25–50% filling); 3—Severe (> 50% filling)

Notes on Implementation: _____

_____

_____

Table 9–2. Compensation Approach to Management

The symptoms of:	Secondary to physiologic abnormality of:	Compensation:
Anterior leakage	Poor orolingual control	Thickened liquid
Inadequate bolus preparation		Chopped or pureed diet
Discoordinated oral transfer		3-second prep
Oral residual		Cyclic ingestion
Pharyngeal pooling to the level of _____		Thickened liquid Volume regulation Chin tuck
	Delayed pharyngeal swallow	Thickened liquid Volume regulation 3-second prep Increased taste-sour bolus Thermal-tactile stimulation Chin tuck*
Nasal regurgitation	Poor pharyngeal motility	Thick consistencies
Inadequate epiglottic deflection	Decreased anterior hyoid movement	No identified compensatory strategy
	Intrinsic structural changes in supportive tissue	
Vallecular residue	Decreased base of tongue to posterior pharyngeal wall approximation	Cyclic ingestion Chin tuck Carbonation—physiology of residual not specified
	Inadequate epiglottic deflection	Cyclic ingestion Carbonation—physiology of residual not specified
Inadequate opening of the UES	Decreased anterior hyoid movement	Head turn
	Intrinsic structural functional changes in cricopharyngeus	
Unilateral pharyngeal residue	Pharyngeal hemiparesis	Head turn to weaker side

continues

Table 9–2. *continued*

Pyriform sinus residue	Inadequate opening of the UES	Cyclic ingestion Carbonation—physiology of residual not specified Head turn
Airway Invasion	Pre-swallow pharyngeal pooling	Thickened liquids Volume regulation 3-second prep Chin tuck* Increased taste-sour bolus Thermal-tactile stimulation
	Inadequate epiglottic deflection	No identified compensatory strategy
	Oral residual	Cyclic ingestion
	Pharyngeal residual	Cyclic ingestion Chin tuck Carbonation
	Reduced laryngeal valving	Super-supraglottic swallow
	Inadequate true vocal fold closure	Supraglottic swallow

*Precaution: use chin tuck only with pooling to valleculae. Use with pooling more inferior may increase airway invasion.
UES = upper esophageal sphincter.

Breath-holding techniques (supraglottic swallow, super-supraglottic swallow—see Chapter 1) have been demonstrated to be effective in reducing aspiration before onset or during the pharyngeal swallow (for review, Logemann, 1998); however, use with the stroke population must be viewed cautiously. These techniques were initially designed for individuals with dysphagia following head and neck cancer. These individuals are frequently younger (and often less frail) than individuals with stroke. Given their relative fitness, they can more readily employ a technique where they are tasked to hold their breath, bear down, swallow, and then cough for each swallow. The less fit stroke patients are more likely to fatigue

using this maneuver during a meal. In addition, research has found increased incidence of arrhythmia when using this technique in individuals with stroke with or without coronary artery disease (Chaudhuri et al., 2002). Given this, the patient's physician should be consulted prior to implementation of the technique.

ETHICAL DILEMMAS

Many stroke patients, particularly those patients evaluated during the acute phase, may have a nasogastric tube (NGT) placed for nutritional support, which would then be present during the initial VFSS. The clinician who is faced with a decision of whether or not to remove the tube during the VFSS is not well guided by the literature as research findings are currently ambiguous. Both large and small-bore NGTs have been reported to affect temporal measures such as stage transit duration and upper esophageal sphincter opening in healthy young adults (Huggins, Tuomi, & Young, 1999). Although not statistically significant, increased temporal measures have been identified in stroke patients who had large-bore NGTs (Wang, Wu, Chang, Hsiao, & Lien, 2006). Moreover, the presence of a manometric catheter in the pharynx has been associated with increased airway invasion in healthy older adults (Robbins, Hamilton, Lof, & Kempster, 1992). Conversely, other research has suggested that aspiration is not increased by the presence of an NGT, regardless of size of the tube (Leder & Suiter, 2008). It should be noted that in that study the authors only evaluated airway invasion and did not assess if an NGT affected bolus flow timing or oropharyngeal clearance.

If an NGT is present during the VFSS, the clinician must determine if the feeding tube is contributing to the dysphagia. Prior to conducting the VFSS, obtaining physician orders for removal of the NGT during the VFSS is recommended. This will allow the clinician the opportunity to remove the feeding tube if the clinician thinks the NGT may be causing or exaggerating any swallowing problem.

Two findings that may arise during the VFSS, and that can lead to the early cessation of the exam, are significant residue with liquids and repeated aspiration early in the study. If swallowing is so impaired that thin liquids are significantly retained in the pharynx, the clinician may question whether barium pudding or a solid should be administered. In these cases implementation of a compensatory strategy to facilitate clearance of the residue could be attempted. If the swallow appears to

be more efficient using the facilitative technique, the examination can proceed with thicker consistencies. If there is a continuation of retention of the bolus, the clinician must weigh the risk for potential further complications during the exam if a thick volume is not swallowed safely or cleared. In these cases, the clinician must carefully balance the value of pushing the patient to the limits by presenting further boluses with the risk of making recommendations for oral intake of bolus volumes and consistencies that were not objectively measured during the evaluation.

The clinician must also consider when to terminate the VFSS when repeated aspiration occurs, even with the implementation of a compensatory strategy. The view is that multiple factors beyond the presence of dysphagia and aspiration influence the development of aspiration pneumonia (Langmore et al., 1998). There is no definitive answer to this. Each patient is different, and the clinician must consider not only the results of VFSS but the medical history of the patient. The volume and depth of travel of aspiration must be considered. In some patients, aspiration that is minimal or that flows just inferior to the true vocal folds may be tolerated, whereas aspiration that is of greater volume or travels into the main stem bronchi may not be tolerated.

MODIFICATION TO THE TECHNIQUE

Administering the liquid barium via a cup was discussed earlier in this chapter. If, however, a patient drinks primarily using a straw, this would be the preferred method for administering the barium. We are unaware of any study that has directly compared the effects of delivery method on swallowing.

Regulating the volume of thin liquid during drinking may reduce the risk of aspiration in some patients. Cups are available that limit the volume that can be taken orally from the cup (i.e., 5ml or 10ml). The effect of this method can be easily assessed during the VFSS. During the cup trials, the clinician can evaluate if hyperextension of the neck is needed to ingest the liquid, and if so, determine how this posture impacts swallowing function. Even if volume regulation is only used to allow the patient to receive thin liquids for pleasure, the effort expended during the VFSS is worth the potential for improving the patient's quality of life.

CLASSIC FINDINGS AND IMAGES

Although patients with lateral medullary stroke may present with an archetypical swallowing pattern, especially during the acute phase, there is no classic or standard presentation of dysphagia for patients with supramedullary strokes. These patients can present with any number of focal or multilayered swallowing impairments of varying severity. Even the most trained clinician cannot look at a VFSS and determine if the medical diagnosis is stroke. What may perhaps shed some light on the diagnosis is cognitive behavior. Poor volume regulation and impulsive bolus control may be evident in individuals with a right hemispheric stroke. However, patients with certain progressive neurologic diseases, for example Huntington's disease, may present with similar bolus control issues. Unilateral pharyngeal hemiparesis may be evident following unilateral supramedullary stroke or a lateral medullary stroke. This swallowing impairment will result in unilateral pharyngeal residue (Figures 9–2A and 9–2B).

The term "apraxia of swallowing" has been applied to patients, particularly those with left hemispheric stroke, who demonstrate "the inability to organize the front-to-back lingual and bolus movement normally characteristic of a swallow or . . . simply holding the bolus without initiating any oral activity" (Logemann, 1998, p. 83). Describing this dis-

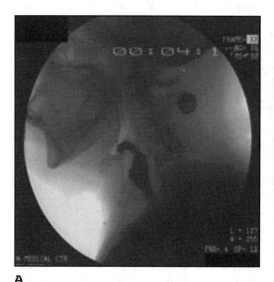
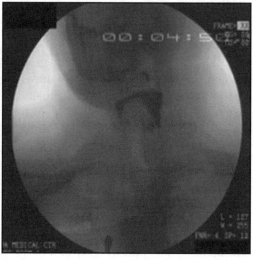

A   **B**

Figure 9–2. *An individual with a right hemisphere stroke with significant pyriform sinus residue (**A**). The anterior-posterior view reveals left unilateral pharyngeal paresis (**B**).*

order as "apraxia," however, implicates specific principles in the act of swallowing. "Apraxia" suggests that swallowing is a learned skilled movement and that the abnormal movement pattern observed is not attributable to sensory or elemental motor deficits. The similarities and differences of apraxia of swallowing with more traditional disturbances of the praxis system (limb apraxia, buccofacial apraxia, apraxia of speech) have previously been reviewed (Daniels, 2000). However, regardless of the semantic or theoretical issues, oral dysmotility disturbances characterized by repetitive, disorganized anterior-posterior bolus movement in the oral cavity, which prolongs oral transfer are evident in stroke patients (Daniels, 2010, Daniels et al., 1999; Robbins & Levine, 1988; Robbins et al., 1993). This can be seen in individuals with cerebral infarction of either cerebral hemisphere as well as other neurological disorders such as Alzheimer's disease.

CONCLUSIONS

Dysphagia is common following stroke. A single, unilateral supramedullary lesion can produce acute and chronic dysphagia. The patient's cognitive and communicative abilities must be considered when performing the evaluation and planning treatment. Treatment begins with the instrumental study, and any recommended compensatory strategy must be tested in the instrumental examination.

REFERENCES

Adams, H. P., Jr., del Zoppo, G., Alberts, M. J., Bhatt, D. L., Brass, L., Furlan, A., . . . Wijdicks, F. M. (2007). Guidelines for the early management of adults with ischemic stroke: A guideline from the American Heart Association/American Stroke Association Stroke Council, Clinical Cardiology Council, Cardiovascular Radiology and Intervention Council, and the Atherosclerotic Peripheral Vascular Disease and Quality of Care Outcomes in Research Interdisciplinary Working Groups: the American Academy of Neurology affirms the value of this guideline as an educational tool for neurologists. *Stroke*, *38*(5), 1655–1711.

Broderick, J., Brott, T., Kothari, R., Miller, R., Khoury, J., Pancioli, A., . . . Shukla, R. (1998). The Greater Cincinnati/Northern Kentucky Stroke Study: Preliminary first-ever and total incidence rates of stroke among blacks. *Stroke*, *29*(2), 415–421.

Butler, S. G., Stuart, A., Markley, L., & Rees, C. (2009). Penetration and aspiration in healthy older adults as assessed during endoscopic evaluation of swallowing. *Annals of Otology, Rhinology, and Laryngology*, *18*(3), 190–198.

Chaudhuri, G., Hildner, C. D., Brady, S., Hutchins, B., Aliga, N., & Abadilla, E. (2002). Cardiovascular effects of supraglottic and super-supraglottic swallowing maneuvers in stroke patients with dysphagia. *Dysphagia*, *17*(1), 19–23.

Chi-Fishman, G., & Sonies, B. C. (2000). Motor strategy in rapid sequential swallowing: New insights. *Journal of Speech, Language, and Hearing Research*, *43*(6), 1481–1492.

Daniels, S. K. (2000). Swallowing apraxia: A disorder of the praxis system? *Dysphagia*, *15*(3), 159–166.

Daniels, S. K. (2010). Apraxia of swallowing. In H. N. Jones & J. C. Rosenbek eds. *Dysphagia in rare conditions*. San Diego, CA: Plural.

Daniels, S. K., Brailey, K., & Foundas, A. L. (1999). Lingual discoordination and dysphagia following acute stroke: Analyses of lesion localization. *Dysphagia*, *14*(2), 85–92.

Daniels, S. K., Brailey, K., Priestly, D. H., Herrington, L. R., Weisberg, L. A., & Foundas, A. L. (1998). Aspiration in patients with acute stroke. *Archives of Physical Medicine and Rehabilitation*, *79*(1), 14–19.

Daniels, S. K., Corey, D. M., Hadskey, L. D., Legendre, C., Priestly, D. H., Rosenbek, J. C., & Foundas, A. L. (2004). Mechanism of sequential swallowing during straw drinking in healthy young and older adults. *Journal of Speech, Language, and Hearing Research*, *47*(1), 33–45.

Daniels, S. K., Corey, D. M., Schulz, P. E., Foundas, A. L., & Rosenbek, J. C. (2007). Effects of evaluation variables on swallowing performance in mild Alzheimer's disease [Abstract]. *Dysphagia*, *22*(4), 386.

Daniels, S. K., & Foundas, A. L. (1999). Lesion localization in acute stroke patients with risk of aspiration. *Journal of Neuroimaging*, *9*(2), 91–98.

Daniels, S. K., & Foundas, A. L. (2001). Swallowing physiology of sequential straw drinking. *Dysphagia*, *16*(3), 176–182.

Daniels, S. K., & Huckabee, M. L. (2008). *Dysphagia following stroke*. San Diego, CA: Plural.

Daniels, S. K., McAdam, C. P., Brailey, K., & Foundas, A. L. (1997). Clinical assessment of swallowing and prediction of dysphagia severity. *American Journal of Speech-Language Pathology*, *6*(4), 7–24.

Daniels, S. K., Schroeder, M. F., DeGeorge, P. C., Corey, D. M., Foundas, A. L., & Rosenbek, J. C. (2009). Defining and measuring dysphagia following stroke. *American Journal of Speech-Language Pathology*, *18*(1), 74–81.

Daniels, S. K., Schroeder, M. F., DeGeorge, P. C., Corey, D. M., & Rosenbek, J. C. (2007). Effects of verbal cue on bolus flow during swallowing. *American Journal of Speech-Language Pathology*, *16*(2), 140–147.

Daniels, S. K., Schroeder, M. F., McClain, M., Corey, D. M., Rosenbek, J. C., & Foundas, A. L. (2006). Dysphagia in stroke: Development of a standard method to examine swallowing recovery. *Journal of Rehabilitation, Research, and Development*, *43*(3), 347–356.

Davalos, A., Ricart, W., Gonzalez-Huix, F., Soler, S., Marrugat, J., Molins, A., Suner, R., & Genis, D. (1996). Effect of malnutrition after acute stroke on clinical outcome. *Stroke*, *27*(6), 1028–1032.

Eisenhuber, E., Schima, W., Schober, E., Pokieser, P., Stadler, A., Scharitzer, M., & Oschatz, E. (2002). Videofluoroscopic assessment of patients with dysphagia: Pharyngeal retention is a predictive factor for aspiration. *AJR American Journal of Roentgenology*, *178*(2), 393–398.

Hind, J. A., Nicosia, M. A., Roecker, E. B., Carnes, M. L., & Robbins, J. (2001). Comparison of effortful and noneffortful swallows in healthy middle-aged and older adults. *Archives of Physical Medicine and Rehabilitation*, *82*(12), 1661–1665.

Huggins, P. S., Tuomi, S. K., & Young, C. (1999). Effects of nasogastric tubes on the young, normal swallowing mechanism. *Dysphagia*, *14*(3), 157–161.

Kuhlemeier, K. V., Palmer, J. B., & Rosenberg, D. (2001). Effect of liquid bolus consistency and delivery method on aspiration and pharyngeal retention in dysphagia patients. *Dysphagia*, *16*(2), 119–122.

Langmore, S. E., Terpenning, M. S., Schork, A., Chen, Y., Murray, J. T., Lopatin, D., & Loesche, W. J. (1998). Predictors of aspiration pneumonia: How important is dysphagia. *Dysphagia*, *13*(2), 69–81.

Lazarus, C. L., Logemann, J. A., Rademaker, A. W., Kahrilas, P. J., Pajak, T., Lazar, R., & Halper, A. (1993). Effects of bolus volume, viscosity, and repeated swallows in nonstroke subjects and stroke patients. *Archives of Physical Medicine and Rehabilitation*, *74*(10), 1066–1070.

Leder, S. B., & Suiter, D. M. (2008). Effect of nasogastric tubes on incidence of aspiration. *Archives of Physical Medicine and Rehabilitation*, *89*(4), 648–651.

Lemen, L. C. (2004). A discussion of radiation in videofluoroscopic swallow studies. *Perspectives on Swallowing and Swallowing Disorders (Dysphagia)*, *13*(3), 5–13.

Logemann, J. A. (1998). *Evaluation and treatment of swallowing disorders* (2nd ed.). Austin, TX: Pro-Ed.

Logemann, J. A., Gensler, G., Robbins, J., Lindblad, A. S., Brandt, D., Hind, J. A., . . . Gardner, P. (2008). A randomized study of three interventions for aspiration of thin liquids in patients with dementia or Parkinson's disease. *Journal of Speech, Language, and Hearing Research*, *51*(1), 173–183.

Logemann, J. A., Pauloski, B. R., Colangelo, L., Lazarus, C., Fujiu, M., & Kihrilas, P. J. (1995). Effects of a sour bolus on oropharyngeal swallowing measures in patients with neurogenic dysphagia. *Journal of Speech and Hearing Research, 38,* 556–563.

Logemann, J. A., Veis, S., & Colangelo, L. (1999). A screening procedure for oropharyngeal dysphagia. *Dysphagia, 14*(1), 44–51.

Mann, G., Hankey, G. J., & Cameron, D. (1999). Swallowing function after stroke: Prognosis and prognostic factors at 6 months. *Stroke, 30*(4), 744–748.

Martin-Harris, B., Brodsky, M. B., Michel, Y., Castell, D. O., Schleicher, M., Sandidge, J., . . . Blair, J. (2008). MBS measurement tool for swallow impairment—MBSImp: Establishing a standard. *Dysphagia, 23*(4), 392–405.

Martin-Harris, B., Brodsky, M. B., Michel, Y., Lee, F. S., & Walters, B. (2007). Delayed initiation of the pharyngeal swallow: Normal variability in adult swallows. *Journal of Speech-Language-Hearing Research, 50*(3), 585–594.

Martino, R., Foley, N., Bhogal, S., Diamant, N., Speechley, M., & Teasell, R. (2005). Dysphagia after stroke: Incidence, diagnosis, and pulmonary complications. *Stroke, 36*(12), 2756–2763.

McCullough, G. H., Rosenbek, J. C., Wertz, R. T., McCoy, S., Mann, G., & McCullough, K. (2005). Utility of clinical swallowing examination measures for detecting aspiration post-stroke. *Journal of Speech, Language, and Hearing Research, 48*(6), 1280–1293.

McCullough, G. H., Rosenbek, J. C., Wertz, R. T., Suiter, D., & McCoy, S. (2007). Defining swallowing by age: Promises and pitfalls of pigeonholing. *Topics in Geriatric Rehabilitation, 23*(4), 290–307.

McCullough, G. H., Wertz, R. T., & Rosenbek, J. C. (2001). Sensitivity and specificity of clinical/bedside examination signs for detecting aspiration in adults subsequent to stroke. *Journal of Communication Disorders, 34,* 55–72.

Murguia, M., Corey, D. M., & Daniels, S. K. (2009). Comparison of sequential swallowing in individuals with acute stroke and healthy adults. *Archives of Physical Medicine and Rehabilitation, 90,* 1860–1865.

Odderson, I. R., Keaton, J. C., & McKenna, B. S. (1995). Swallow management in patients on an acute stroke pathway: Quality is cost effective. *Archives of Physical Medicine and Rehabilitation, 76*(12), 1130–1133.

Parker, C., Power, M., Hamdy, S., Bowen, A., Tyrrell, P., & Thompson, D. G. (2004). Awareness of dysphagia by patients following stroke predicts swallowing performance. *Dysphagia, 19*(1), 28–35.

Pelletier, C. A., & Lawless, H. T. (2003). Effect of citric acid and citric acid-sucrose mixtures on swallowing in neurogenic oropharyngeal dysphagia. *Dysphagia, 18*(4), 231–241.

Perlman, A. L., Booth, B. M., & Grayhack, J. P. (1994). Videofluoroscopic predictors of aspiration in patients with oropharyngeal dysphagia. *Dysphagia, 9,* 90–95.

Robbins, J., Hamilton, J. W., Lof, G. L., & Kempster, G. B. (1992). Oropharyngeal swallowing in normal adults of different ages. *Gastroenterology, 103*(3), 823–829.

Robbins, J., & Levine, R. L. (1988). Swallowing after unilateral stroke of the cerebral cortex: Preliminary experience. *Dysphagia, 3*(1), 11–17.

Robbins, J., Levine, R. L., Maser, A., Rosenbek, J. C., & Kempster, G. B. (1993). Swallowing after unilateral stroke of the cerebral cortex. *Archives of Physical Medicine and Rehabilitation, 74*(12), 1295–1300.

Rosenbek, J. C., McCullough, G. H., & Wertz, R. T. (2004). Is the information about a test important? Applying the methods of evidence-based medicine to the clinical examination of swallowing. *Journal of Communication Disorders, 37*(5), 437–450.

Rosenbek, J. C., Robbins, J. A., Roecker, E. B., Coyle, J. L., & Wood, J. L. (1996). A penetration-aspiration scale. *Dysphagia, 11*(2), 93–98.

Shanahan, T. K., Logemann, J. A., Rademaker, A. W., Pauloski, B. R., & Kahrilas, P. J. (1993). Chin-down posture effect on aspiration in dysphagic patients. *Archives of Physical Medicine and Rehabilitation, 74*(7), 736–739.

Splaingard, M. L., Hutchins, B., Sulton, L. D., & Chaudhuri, G. (1988). Aspiration in rehabilitation patients: Videofluoroscopy vs. bedside clinical assessment. *Archives of Physical Medicine and Rehabilitation, 69*(8), 637–640.

Stephen, J. R., Taves, D. H., Smith, R. C., & Martin, R. E. (2005). Bolus location at the initiation of the pharyngeal stage of swallowing in healthy older adults. *Dysphagia, 20*(4), 266–272.

Thorvaldsen, P., Asplund, K., Kuulasmaa, K., Rajakangas, A. M., & Schroll, M. (1995). Stroke incidence, case fatality, and mortality in the WHO MONICA project. World Health Organization monitoring trends and determinants in cardiovascular disease. *Stroke, 26*(3), 361–367.

Theurer, J. A., Johnston, J. L., Taves, D. H., Bach, D., Hachinski, V., & Martin, R. E. (2008). Swallowing after right hemisphere stroke: Oral versus pharyngeal deficits. *Canadian Journal of Speech-Language Pathology and Audiology, 32*(3), 114–122.

Wang, T. G., Wu, M. C., Chang, Y. C., Hsiao, T. Y., & Lien, I. N. (2006). The effect of nasogastric tubes on swallowing function in persons with dysphagia following stroke. *Archives of Physical Medicine and Rehabilitation, 87*(9), 1270–1273.

Wolfe, C. D. A. (2000). The impact of stroke. *British Medical Bulletin, 56*, 275–286.

Zammit-Maempel, I., Chapple, C. L., & Leslie, P. (2007). Radiation dose in videofluoroscopic swallow studies. *Dysphagia, 22*, 13–15.

Chapter

10

NEUROMUSCULAR CONDITIONS

Julie Regan and Margaret Walshe

INTRODUCTION

Individuals with neuromuscular conditions (NMC) constitute a very heterogeneous group in terms of incidence, inheritance, etiology, clinical presentation, and prognosis (Table 10–1). Typical features of NMC relate to progressive muscle impairment and include loss of ambulation, swallowing difficulties and respiratory failure. Dysphagia presents at the oral preparatory, oral, pharyngeal, and upper esophageal stages of swallowing due to muscle weakness of the tongue, jaw, palate, pharynx, larynx, and suprahyoid muscles (see Chapter 4). Furthermore, respiratory weakness can compromise airway protection including the cough reflex in response to material penetrating the laryngeal inlet or aspirated beyond the level of the vocal folds. Dysphagia associated with NMC often leads to weight loss, malnutrition, dehydration, and aspiration pneumonia. Although one study purported a 35% prevalence rate of dysphagia in NMCs (Willig, Paulus, Lacau, Béon, & Navarro, 1994), exact prevalence remains unclear due to variation in diagnostic methods, underreporting of dysphagia and variation between participant groups across studies (Hill, Hughes, & Milford, 2004). This chapter reviews a selection of both rapidly and slowly progressive neuromuscular conditions commonly associated with oropharyngeal dysphagia and hence regularly encountered in the VFSS clinic.

MOTOR NEURON DISEASE/ AMYOTROPHIC LATERAL SCLEROSIS

Introduction, Incidence, and Pathophysiology

Motor neuron disease (MND) (also termed amyotrophic lateral sclerosis [ALS] and Lou Gehrig's disease) is a rapidly progressive disease of the upper and lower motor neurons in the cortex, brainstem, and spinal cord. With the exception of some familial cases (about 5%) (Byrne et al., 2011), the etiology of MND remains unknown. The incidence of MND ranges between 0.6 and 2.6 per 100,000 population (Cronin, Hardiman, & Traynor, 2007) leading to a lifetime risk of developing MND of 1 per 800 (Cleveland & Rothstein, 2001). Age is the most significant

Table 10–1. *Overview of Neuromuscular Conditions*

Category	Neuromuscular Conditions
Muscular dystrophies	Duchenne muscular dystrophy
	Becker muscular dystrophy
	Limb-girdle muscular dystrophy
	Oculopharyngeal muscular dystrophy
	Congenital muscular dystrophy
	Emery-Dreifuss muscular dystrophy
	Facioscapulohumeral muscular dystrophy
	Distal muscular dystrophy
	Myotonic dystrophy
Motor neuron diseases	Amyotrophic lateral sclerosis
	Spinal muscular atrophy
	Spinal bulbar muscular atrophy
Metabolic disease of muscle	McArdle's disease
	Pompe disease
	Tarui disease
Peripheral nerve diseases	Charcot-Marie-Tooth disease
	Friedrich's ataxia
Inflammatory myopathies	Dermatomyositis
	Polymyositis
	Inclusion body myositis
Diseases of neuromuscular junction	Myasthenia gravis
	Lambert-Eaton syndrome
	Congenital myasthenic syndrome
Myopathies due to endocrine abnormalities	Hyperthyroid myopathy
	Hypothyroid myopathy
Other myopathies	Myotonia congenital
	Periodic paralysis

predictor of MND: the highest rate of onset occurs between 55 and 75 years of age. MND is more common in males than females (1.3 to 1.6:1) but this disparity decreases over the age of 70 (Nelson, 1995). Other suggested risk factors include excessive physical activity, military service, smoking, electric shock, and exposure to pesticides, although larger studies are required to confirm this (Weisskopf et al., 2005). Although a small percentage (8–16%) of patients will survive over 10 years, the majority of patients die within 3 to 5 years from the time of diagnosis (Phukan & Hardiman, 2009).

The time from symptom onset to the diagnosis of MND is often over a year (Traynor, Alexander, Corr, Frost, & Hardiman, 2003). The diagnosis is based on clinical criteria that include the presence of upper motor neuron (UMN) and lower motor neuron (LMN) signs, progression of disease, and the absence of an alternative explanation. No single diagnostic test can confirm or entirely exclude the diagnosis of MND. The "El Escorial criteria" have been shown to be sensitive and specific and have been validated pathologically (Chaudhuri, Crump, Al-Sarraj, Anderson, Cavanagh, & Leigh, PN. (1995). There currently is no cure for MND. Riluzole is the only drug licensed to treat MND although its precise mechanism is unknown. It has been proven to prolong survival for two to four months (Simmons, 2005). The mainstay of management is symptomatic treatment in MND. Patients receiving multidisciplinary care have been found to have a better prognosis than patients attending a general neurology clinic (Traynor et al., 2003). Median survival was up to 7.5 months longer for the former group and was up to 2 months more for patients with bulbar (i.e., medulla and/or brainstem) dysfunction. Recent advances in MND care have included noninvasive ventilation and alternative feeding options.

Clinical Presentation

Most individuals with MND initially experience limb weakness due to involvement of the spinal system. Dysarthria, dysphonia (voice loss), and/or dysphagia (i.e., bulbar onset MND) are the presenting symptoms in 20 to 30% of patients when the disease process involves the motor neurons in the brainstem that innervate muscles of the face, tongue, pharynx, and larynx (Rosen, 1978). Respiratory onset MND is the least common initial presentation. Upper motor neuron involvement results in weakness, increased tone, spas-

ticity, hyperreflexia, plantar extensor responses, and, in some cases, emotional lability (involuntary laughing or crying). Lower motor neuron involvement is manifested by weakness, flaccid muscle tone with muscle atrophy, hyporeflexia, plantar flexor response and fasciculation (involuntary muscle twitches) (Yorkston, Miller, & Strand, 2004). As the disease progresses, patients will demonstrate involvement of essentially all skeletal muscles except the ocular muscles. Up to 60% of those diagnosed with MND present with cognitive decline (Phukan, Hardiman, Jordan, Gallagher, & Pender, 2010). Most patients die of progressive respiratory failure (Simmons, 2005).

Up to 30% of individuals with dysphagia present with bulbar symptoms at diagnosis and almost all patients present with dysphagia in the advanced stages of the disease (Haverkamp, Appel, & Appel, 1995). Dysphagia can result from flaccidity (low tone) or spasticity (high tone) of the muscles involved in swallowing that are innervated by trigeminal, facial, hypoglossal, glossopharyngeal, or vagal nerves (see Chapter 5). Symptoms of oral stage dysphagia include poor lip closure, drooling of saliva, weak lingual movement and bolus formation, poor mastication, weak bolus propulsion, and residue post-swallow in the anterior and lateral sulci (Kawai et al., 2003). Premature spillage of fluid into the pharynx can cause aspiration before swallowing (Kawai et al., 2003). Pharyngeal stage symptoms include a delay in initiating the pharyngeal swallow, poor tongue base retraction, weak pharyngeal contraction, disordered upper esophageal sphincter (UES) opening and poor hyolaryngeal excursion (Graner & Strand, 2010; Leder, Novella, & Patwa, 2004). This leads to residue post-swallow in the valleculae and pyriform sinuses, resulting in aspiration post-swallow (Kawai et al., 2003; Leder et al., 2004) (see Table 10–2).

As dysphagia progresses, impairment becomes more pronounced in both the oral and pharyngeal stages of swallowing (Kühnlein et al., 2008). As the respiratory status declines, the weakened cough makes it more difficult to clear material from the airway. This can be exacerbated by the presence of thick secretions and excess phlegm in the pharynx and airway. Many individuals with MND will reach a point where eating and drinking becomes too effortful or unsafe. Mealtimes become prolonged and choking episodes may be traumatic for both the patient and family. When managing swallowing in individuals with MND, the goals are to maximize function and safety through the use of compensatory strategies, energy conservation, and patient and caregiver education and counseling (Palovcak, 2009). The ALS Severity Scale (ALSSS) (Hillel, Miller, Yorkston, McDonald, Norris, & Konikow, 1989) can be used to rate progression of dysphagia severity (among other parameters) and to guide feeding decisions. The decision to proceed with percutaneous endoscopic gastrostomy (PEG) placement should be multidisciplinary and based on swallowing symptoms (i.e., safety and efficiency), weight loss, hydration status, ability to swallow medications, and quality of life. Advantages to PEG placement include improved nutrition and hydration, although the survival effect is likely to be marginal (Forbes, Colville, & Swingler, 2004). Morbidity relating to PEG placement increases with worsening respiratory function. Patients with significant respiratory insufficiency (i.e., vital capacity of less than 50%) should have their gastrostomy inserted under radiological guidance (radiologically inserted gastrostomy or RIG) (Phukan & Hardiman, 2009).

Role of VFSS in the Management of This Patient Group

Bulbar symptoms of MND can present similarly to other neurodegenerative conditions, such as myasthenia gravis, inclusion body myositis, or Kennedy's disease. VFSS at initial presentation can therefore aid in differential diagnosis of the condition. At this point, the safety and efficiency of current oral diet and effectiveness of cough in response to penetration or aspiration can also be determined. A repeat VFSS within a designated time period can be useful to ascertain the rate of progression of dysphagia and the appropriate timing for non-oral feeding methods (i.e., PEG or RIG, depending on respiratory status). During each procedure, the effectiveness of compensatory strategies (e.g., head postures, voluntary maneuvers, bolus volume, or consistency changes) in eliminating aspiration or clearing residue can be examined or reviewed. This is particularly relevant as, due to the rapidly progressive nature of the condition, dysphagia rehabilitation is not indicated in individuals with MND. Despite the reliance on compensation, few studies have evaluated the effects of postures and maneuvers on swallowing in MND. VFSS can also act as a useful biofeedback tool for the multidisciplinary team in demonstrating the need for diet modification or tube feeding to individuals and their families or carers. In some instances, VFSS can help in advanced stages of the disease to establish any safe consistencies for quality of life purposes when tube feeding is in place.

Ethical Dilemmas

Ethical dilemmas are rife in the management of MND and include decision making around continuing oral intake and the initiation of tube feeding. VFSS is crucial to these decisions as management plans are regularly based on this instrumental examination. Use of rating scales, such as the ALS Severity Scale (ALSSS) (Hillel et al., 1989), which guide clinical decision making, can be useful. Decisions made on these issues by the multidisciplinary team should be patient-centered with consideration of quality of life as well as clinical status. Often, the completion of a VFSS at the time of feeding tube insertion establishes if an individual can continue to take a limited oral diet for quality of life purposes.

Modification to the Technique

Please refer to Table 10–3 for full details of modifications to the standard VFSS for patients with motor neuron disease.

Classic Findings and Images

Typically, both oral and pharyngeal stages of swallowing are disordered on videofluoroscopy. As the oral preparatory phase is frequently prolonged, anterior spillage and loss of bolus to the anterior and lateral sulci tend to be observed. A delay in the initiation of the pharyngeal swallow may be evident, coupled with inadequate velopharyngeal seal to prevent nasal regurgitation of material. Hyolaryngeal excursion may be disordered, which can compromise airway protection and upper esophageal sphincter opening. Consequently, aspiration and pharyngeal retention may present. Depending on the stage of disease, a reflexive cough may not be adequate to clear aspirated material (Figure 10–1).

MYASTHENIA GRAVIS

Introduction, Incidence, and Pathophysiology

Myasthenia gravis (MG) (Latin for "grave muscle weakness") is an antibody-mediated autoimmune disorder of the neuromuscular junctions (Drachman, 1994). It is caused by auto-antibodies which block receptors for skeletal muscle acetylcholine. The cause of MG is unknown, although it frequently presents alongside thymus gland pathology (Berrih, Morel, Gaud, Raimond, Brigand, & Bach, 1984). The prevalence of MG is 20 per 100,000 in the United States population (Phillips, 2004) and the incidence is up to 21 per million (Aragones et al., 2003). Women are affected nearly three times more often in early adulthood (second to third decade). After 50 years of age, incidence is higher in men (Grob, Brunner, Namba, & Pagala, 2008).

Clinical Presentation

MG is characterized by fluctuating skeletal muscle weakness that increases with effort and improves after periods of rest. Clinical features include a fatigable ptosis (drooping of one or both eyelids), diplopia, flaccid dysarthria, dysphagia, dyspnea, facial weakness (termed a "myasthenic snarl"), and fatigable limb or axial weakness (Meriggioli & Sanders, 2009). Six subtypes of MG have been identified based on disease distribution (ocular versus generalized), age of onset, thymic abnormalities, and autoantibody profiles (Meriggioli & Sanders, 2009). Ocular features are the initial symptom in 85% of patients, whereas bulbar weakness is the initial symptom in 15% of MG patients (Grob et al., 2008). If bulbar features present in the absence of ocular symptoms, MG can present similarly to motor neuron disease. The course of MG is variable, although maximum severity is usually reached within 2 years (Grob et al., 2008). Factors that may worsen myasthenic symptoms include emotional upset, systemic illness, pregnancy, the menstrual cycle, increased body temperature, or any drugs that affect neuromuscular transmission (Meriggioli & Sanders, 2009). Patients need to be monitored for myasthenic crisis (not enough anticholinesterase medication)

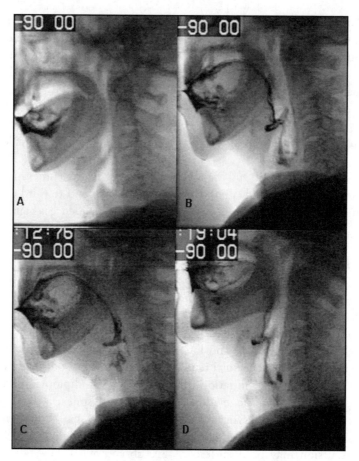

Figure 10–1. *Videofluoroscopic images of 56-year-old male with MND/ALS and moderate to severe oropharyngeal dysphagia. Note in image A, difficulty with bolus formation is evident as material remains in the anterior sulcus and is lost to the lateral sulci. Overspill into the pharynx is evident in image B as the bolus is divided, and approximately half of it remains in the oral cavity, and half falls below the level of the valleculae and into the pyriform sinuses. The hyoid bone can be seen to have moved from its resting position upon initiation of the pharyngeal swallow secondary to suprahyoid muscle contraction. In image C, hyolaryngeal excursion continues as the bolus passes through the pharynx toward the UES. However, base of tongue retraction is weak and laryngeal elevation is reduced. A small amount of contrast can also be seen coating the posterior epiglottis and entering the laryngeal vestibule. In image D, the hyoid bone and epiglottis have returned to their resting positions. Mild residue is seen in the valleculae as a result of weak tongue base retraction toward the posterior pharyngeal wall during swallowing, with coating of the arytenoids. Mild to moderate residue in the pyriform sinuses indicates poor UES opening during swallowing. Anterior spillage from the mouth is also seen, indicating poor lip seal.*

or cholinergic crisis (too much anticholinesterase medication).

There frequently is a diagnostic delay in MG. Diagnosis tests include an edrophonium (Tensilon) test conducted at the bedside to observe for transient relief from visible MG symptoms (Pascuzzi, 2003). Tensilon is a rapid, short-acting anticholinesterase that blocks the breakdown of acetylcholine by cholinesterase and temporarily increases acetylcholine levels at the neuromuscular junction. Electrophysiological (repetitive nerve stimulation and single-fiber electromyography), immunological (autoantibodies such as Anti-AChr, Anti-MUSK), thyroid function and CT/MRI thorax tests are also completed to confirm MG diagnosis (Meriggioli & Sanders, 2005). Generally, symptoms of MG can be well controlled pharmacologically. Cholinesterase inhibitors (e.g., pyridostigmine bromide) increase the amount of acetylcholine available at the neuromuscular junction and are the first-line treatment in MG (Drachman, 1994). They can be taken 30 to 60 minutes before meals to optimize swallowing in patients with bulbar symptoms (Meriggioli & Sanders, 2009). Other treatments include immune therapies (i.e., plasma exchange or intravenous immunoglobulin (Zinman, Ng, & Bril, 2007)) and corticosteroids (Evoli, Batocchi, Palmisani, Lo Monaco, & Tonali, 1992).

Features of dysphagia typically present secondary to fatigue toward the end of a meal. Swallowing difficulties observed on VFSS are predominantly pharyngeal in nature, justifying the need for instrumental examination. However, oral preparatory and oral phase features have been reported including weak lip seal, poor bolus formation, prolonged mastication, piecemeal deglutition, and residue post-swallow (Colton-Hudson, Koopman, Moosa, Smith, Bach, & Nicolle, 2002). In fact, patients with bulbar MG are often observed holding their jaws when masticating to chew more efficiently as meals progress (see Table 10–2).

Pharyngeal phase features observed on VFSS include aspiration, which has frequently been reported to be silent in nature (Colton-Hudson et al, 2002; Koopman et al., 2004). Disturbance of hyolaryngeal excursion and incomplete upper esophageal sphincter (UES) opening are evident in the literature (Higo, Nito, & Tayama, 2005). Other symptoms observed include slow or labored bolus transport from the oral cavity to the pharynx, pharyngeal constriction, or pyriform sinus stasis (Higo et al., 2005) (see Table 10–2).

Role of VFSS in the Management of This Patient Group

As in MND, VFSS aids in differential diagnosis of MG as, clinically, bulbar symptoms of MG can present similarly to other neurological conditions (e.g., MND, inclusion body myositis, or Guillain-Barré syndrome). Once the nature of dysphagia is established, any fatigue element can be detected on VFSS. Typically, this is done using rating scales (e.g., penetration-aspiration scale (Rosenbek, Robbins, Roecker, Coyle, & Wood, 1996) to determine changes in aspiration, residue or timing of swallowing at the beginning and the end of the VFSS procedure. Where individuals present with dysphagia as a sole presentation of MG, Tensilon injections can be administered by medical staff during VFSS and its immediate effects on swallowing observed and evaluated. From a management viewpoint, VFSS can assist in establishing a safe quantity of oral intake for individuals before fatigue of oropharyngeal musculature is induced. As rehabilitation is not indicated in these patients, the effectiveness of compensatory strategies (e.g. chin tuck, head turn, supraglottic swallow) and diet modification should be identified in those who have impaired safety and efficiency of swallowing.

Ethical Dilemmas

There are no specific ethical dilemmas in the management of dysphagia in MG. As direct dysphagia rehabilitation (e.g., oromotor exercises) exacerbates symptoms, dysphagia management typically involves monitoring the effects of pharmacological interventions on swallowing, patient education and the development of compensatory strategies to optimize swallow safety and efficiency. Care should be taken in differentiating between a myasthenic and cholinergic crisis, both of which frequently involve intensive care management.

Modification to the Technique

Please refer to Table 10–3 for full details of modifications to the standard VFSS for patients with myasthenia gravis.

Classic Findings and Images

One of the main difficulties that a patient with MG has when swallowing is controlling the bolus both anteriorly and posteriorly. This can result in spillage from the lips, or pre-swallow overspill into the pharynx due to poor tongue base retraction (Figure 10–2). Further descriptions of the characteristics of dysphagia in MG can be found in Table 10–2.

INCLUSION BODY MYOSITIS

Introduction, Incidence, and Pathophysiology

Inflammatory myopathies (IM) are a heterogeneous group of rare immune-mediated diseases that involve chronic muscle inflam-

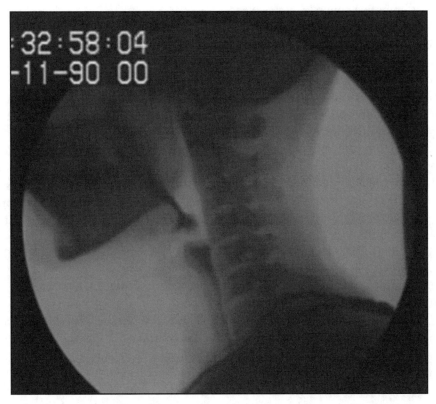

Figure 10–2. *Lateral view of a 35-year-old female with myasthenia gravis clearly showing the tongue base not retracting to meet the posterior pharyngeal wall in order to control and propel the bolus through the pharynx and through the upper esophageal sphincter. In addition, the soft palate is not elevated to block off the nasal cavity, and epiglottic inversion to meet the arytenoid cartilages is incomplete, leaving the airway at risk.*

mation, accompanied by muscle weakness. They include inclusion body myositis (IBM), dermatomyositis (DM), polymyositis (PM), and an overlap syndrome with mixed characteristics (Mastaglia, 2008). The incidence of IM has been reported as between 3.7 and 7.7 per million (Mastaglia, 2008). In general, the incidence rates of PM and DM are higher in women, whereas the prevalence rates of IBM are higher in men. The reasons for gender differences are not known (Needham et al., 2008). IBM also presents most frequently in patients over age 50 years (Needham et al., 2008).

Clinical Presentation

Symptoms include slow but progressive muscle weakness starting in the proximal muscles, fatigue after walking/standing, tripping or falling and difficulty swallowing or breathing. Each subtype of inflammatory myopathy also has distinct clinical and histopathalogical features. Specific diagnostic criteria for each IM have been developed (Mastaglia, Garlepp, Phillips, & Zilko, 2003). Diagnosis of an IM is based on medical history, physical examination, muscle and skin biopsy, neurophysiological (EMG/nerve conduction) tests, ultrasound, and blood (antibody) tests. IM treatment remains largely empirical with use of corticosteroids, immunosuppressant agents, and intravenous immunoglobulin (Mastaglia et al., 2003).

Specific research found that 94% of patients with IM (17/18: 4 DM; 6 PM; 8 IBM) reported some form of dysphagia (Mulcahy, Langdon, & Mastaglia, 2011). The highest incidence of dysphagia is reported in IBM, with 65 to 86% of IBM patients demonstrating dysphagic symptoms (Cox, Verschuuren, Verbist, Niks, Wintzen, & Badrising, 2009; Needham & Mastaglia, 2007; Oh, Brumfield, Hoskin, Stolp, Murray, & Basford, 2007; Williams, Grehan, Hersch, Andre, & Cook, 2003). Cox et al. (2009) found that women with IBM reported swallowing difficulty more frequently than men (88% vs. 56%). However, dysphagia does not appear to be correlated with age or duration of disease (Mulcahy et al., 2011).

Mulcahy et al. (2011) found that 78% of participants with IM (14/18) had abnormal videofluoroscopy studies (Mulcahy et al., 2011). All eight (100%) participants with IBM were found to have impaired swallowing. The most frequent VFSS findings reported are pharyngeal in nature, with no reports of oral preparatory or oral stage symptoms of dysphagia (see Table 10–2). The most frequently reported dysphagia-related symptom is difficulty swallowing solid and dry food (72–85%) (Badrising et al., 2005; Mulcahy et al, 2011; Oh, Brumfield, Hoskin, Kasperbauer, & Basford, 2008; Oh, Brumfield, Hoskin, Stolp, Murray, & Basford, 2007). Other reports include "food sticking in the throat" and "coughing while eating" (75%). Less frequently reported symptoms include difficulty with liquids (50%, 9/18); 44% (8/18) reported difficulty swallowing saliva/secretions and 39% (7/18) reported problems swallowing medications (Mulcahy et al., 2011). VFSS studies have found that the primary impairment observed in all IMs is upper esophageal sphincter (UES) or cricopharyngeal (CP) dysfunction (Oh, 2007) (see Table 10–2), preventing efficient bolus clearance through the UES during swallowing. Individuals are therefore at risk of aspiration on pharyngeal residue post-swallow (see Table 10–2).

Dysphagia in IBM is associated with nutritional deficits, aspiration pneumonia, decreased quality of life, and poor prognosis (Oh, Brumfield, Hoskin, Kasperbauer, & Basford, 2008; Williams, Grehan, Hersch, Andre, & Cook, 2003). Furthermore, patients with IM and dysphagia are reported to have a 1-year mortality rate of 31% (Williams et al.,

2003). Invasive procedures to treat dysphagia have been frequently reported in IM, perhaps due to the commonly localized region of dysfunction in the UES region. In a retrospective review of IM patients over a 5-year period, Oh et al. (2007) report that surgical interventions were performed in 24 patients (39%) with IM. They were most frequently completed in patients with IBM (62%), with cricopharyngeal myotomy (surgical sectioning of the cricopharyngeus [CP] muscle) being most beneficial. Other invasive procedures reported in IM include botulinum toxin A injections into the CP muscle in individuals with IM (Liu, Tarnopolsky, & Armstrong, 2004). Additionally, UES dilatation has been reported in IM with varying benefit (Oh et al., 2007).

Role of VFSS in the Management of This Patient Group

Dysphagia is frequently the initial or sole presenting symptom in IBM (Cox et al., 2009). Information provided from VFSS can therefore contribute significantly to the medical diagnosis. Individuals with IBM who experience dysphagia frequently do not report swallowing difficulties to their physicians (Cox et al., 2009). VFSS can therefore rule out any swallowing difficulty and minimize the risk of any clinical sequelae of dysphagia. As individuals with IBM frequently rely on alternative feeding methods, VFSS can establish the effect of medical treatment (e.g., corticosteroids, immunosuppressant agents), dysphagia compensatory strategies (e.g., head turn) or rehabilitation (e.g., Shaker head lifting exercises or Mendelsohn maneuver) on swallowing. Where these interventions are unsuccessful, VFSS is often required to establish candidacy for more invasive dysphagia interventions to improve UES opening (e.g., dilatation, Botox, myotomy).

Ethical Dilemmas

There are no specific ethical issues in the management of dysphagia in this diagnostic group. Until further research is available, the evidence base for invasive dysphagia interventions (e.g. dilatations, myotomy, Botox injections) to treat poor UES opening in IBM remains limited. Considering the adverse events associated with some of these interventions, candidacy needs to be ascertained clearly in each individual case.

Modification to This Technique

Please refer to Table 10–3 for full details of modifications to standard VFSS for patients with inclusion body myositis.

Classic Findings and Images

The main swallowing difficulties experienced by a patient suffering from IBM occur at the pharyngeal stage of deglutition. Impaired UES opening during the swallow often prevents bolus passage into the esophagus, and impaired hyolaryngeal excursion reduces airway closure leading to a potential risk of aspiration. Post-swallow pooling in the pyriform sinuses and difficulty clearing the residue may also lead to aspiration post-swallow (Figure 10–3). Further descriptions of the characteristics of dysphagia in IBM can be found in Table 10–2.

DUCHENNE MUSCULAR DYSTROPHY

Introduction, Incidence, and Pathophysiology

Duchenne muscular dystrophy (DMD) is an inherited X-linked recessive neuromuscular

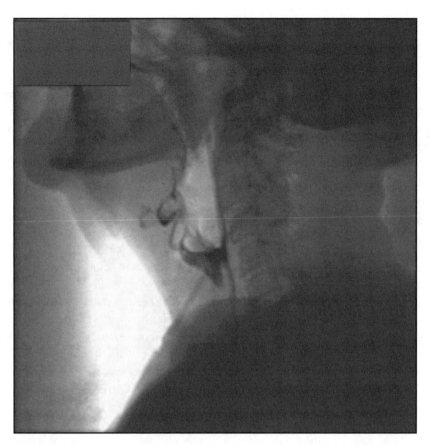

Figure 10-3. *Lateral view of a 62-year-old female with inclusion body myositis. A nasogastric tube was passed to address her nutrition requirements prior to the VFSS. The post-swallow image clearly shows that only a small percentage of the bolus actually passed through the UES into the esophagus during the swallow. Significant residue in the pyriform sinuses is evident secondary to impaired opening of the UES. To a lesser extent, some residue remains in the valleculae.*

disorder. It is one of a heterogeneous group of 30 or more inherited genetic myopathies that are characterized by wasting and weakness of the skeletal muscles. Other muscular dystrophy groups include: Becker muscular dystrophy, congenital muscular dystrophy, Emery-Dreifuss muscular dystrophy, facioscapulohumeral muscular dystrophy, limbgirdle muscular dystrophy, distal muscular dystrophy, myotonic dystrophy, and oculopharyngeal muscular dystrophy. Some forms of muscular dystrophy begin in childhood, whereas others only become apparent in adulthood. DMD, with onset in childhood, is the most common form of childhood muscular dystrophy, affecting up to 1 in 3,600 to 4,700 live male births (Muntoni, Torelli, & Ferlini, 2003). DMD primarily affects boys but females who carry the gene may also show symptoms. The condition is caused by a lack of dystrophin, a protein important for muscle function. DMD is characterized by progressive symmetric muscle weakness and gait disturbance.

Clinical Presentation

The first symptoms may become apparent between 2 to 5 years. Affected children present with gait problems, hypertrophy of the calf muscles, difficulty rising from the floor and climbing stairs. Deterioration begins between 6 to 8 years. Upper limb function is preserved longer than lower limb function. Between 9 to 12 years the majority of children become wheelchair bound.

Respiratory difficulties arise as a result of respiratory muscle weakness and kyphoscoliosis. There is occasional involvement of the facial muscles (Perrin, Unterborn, Ambrosio, & Hill, 2004). Gastrointestinal difficulties can arise as a result of involvement of the gastrointestinal smooth muscle (Jaffe, 1990). Cardiorespiratory complications appear during the second decade and respiratory failure is reported to be one of the leading causes of death (Bushby et al., 2010). Advances in clinical medicine and rehabilitation result in increased survival rates. People with DMD are now surviving later into the second decade and in some instances into the fourth decade (Eagle et al., 2007). Glucocorticoid corticosteroids remain the most effective treatment for DMD with noninvasive ventilation used to improve respiratory function.

Prevalence of dysphagia in DMD is difficult to determine as few studies have systematically examined the characteristics of dysphagia. Pane et al. (2006) surveyed 118 people with DMD and found that less than 28% reported feeding and swallowing difficulties. Chewing difficulty was reported as the most frequent symptom and this was reported in 20% of participants. The involvement of respiratory muscles results in ineffective cough and compromised respiratory status (see Table 10–2).

Prolonged mealtimes, problems positioning food in the mouth, choking episodes, and weight loss are common features of dysphagia in people with DMD particularly as they grow older (Aloysius, Born, Kinali, Davis, Pane, & Mercuri, 2008; Hanayama et al., 2008; Shinonaga et al., 2008). Pane et al. (2006) found that complaints of feeding and swallowing problems were relatively uncommon in people with DMD below 18 years of age but Hanayama et al. (2008) found difficulties amongst teenagers with DMD. Problems with gastroesophageal reflux can also exist. One study showed that as many as 47% of sufferers reported gastrointestinal symptoms (Pane et al., 2006).

Studies that have looked at the history of feeding and swallowing difficulties coupled with VFSS (Aloysius et al., 2008; Hanayama et al., 2008; Shinonaga et al., 2008) have found discrepancies between reported swallowing difficulties and presentation on VFSS. Using VFSS, Aloysius et al. (2008), Hanayama et al. (2008) and Shinonaga et al. (2008) all found swallowing difficulties at the oral preparatory, oral, and pharyngeal phases (see Table 10–2). All three studies found no consistent evidence of pharyngeal delay or aspiration although laryngeal penetration was noted by Aloysius et al. (2008).

Role of VFSS in the Management of This Patient Group

Close monitoring of feeding and swallowing problems is particularly important as the person with DMD ages. Given the discrepancies between verbal reports of dysphagia and VFSS findings, it is important to incorporate VFSS into assessment. The DMD Care Considerations Working Group (Bushby et al., 2010) recommends VFSS for patients with clinical indicators of possible aspiration and pharyngeal dysmotility. An already compromised respiratory status suggests that early detection of aspiration is important. VFSS may also help allay fears of choking, reported to be common in this population.

Table 10–2. *Characteristics of Oropharyngeal Dysphagia on Videofluoroscopy Across Neuromuscular Conditions*

Symptoms of Dysphagia on Videofluoroscopy	Motor Neuron Disease	Myasthenia Gravis (symptoms are fatigue-dependent)	Inclusion Body Myositis	Duchenne Muscular Dystrophy
Oral Preparatory/ Oral Phase	Reduced lip closure during oral stage of swallow leading to bilateral anterior spillage of material	Weak lip seal and anterior spillage of material (bilateral)		Macroglossia leads to biting of tongue
	Difficulty collecting material from anterior and lateral sulci in oral cavity leading to oral residue post-swallow	Poor bolus formation and propulsion upon fatigue		Dry oral mucosa, malocclusion, weak masticatory muscles and bilateral facial weakness cause difficulty chewing
	Difficulty forming and propelling bolus and prolonged mastication on solid foods	Fatigue on chewing solid foods—hand often used to support mandible when chewing solids		
	Premature spillage of material into pharynx often leading to aspiration pre-swallow	Premature spillage of material into pharynx pre-swallow		Weak tongue muscles cause effortful bolus transit and premature loss of bolus into pharynx
	Piecemeal deglutition to minimize risk of aspiration	Piecemeal deglutition		

continues

Table 10–2. *continued*

Symptoms of Dysphagia on Videofluoroscopy	Motor Neuron Disease	Myasthenia Gravis (symptoms are fatigue-dependent)	Inclusion Body Myositis	Duchenne Muscular Dystrophy
Pharyngeal Phase	Nasal regurgitation of material due to weak velar elevation to block off nasal cavity or due to mis-timing of pharyngeal swallow	Nasal regurgitation	Impaired UES opening/CP dysfunction during swallowing preventing bolus transport into the esophagus	Reduced bolus manipulation and control can result in penetration and choking
	Reduced pharyngeal propulsion including weak tongue base retraction toward posterior pharyngeal wall leading to residue in valleculae	Poor contact between tongue base and posterior pharyngeal wall during swallow leading to residue in valleculae and on posterior pharyngeal wall post-swallow	Impaired hyolaryngeal excursion	Weak bolus pressure leading to vallecular residue post-swallow
	Delay in initiating pharyngeal swallow leading to risk of aspiration pre-swallow		Pooling in the pyriform sinuses leading to aspiration post-swallow	
	Reduced superior and anterior hyolaryngeal excursion leading to poor airway protection and residue in pyriform sinuses post-swallow	Weak superior and anterior hyolaryngeal excursion leading to pyriform residue and risk of aspiration post-swallow	Impaired tongue base retraction leading to residue in valleculae post-swallow	Weak pharyngeal peristalsis and reduced bolus pressure leading to pharyngeal residue post-swallow
	Impaired UES opening (disordered relaxation of CP muscle)			

Table 10–2. *continued*

Symptoms of Dysphagia on Videofluoroscopy	Motor Neuron Disease	Myasthenia Gravis (symptoms are fatigue-dependent)	Inclusion Body Myositis	Duchenne Muscular Dystrophy
Pharyngeal Phase *continued*	Weak inefficient protective cough in response to aspiration Multiple swallows to clear pharyngeal residue	Poor airway protection due to reduced epiglottic tilt toward arytenoid cartilage secondary to weak hyolaryngeal excursion and due to weak vocal fold adduction	Multiple effortful swallows to clear material through UES	Poor UES opening can lead to voluntary pharyngo-oral regurgitation as a compensatory strategy

Ethical Dilemmas

There are no specific ethical issues pertaining to dysphagia management in Duchenne muscular dystrophy. As with other conditions, decision making regarding non-oral feeding based on VFSS findings should be patient centered and with quality of life in mind.

Modifications to the Technique

See Table 10–3 for full modification techniques.

Classic Findings

Dry oral mucosa, malocclusion, weak masticatory muscles, and bilateral facial weakness cause difficulty chewing at the oral stage of swallowing. Poor UES opening during swallowing can lead to voluntary pharyngo-oral regurgitation as a compensatory strategy.

CONCLUSION

Dysphagia is frequently observed across NMCs and can contribute substantially to both clinical status and quality of life. Each of the neuromuscular conditions outlined in this chapter have very precise features of dysphagia on videofluoroscopy. Considering that dysphagia can frequently be the initial presenting feature across numerous NMCs, knowledge of these various features is imperative in order to contribute to the diagnostic process. Awareness is also paramount in order to trial appropriate strategies during the VFSS protocol. The limited evidence base for dysphagia interventions in this clinical group is apparent and highlights the need for future research in this area.

Table 10–3. *Modification to VFSS Protocol Across Neuromuscular Conditions*

Neuromuscular Condition	Modifications to VFSS Protocol
MND	Repeat fluid trials at end of procedure to rule out fatigue element
	Establish effectiveness of postural strategies (e.g., chin tuck, head turn), voluntary maneuvers (e.g., effortful swallow) and bolus volume changes before altering fluid consistency due to risk of dehydration in this clinical group.
	Where dysphagia is severe and chest status is compromised, begin protocol with soft food consistency. Ensure oral suctioning equipment is on-site if necessary.
	If individual is unable to self-feed due to bilateral upper limb weakness, ask regular carer to feed during procedure to replicate typical feeding process.
	Use any feeding equipment which is being employed on a day to day basis (e.g., volume control beaker, Neater-Eater, one-way valve straw).
Myasthenia Gravis	Complete fatigability test (stop screening during procedure and ask individual to chew gum/eat an apple. Start screening once person has chewed considerably and observe for any evidence of fatigue during swallow). Compare aspiration or temporal outcomes pre- and post-fatigue to establish changes in presentation.
	Include chewy solids in protocol to induce and observe effects of muscle fatigue.
	Retry liquids at end of examination (may aspirate when fatigued).
	AP view to assess vocal fold adduction.
	Ask person to take relevant medications (e.g., Mestinon) pre-procedure to optimize swallow for eating and drinking.
Inclusion Body Myositis	Complete compensatory strategies (e.g., head turn) and voluntary maneuvers (e.g., Mendelsohn maneuver) on controlled bolus volumes and consistencies and establish their effectiveness in optimizing UES opening during swallowing.
	Adhere to a standardized protocol (i.e., standardized volumes and consistencies) in order to determine the effect of medical treatment (e.g., corticosteroids, immnosuppressant agents), dysphagia rehabilitation (e.g., shaker exercises), or surgical intervention (e.g., UES dilatation, myotomy) on swallowing difficulties.
Duchenne Muscular Dystrophy	The presence of skeletal abnormalities including kyphoscoliosis can result in difficulties with physical positioning for VFSS. Use seating support system (e.g., VIC chair or VESS chair) where possible.
	The patient should be encouraged to self-feed where possible using adapted feeding utensils. If regular carer who assists with feeding present, involve them to replicate feeding process.
	Use any equipment which is being employed on a day to day basis (e.g., volume control beaker, Neater-Eater, valved straw).

REFERENCES

Aloysius, A., Born, P., Kinali, M., Davis, T., Pane, M., & Mercuri, E. (2008). Swallowing difficulties in Duchenne muscular dystrophy: Indications for feeding assessment and outcome of video-fluoroscopic swallow studies. *European Journal of Paediatric Neurology, 12*(3), 239–245.

Aragones, J., Bolibar, I., Bonfill, X., Bufill, E., Mummany, A., Alonso, F., & Illa, I. (2003). Myasthenia gravis. *Neurology, 60*(6), 1024–1026.

Badrising, U. A., Maat-Schieman, M. L. C., Van Houwelingen O, J. C., Van Doorn, P. A., Van Diunen, S. G., Van Engelen, B. G. M., . . . Koehler, P. J. (2005). Inclusion body myositis: Clinical features and clinical course of the disease in 64 patients. *Journal of Neurology, 252*(12), 1448–1454.

Berrih, S., Morel, E., Gaud, C., Raimond, F., Brigand, H. L., & Bach, J. F. (1984). Anti-AChR antibodies, thymic histology, and T cell subsets in myasthenia gravis. *Neurology, 34*(1), 66–71.

Bushby, K., Finkel, R., Birnkrant, D. J., Case, L. E., Clemens, P. R., Cripe, L., . . . Pandya, S. (2010). Diagnosis and management of Duchenne muscular dystrophy, part 1: Diagnosis, and pharmacological and psychosocial management. *The Lancet Neurology, 9*(1), 77–93.

Byrne, S., Walsh, C., Lynch, C., Bede, P., Elamin, M., Kenna, K., . . . Hardiman, O. (2011). Rate of familial amyotrophic lateral sclerosis: A systematic review and meta-analysis. *Journal of Neurology, Neurosurgery, and Psychiatry, 82*(6), 623–627.

Chaudhuri, K. R., Crump, S., al-Sarraj, S., Anderson, V., Cavanagh, J., & Leigh, P. N. (1995). The validation of El Escorial criteria for the diagnosis of amyotrophic lateral sclerosis: A clinicopathological study. *Journal of Neurological Science, 129*(Suppl.), 11–12.

Cleveland, D. W., & Rothstein, J. D. (2001). From Charcot to Lou Gehrig: Deciphering selective motor neuron death in ALS. *Nature Reviews Neuroscience, 2*(11), 806–819.

Colton-Hudson, A., Koopman, W. J., Moosa, T., Smith, D., Bach, D., & Nicolle, M. (2002). A prospective assessment of the characteristics of dysphagia in myasthenia gravis. *Dysphagia, 17*(2), 147–151.

Cox, F. M., Verschuuren, J. J., Verbist, B. M., Niks, E. H., Wintzen, A. R., & Badrising, U. A. (2009). Detecting dysphagia in inclusion body myositis. *Journal of Neurology, 256*(12), 2009–2013.

Cronin, S., Hardiman, O., & Traynor, B. J. (2007). Ethnic variation in the incidence of ALS. *Neurology, 68*(13), 1002–1007.

Drachman, D. B. (1994). Medical progress: Myasthenia gravis. *New England Journal of Medicine, 330*(25), 1797–1810.

Eagle, M., Bourke, J., Bullock, R., Gibson, M., Mehta, J., Giddings, D., . . . Bushby, K. (2007). Managing Duchenne muscular dystrophy: The additive effect of spinal surgery and home nocturnal ventilation in improving survival. *Neuromuscular Disorders, 17*(6), 470–475.

Evoli, A., Batocchi, A. P., Palmisani, M. T., Lo Monaco, M., & Tonali, P. (1992). Long-term results of corticosteroid therapy in patients with myasthenia gravis. *European Neurology, 32*(1), 37–43.

Forbes, R. B., Colville, S., & Swingler, R .J. (2004). Frequency, timing and outcome of gastrostomy tubes for amyotrophic lateral sclerosis/motor neurone disease. *Journal of Neurology, 251*(7), 813–817.

Graner, D. E., & Strand, E. A. (2010). Management of dysarthria and dysphagia in patients with amyotrophic lateral sclerosis. *Perspectives on Neurophysiology and Neurogenic Speech and Language Disorders, 20*(2), 39–44.

Grob, D., Brunner, N., Namba, T., & Pagala, M. (2008). Lifetime course of myasthenia gravis. *Muscle and Nerve, 37*(2), 141–149.

Hanayama, K., Liu, M., Higuchi, Y., Fujiwara, T., Tsuji, T., Hase, K., & Ishihara, T. (2008). Dysphagia in patients with Duchenne muscular dystrophy evaluated with a questionnaire and videofluorography. *Disability and Rehabilitation, 30*(7), 517–522.

Haverkamp, L. J., Appel, V., & Appel, S. H. (1995). Natural history of amyotrophic lateral sclerosis in a database population: Validation of a scoring system and a model for survival prediction. *Brain, 118*(3), 707–719.

Higo, R., Nito, T., & Tayama, N. (2005). Videofluoroscopic assessment of swallowing function in patients with myasthenia gravis. *Journal of the Neurological Sciences, 231*(1–2), 45–48.

Hill, M., Hughes, T., & Milford, C. (2004). Treatment for swallowing difficulties (dysphagia) in chronic muscle disease. *Cochrane Database of Systematic Reviews, Issue 2.* CD004303. CD004303.

Hillel, A., Miller, R., Yorkston, K., McDonald, E., Norris, F., & Konikow, N. (1989). Amyotrophic lateral sclerosis severity scale. *Neuroepidemiology, 8*(3), 142–150.

Jaffe, K. M., McDonald, C. M., Ingham, E., & Haas, J. (1990). Symptoms of upper gastrointestinal dysfunction: Case-control study. *Archives of Physical Medical Rehabilitation, 71,* 742–744.

Kawai, S., Tsukuda, M., Mochimatsu, I., Enomoto, H., Kagesato, Y., Hirose, H., . . . Suzuki, Y. (2003). A study of the early stage of dysphagia in amyotrophic lateral sclerosis. *Dysphagia, 18*(1), 1–8.

Koopman, W. J., Wiebe, S., Colton Hudson, A., Moosa, T., Smith, D., Bach, D., & Nicolle, M. W. (2004). Prediction of aspiration in myasthenia gravis. *Muscle and Nerve, 29*(2), 256–260.

Kühnlein, P., Gdynia, H. J., Sperfeld, A. D., Lindner-Pfleghar, B., Ludolph, A. C., Prosiegel, M., & Riecker, A. (2008). Diagnosis and treatment of bulbar symptoms in amyotrophic lateral sclerosis. *Nature Clinical Practice Neurology, 4*(7), 366–374.

Leder, S. B., Novella, S., & Patwa, H. (2004). Use of fiberoptic endoscopic evaluation of swallowing (FEES) in patients with amyotrophic lateral sclerosis. *Dysphagia, 19*(3), 177–181.

Liu, L. W., Tarnopolsky, M., & Armstrong, D. (2004). Injection of botulinum toxin A to the upper esophageal sphincter for oropharyngeal dysphagia in two patients with inclusion body myositis. *Canadian Journal of Gastroenterology, 18*(6), 397–399.

Mastaglia, F. L. (2008). Inflammatory muscle diseases. *Neurology India, 56*(3), 263–270.

Mastaglia, F. L., Garlepp, M. J., Phillips, B. A., & Zilko, P. J. (2003). Inflammatory myopathies: clinical, diagnostic and therapeutic aspects. *Muscle and Nerve, 27*(4), 407–425.

Meriggioli, M. N., & Sanders, D. B. (2005). Advances in the diagnosis of neuromuscular junction disorders. *American Journal of Physical Medicine and Rehabilitation, 84*(8), 627–638.

Meriggioli, M. N., & Sanders, D. B. (2009). Autoimmune myasthenia gravis: emerging clinical and biological heterogeneity. *The Lancet Neurology, 8*(5), 475–490.

Mulcahy, K. P., Langdon, P. C., & Mastaglia, F. (2011). Dysphagia in inflammatory myopathy: self-report, incidence, and prevalence. *Dysphagia, Online First March 2011,* 1–6.

Muntoni, F., Torelli, S., & Ferlini, A. (2003). Dystrophin and mutations: One gene, several proteins, multiple phenotypes. *The Lancet Neurology, 2*(12), 731–740.

Needham, M., Corbett, A., Day, T., Christiansen, F., Fabian, V., & Mastaglia, F. L. (2008). Prevalence of sporadic inclusion body myositis and factors contributing to delayed diagnosis. *Journal of Clinical Neuroscience, 15*(12), 1350–1353.

Needham, M., & Mastaglia, F. L. (2007). Inclusion body myositis: current pathogenetic concepts and diagnostic and therapeutic approaches. *The Lancet Neurology, 6*(7), 620–631.

Nelson, L.M. (1995). Epidemiology of ALS. *Clinical Neuroscience, 3*(6), 327–331.

Oh, T. H., Brumfield, K. A., Hoskin, T. L., Kasperbauer, J. L., & Basford, J. R. (2008). Dysphagia in inclusion body myositis: Clinical features, management, and clinical outcome. *American Journal of Physical Medicine and Rehabilitation, 87*(11), 883–889.

Oh, T. H., Brumfield, K. A., Hoskin, T. L., Stolp, K. A., Murray, J. A., & Basford, J. R. (2007). Dysphagia in inflammatory myopathy: Clinical characteristics, treatment strategies, and outcome in 62 patients. *Mayo Clinic Proceedings, 82*(4), 441–447.

Pane, M., Vasta, I., Messina, S., Sorleti, D., Aloysius, A., Sciarra, F., . . . Mercuri, E. (2006). Feeding problems and weight gain in Duchenne muscular dystrophy. *European Journal of Paediatric Neurology, 10*(5–6), 231–236.

Pascuzzi, R. M. (2003). The edrophonium test. *Seminars in Neurology, 23*(1) 83–88.

Palovcak, M., Mancinelli, J. M., Elman, L. B., & McCluskey, L. (2007). Diagnostic and therapeutic methods in the management of dysphagia in the ALS population: Issues in efficacy for the out-patient setting. *NeuroRehabilitation, 22*(6), 417–423.

Perrin, C., Unterborn, J. N., Ambrosio, C. D., & Hill, N. S. (2004). Pulmonary complications of chronic neuromuscular diseases and their management. *Muscle and Nerve, 29*(1), 5–27.

Phillips, L. H. (2004). The epidemiology of myasthenia gravis. *Seminars in Neurology, 24*(1), 17–20.

Phukan, J., & Hardiman, O. (2009). The management of amyotrophic lateral sclerosis. *Journal of Neurology, 256*(2), 176–186.

Phukan, J., Hardiman, O., Jordan, N., Gallagher, L., & Pender, N. P. (2010). PATU4 A population-based longitudinal study of cognitive and behavioural impairment in amyotrophic lateral sclerosis. *Journal of Neurology, Neurosurgery, and Psychiatry, 81*(11), e25.

Rosen, A. D. (1978). Amyotrophic lateral sclerosis. *Archives of Neurology, 35*(10), 638–642.

Rosenbek, J. C., Robbins, J. A., Roecker, E. B., Coyle, J. L., & Wood, J. L. (1996). A penetration-aspiration scale. *Dysphagia, 11*(2), 93–98.

Shinonaga, C., Fukuda, M., Suzuki, Y., Higaki, T., Ishida, Y., Ishii, E., . . . Sano, N. (2008). Evaluation of swallowing function in Duchenne muscular dystrophy. *Developmental Medicine and Child Neurology, 50*(6), 478–480.

Simmons, Z. (2005). Management strategies for patients with amyotrophic lateral sclerosis from diagnosis through death. *The Neurologist, 11*(5), 257–270.

Traynor, B. J., Alexander, M., Corr, B., Frost, E., & Hardiman, O. (2003). Effect of a multidisciplinary amyotrophic lateral sclerosis (ALS) clinic on ALS survival: A population based study, 1996–2000. *Journal of Neurology, Neurosurgery, and Psychiatry, 74*(9), 1258–1261

Weisskopf, M., O'Reilly, E., McCullough, M., Calle, E., Thun, M., Cudkowicz, M., & Ascherio, A. (2005). Prospective study of military service and mortality from ALS. *Neurology, 64*(1), 32–37.

Williams, R. B., Grehan, M. J., Hersch, M., Andre, J., & Cook, I. J. (2003). Biomechanics, diagnosis, and treatment outcome in inflammatory myopathy presenting as oropharyngeal dysphagia. *Gut, 52*(4), 471–478.

Willig, T. N., Paulus, J., Lacau, S. G. J., Béon, C., & Navarro, J. (1994). Swallowing problems in neuromuscular disorders. *Archives of Physical Medicine and Rehabilitation, 75*(11), 1175–1181.

Yorkston, K., Miller, R., & Strand, E. (2004). *Management of speech and swallowing in degenerative diseases* (2nd ed.). Austin, TX: Pro-Ed.

Zinman, L., Ng, E., & Bril, V. (2007). IV immunoglobulin in patients with myasthenia gravis. *Neurology, 68*(11), 837–841.

Chapter

11

PEDIATRIC VIDEOFLUOROSCOPY

Joanne Marks and Rebecca Howarth

INTRODUCTION

Videofluoroscopic swallowing studies (VFSS) have long been considered the "gold standard" for the assessment of dysphagia (Logemann, 1993). In order to evaluate the role of VFSS in the assessment and management of pediatric dysphagia we first need to define terminology used, as well as considering how VFSS has developed in pediatrics to become the considered "gold standard."

The reliability of bedside (noninstrumental) swallow assessment has been frequently researched and it is known that its sensitivity for detecting silent aspiration is poor (Splaingard, Hutchins, Sulton, & Chaudhuri (1998). Splaingard et al. (1988) established that 70% of severe aspirators were missed on bedside swallowing assessment.

VFSS refers to the ability to pair fluoroscopic imaging with video (and, more recently, DVD) recording of the images. The aim of the procedure is to evaluate the pediatric oral and pharyngeal stages of swallowing, the presence or absence of aspiration and identify any potential risk of aspiration. There is also the opportunity to trial therapeutic techniques with the children during the procedure. How-

ever, one of the striking differences between adult and pediatric VFSS is the appreciation of significant anatomical differences. The changes in anatomy and function in the pediatric population, which occurs with maturation of structures, is an important consideration discussed in this chapter.

The application of the VFSS in pediatrics developed from extensive experience of use in the adult dysphagia population. The theory and procedure of VFSS has been thoroughly documented by Logemann (1986, 1993) in a general VFSS text, as well as by Arvedson and Lefton-Greif (1998) in a text related specifically to pediatric VFSS. Whereas the aims for completing the procedure and the rationale and aims for requesting a VFSS in pediatrics may be similar to that in adults, the procedural changes with regard to food preparation, presentation, and acceptance are significant and are also discussed in this chapter.

Incidence

There are a wide range of pediatric etiologies that can result in oropharyngeal dysphagia. For example, there is documented incidence of dysphagia in 60 to 61% of the cerebral palsy population (Bader & Niemann, 2010; Ota-powicz et al., 2010). Moderate to severe traumatic brain injury (TBI) also has a reported incidence of dysphagia of 68 to 76% in the pediatric population (Morgan, 2010).

Estimations from data collected in 2001 are that 23,000 children were admitted to United Kingdom hospitals with a head injury (NICE, 2007). Of this population, those with moderate to severe injuries will present with a high risk for dysphagia and are potential VFSS candidates. The use of VFSS to objectively diagnose dysphagia in such patients is common practice within the remit of speech-language pathologists (SLP).

However, the evidence base for the use of VFSS to assess swallowing in children is limited by a lack of documented or standardized quality assessment, as noted within a Cochrane Review (McNair & Reilly, 2007).

The authors' hospital is a tertiary center accepting regional and national referrals, with average referral rates for outpatients of 12 to 15 patients per month. These are distributed between three outpatient clinics each month (five appointments per clinic). Waiting times from referral can then be maintained at a maximum of six weeks taking into account staff annual leave. Acute inpatients can be managed via separate clinic appointments due to the fluctuating nature of referral rates. A realistic aim for inpatients at the authors' center is to perform a VFSS within five working days from referral. Tertiary units accepting referrals nationally will expect referral rates ranging from 5 to 15 per month for outpatients and 1 to 6 per month for inpatients (unpublished data, Royal Manchester Children's Hospital and Birmingham Children's Hospital). Pediatric videofluoroscopy is typically performed at a tertiary center, although some secondary level hospitals have a smaller service for non-complex patients, and report referral rates ranging from 1 to 5 per month. Based on these numbers we can calculate that a specialist center will perform approximately 180 out-patient procedures plus 72 inpatient procedures per annum.

PATHOPHYSIOLOGY

Embryological Development

The facial structures of the embryo develop between the 5th and 8th week of fetal life. Initially the nasal and oral cavities communicate directly, but the hard palate develops followed by the soft palate. The uvula is normally the last structure to develop at about the 11th week of gestation (Tuchman & Walter, 1994).

The oral cavity develops from the cephalic end of the primitive foregut between the 4th and 8th week of fetal life, with the pharynx arising from multiple structures including the branchial arches, the cephalic end of the foregut, and the pharyngeal pouches (Tuchman & Walter, 1994). By the 5th week of gestation the oropharyngeal membrane ruptures, allowing communication between the digestive tract and the amniotic fluid.

The esophagus begins to develop by the end of week 4, arising from the embryonic foregut. It begins as a short tube, extending in length as the heart and diaphragm descend. The esophagus is initially lined by stratified epithelium, which proliferates rapidly forming an almost solid core, but the lumen becomes re-canalized by approximately the 10th week. By the 7th month, the esophagus has replaced columnar epithelium with mainly squamous epithelium. The combined oesophageal/tracheal/laryngeal tube begins to separate, with the primitive airway and food passages separated below the oropharynx by 33 days gestation (Tuchman & Walter, 1994).

Development Following Birth

In the infant the processes of sucking, swallowing and breathing are related both functionally and anatomically. At birth there is close approximation of structures, with the tongue, lower lip, mandible, and hyoid acting as a single unit. This configuration is summarized as follows (Figure 11–1):

1. The tongue is large in comparison to the oral cavity and is in approximation with the cheeks, hard palate, and soft palate.
2. The tongue tip maintains contact with lower lip.
3. Sucking pads in the cheeks stabilize mandibular movement and facilitates intraoral suction.
4. The larynx is in a more elevated position thus there is a small oropharynx and less laryngeal elevation is required to protect the airway.

These close approximations facilitate the relationship between suck, swallow, and breathing and are present until around six months of age, when anatomical growth moves the soft palate and epiglottis apart, and the larynx descends from cervical vertebral (CV) level CV1 to CV3. As a child matures, the larynx will descend to between CV3 and CV6 by adulthood. Between 2 and 4 years of age, the tongue begins to descend so that by age 9 the posterior third is located in the neck (Tuchman & Walter, 1994).

Sucking and Swallowing

Newborn feeding is predominantly reflexive, namely, rooting, latching, sucking, and swallowing, all of which originate in the brainstem.

- *Rooting:* process of moving head toward a stimulus and "latching on"—primitive rooting is observed at 14 weeks gestation and is refined during the period up to birth. It tends to disappear by 3 to 4 months, possibly later in breast-fed infants (Tuchman & Walter, 1994).
- *Nutritive Sucking:* a reflex feeding activity initially observed in utero at 15 weeks; however, a rhythmical and coordinated suck is not developed until 33 to 36 weeks gestation. Preterm infants exhibit mouthing movements which are not associated with effective sucking. Immature suck-swallow patterns are seen after birth, with mature patterns with multiple swallows seen to occur several days after birth in full-term infants (Tuchman & Walter, 1994).
- *Nonnutritive sucking* occurs when there is no milk flow (for example on a dummy/finger) and is characterized by short bursts of rhythmic sucking and brief pauses.
- *Swallowing:* from 13 weeks gestation, the fetus is observed to swallow amniotic fluid. In utero swallowing assists with maintenance of normal amniotic fluid volume, and growth and development of the gut (Tuchman & Walter, 1994).

At around 6 months of age, feeding moves from a reflexive process under brainstem control, to a process with cortical control enabling more sophisticated oral movements. As weaning through solids progresses (6–18 months) oral skills such as biting and chewing are refined, and by 3 years of age oral skills are similar to that of an adult (Morris & Klein 2000). Children older than 3 years typically are eating regular meals at a table and are drinking from a cup. Beyond this age they continue to refine their eating and swallowing skills, but do not attain any new skills. Efficiency of chewing reaches maximum levels at approximately 16 years of age.

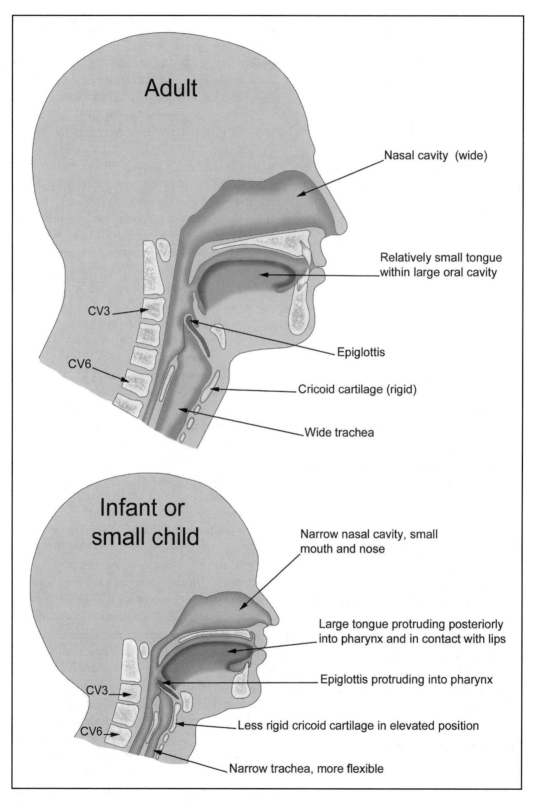

Figure 11–1. *Anatomical development of structures associated with swallowing: Comparison between an infant/small child, and an adult. (Image courtesy of Graham Nightingale.)*

Swallowing Difficulties

Problems may arise in the oral, pharyngeal, and esophageal phases of the swallow and in how the phases interact with each other. Behavioral or aversive patterns may also be encountered, for example as a result of severe gastroesophageal reflux disease (GERD). This condition can result in food refusal, food selectivity by type or texture, delayed feeding development and reliance on enteral feeding, all within the context of a normal physiological swallow.

Common reported signs of difficulty are shown in Table 11–1, and may be specific to certain textures or generalized across solids and fluids. Not all these symptoms are indicative of aspiration and as such do not necessarily require a videofluoroscopy. However, several signs are of most concern and the use of VFSS in these cases should be considered.

CLINICAL PRESENTATIONS IN PEDIATRICS

The use of VFSS in pediatrics continues to increase with a wide clinical presentation occurring within both tertiary centers and local services. There is a limited evidence base looking at the use of VFSS in pertinent clinical groups within pediatrics, but these include the cerebral palsy population (Baikie et al., 2005) and neuromuscular disorders (O'Donoghue & Bagnall, 1999). There are many etiologies that present within pediatric VFSS clinics as discussed later in this chapter. On review of the authors' tertiary VFSS service, core clinical presentations identified include the following (Table 11–2).

Respiratory Conditions

Infants with respiratory conditions are at increased risk of swallowing difficulties due to the integral interplay between the swallow and the respiratory system. This category covers those infants born preterm with chronic lung disease and bronchopulmonary dysplasia. It also includes infants with acute conditions, for example, bronchiolitis, and those infants with chronic chest status including possible repeated aspirations, asthma, and other airway obstructions.

Table 11–1. *Signs of Swallowing Difficulty in Pediatrics*

Signs That May Indicate VFSS	Signs Strongly Indicative for VFSS
Excessive gagging with solid feeds	Coughing during feeds
Food/fluid refusal	Wet or gurgly voice during or post feeds
Slow feeding (e.g., bottle feeds taking longer than 30 mins)	Recurrent chest infections
Failure to thrive	Change in vital signs during feeds
Aversive behaviors when offering feeds — pulling away from teat	
Slow weaning development	

Table 11–2. VFSS Findings and Their Possible Implications

Stage of Swallow	Finding Observed on VFSS	Implications
Oral	Disordered/disorganized/absent suck (nutritive)	• Reduced intake, excessive feeding times, poor preparation for swallow, leading to penetration/aspiration pre-swallow
	Reduced/slow anterior to posterior bolus transition to posterior pharyngeal wall (with fluid and/or solid bolus).	• Excessive feeding times • Nasopharyngeal regurgitation • Premature spillage over back of tongue • Pre-swallow penetration/aspiration (see Figure 11–3)
	Anterior loss of bolus	• Drooling/dribbling • Poor bolus transition
Pharyngeal	Nasopharyngeal reflux	• Discomfort with feeds. Food refusal.
	Delay in hyoid excursion	• Pre-swallow aspiration and/or post-swallow aspiration
	Reduced/incomplete laryngeal elevation	• Penetration and/or aspiration during the swallow
	Residue in valleculae and/or pyriform sinus post-swallow	• Laryngeal penetration and/or aspiration of residue after the swallow

Neurological Conditions

This group spans a wide range of presenting etiologies including those infants with congenital presentation, birth asphyxia, and acquired brain trauma. Damage to the neurological system may affect all stages of the swallow (Figures 11–2 and 11–3).

Ear, Nose, and Throat (ENT) and Structural Conditions

Infants with significantly compromised airway including stridor, tracheolaryngomalacia (a common neonatal deficit comprising expiratory collapse of the airway, due to defective cartilaginous support), and structural abnormalities to airway including tumors and laryngeal clefts are a complex population requiring objective VFSS assessment alongside alternate ENT investigations. A baby may also be born with a cleft lip and/or palate, whereby incomplete fusion of the hard palate will have significant impact upon the success of suck-swallow, and repeated VFSS may be necessary to ascertain any appropriate feeding modifications early in the child's life.

Gastroenterological Presentation

The interplay between GERD and feeding in pediatrics is complex and should not be

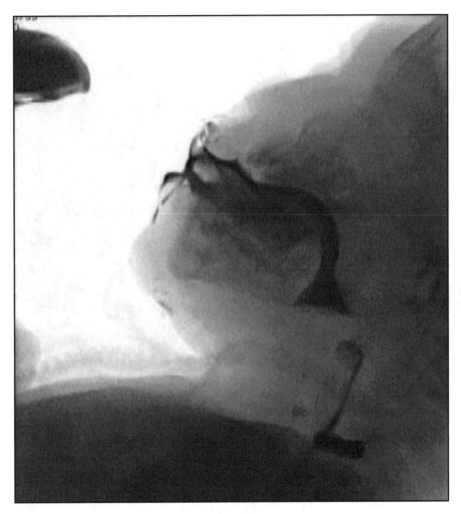

Figure 11–2. *Child with severe cerebral palsy. Intraesophageal reflux aspiration.*

underestimated. Other structural gastrointestinal conditions that have a great impact on the feeding process include infants with tracheoesophageal fistulas and esophageal webs (Figure 11–4).

Cardiac Presentation

Although physiologically this population feed well, the effects of fatigue are significant, at times warranting objective measures to give clear boundaries within timings of oral feeding and endurance.

Long-Term Tracheostomy/Ventilation Population

The interplay between complex respiratory status and structural component means this population is at significant risk of aspiration requiring objective assessments such as the VFSS.

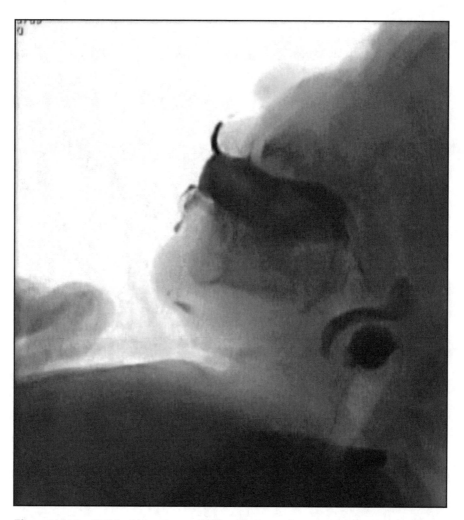

Figure 11–3. *Child with severe cerebral palsy. Nasopharyngeal reflux evident during the swallow.*

The use of a speech and swallow valve (Passy-Muir valve) may require objective assessment to fully assess its impact on the safety of feeding (Figure 11–5).

Degenerative Conditions

Although safety versus quality of life is an ongoing theme in this population, there is often a need for an objective baseline used to monitor deterioration in certain conditions such as metabolic disorders. The deterioration of motor control, respiratory status, and neurological condition results in this population requiring close monitoring of oral intake balanced with risks presented.

Sensory-Based Feeding Disorders/ Learned Aversive Patterns

There is on occasion a need to undergo the VFSS procedure with those infants who pre-

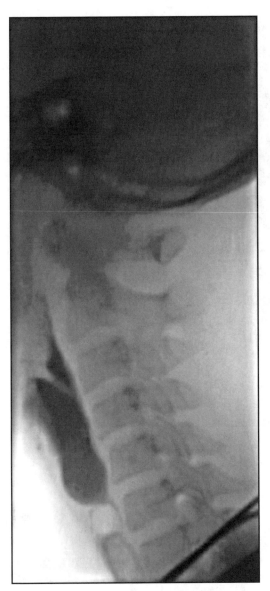

Figure 11–4. *Patient complaining of "food getting stuck." History of weight loss and discomfort with feeds. Referred for videofluoroscopy. An esophageal web has been identified.*

the rationale for this investigation should be clear as to the reason for request and the subsequent outcome of procedure.

As a general rule, the VFSS is not the appropriate investigation for those children whose "behavioral" feeding patterns are part of their condition, for example the autistic spectrum disorder population. The clinical presentation of this client group is often complex in nature crossing the boundaries of a number of "clinical" areas.

ROLE OF VFSS IN THE MANAGEMENT OF PEDIATRICS

While the importance of a skilled bedside feeding examination cannot be underestimated alongside the use of other tools (e.g., cervical auscultation; pulse oximetry), the need for further detailed objective assessment is often essential to identify or confirm difficulties at both oral and pharyngeal stages, and to further enhance the management of this often vulnerable population.

Evidence reported by DeMatteo, Matovich, and Hjartarson (2005) suggests that experienced therapists are reliable at identifying penetration/aspiration with fluids on clinical bedside assessment; however, they are unreliable with solids. They go on to explain that "experienced therapists should use their uncertainty about the presence or absence of penetration or aspiration as an indicator that further diagnostic tests are required, specifically VFSS" (DeMatteo et al., 2005, p. 155).

As already stated within pediatrics, VFSS is still recognized as the "gold standard" (Logemann, 1993). There is, however, a great challenge within this area as the evidence base is driven from an adult field, with the procedure being applied to pediatric population. This shall be discussed later in the section Modification to the Technique.

sent primarily with a sensory-based feeding disorder. These patterns of feeding can be a result of early negative experiences from invasive medical interventions, long-term tube feeding, or significant history of GERD, but

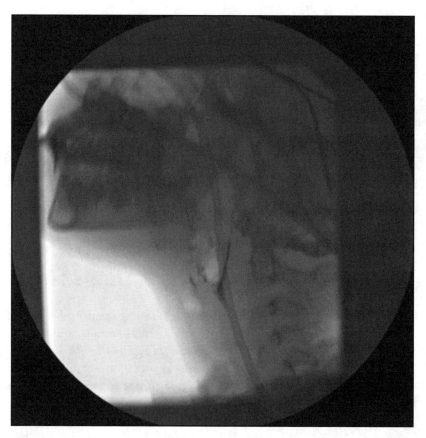

Figure 11–5. *Absent swallow: dysphagia in neuromuscular disease, exacerbated by long-term ventilation and tracheostomy, resulting in a desensitized glottis/ reduced cough. NB. Use of closed position valve, for example, Passy–Muir, may offer some improvement in this situation with sensation*

Nevertheless, videofluoroscopy provides us with our most objective data. Often, when the referral is driven by our medical colleagues, the answer to the clinical question "Is this infant aspirating?" is of paramount importance. However, with the combined skill of the SLP and radiological team, VFSS allows us to identify further risk parameters of aspiration, assessment of different textures, implementation of therapeutic techniques and to make long-term plans for oral feeding alongside developmental stages. VFSS in pediatrics allows the experienced SLP to observe the interplay between the oral and pharyn-geal stage related to the child's developmental stage. Great effort is made to replicate as "normal" a feeding pattern as possible.

Although VFSS clearly has benefits for the investigation of a whole range of pediatric swallowing disorders it should not replace clinical bedside assessment and it should not be used as a last resort. Often, it is used within a "batch" of respiratory assessments, not always with a clear justification from SLP bedside assessment. The importance of limiting radiation exposure in the infant population is a factor that should be high priority in the consideration of performing this procedure

(Cohen, 2009). The VFSS examination should be led by an experienced SLP, supported by a second SLP and a consultant radiologist and/or a specialist radiographer to manage the imaging aspects. On occasion other colleagues from the multidisciplinary team may be present including community SLP, occupational therapist, physiotherapist, nursing team, or play therapist. This enables this objective measure to be optimized in both assessment and determining future patient management.

ETHICAL DILEMMAS

Consent

Individual consent and parental consent is required (see Chapter 3 for further information). In all cases, parental consent should be fully informed but this is particularly necessary in cases of palliative care or where decisions are being made regarding instigation of nonoral feeding.

Compliance

Compliance with the results of the VFSS and any feeding recommendations provided is required from the parents and the child. The purpose and implications of performing the procedure should be discussed with the carers/family prior to the procedure. It is expected that in most instances the Community team will fulfill this role and that the SLP will have a key role in the discussions.

In some cases, children may have to be positioned or fed differently for the purpose of the procedure. It should be made clear to carers that this should not affect the results obtained with regard to the presence or absence of aspiration. As such, repeat procedures in alternative positions are not advised.

Risk of the Procedure/ Exposure to Radiation

Recent analysis of the average exposure times for pediatric VFSS procedures in the author's Tertiary center indicate an average radiation exposure (screening) time per client of 188 seconds (range = 56 to 332 seconds). A previous study of 80 children identified a reasonably comparable mean fluoroscopic time of 2.48 minutes (Weir et al, 2007). Reported fluoroscopic times in the adult population include 18 to 564 seconds (Zammit-Maempel, Chapple, & Leslie, 2007) and 263 seconds (Chau & Kung, 2009). There are currently no national benchmarks (Diagnostic Reference Levels or DRLs) for videofluoroscopy radiation doses within the U.K., but each hospital should set local DRLs, and work toward dose optimization strategies as required within the country's radiation protection legislation. In the U.K., the operator (a radiographer or radiologist) will have a responsibility to ensure that the dose is as low as reasonably practicable (ALARP), as required by the Ionising Radiation (Medical Exposure) Regulations (2000). Similarly, in the United States, the Alliance for Radiation Safety in Pediatric Imaging launched the Image Gently campaign in 2008, which is an alliance of medical societies focusing on efforts to ensure that medical protocols for imaging children keep pace with advances in technology. The campaign concludes that the techniques used in pediatric imaging are not necessarily always tailored to children's smaller bodies, resulting in radiation exposures that are greater than needed (SCoR, 2009). The fourth phase of the Image Gently campaign has recently been launched, centered on reducing doses in pediatric fluoroscopy. This campaign urges the use of pulsed fluoroscopy with lower frame rates for imaging children, which can have significant dose savings (ACR, 2012). However, caution should be urged when considering this strategy in VFSS, as research findings have demonstrated that attempts to reduce the pulse rate below 30 frames per second in small children will miss important abnormalities of the rapidly occurring swallow (Cohen, 2009).

There are many strategies for reducing dose, including the use of *distance from the source* (staff and carers); *shielding* (lead rubber aprons and gloves for staff and carer, and use of lead rubber over the child's abdomen); *collimation* (reducing the image field size to the minimum required, which has an added value of improving image quality); *centering* (centering the beam over the required anatomy and reducing exposure to sensitive tissues); and *time* (limiting the fluoroscopic time to record only the required swallows). Although a range of dose-reducing strategies as mentioned above can also be employed for adult examinations, the importance of ALARP for infants and children cannot be underestimated. Rapidly dividing cells in infants and children are more three to five times more susceptible than adults to damage by radiation (SCoR, 2009), and their potentially long life span and possible cumulative exposures gives a higher likelihood of seeing the effects of any radiation damage in the future (e.g., cancer).

With the above concerns in mind, even though exposure times and rates are within accepted limits set locally, the practitioner should always consider the potential risk of further exposure to radiation to both client and clinicians. There should be a clear rationale for referral with the expectation that results obtained will alter management. All SLPs who are routinely involved in VFSS procedures should have personal radiation monitoring or be subject to environmental monitoring in line with local policy.

Some children present with a significant risk of aspiration during the procedure and as such the risk on their respiratory system of aspiration of barium should be seriously con-sidered. In some cases, the results of a bedside swallowing assessment may indicate that the child is not a suitable candidate for the procedure. Alternatively, water-soluble contrast agents may be utilized.

Cooperation During the Procedure

For some children, feeding is a stressful experience and they do not react well to the hospital environment. In cases where a child is refusing to eat or drink, there should be discussion with the parents as to how much restraint is deemed appropriate. Radiographers are guided to differentiate between immobilization (e.g., swaddling by a blanket or supported by foam pads) and active restraint, and identify alternative means of gaining cooperation, including the use of distraction techniques (SCoR, 2005). In some cases the need for a definitive diagnosis regarding aspiration may result in delivering a bolus in an unconventional manner against agreed practice, for example, syringe feeding. In other cases the clinical indicators for aspiration are not sufficiently strong to justify any degree of active restraint. In all cases the parents will lead the decision.

End of Life/Consideration for Non-Oral Feeding

Often children with degenerative diseases are referred for VFSS. This procedure can serve to provide a baseline as a reference point in the deteriorating condition. However, in such cases there needs to be a clear plan agreed by the medical team prior to the procedure with regard to how feeding is to be managed, particularly in the event of aspiration on all consistencies, and in balance with quality of life decisions.

MODIFICATION TO THE TECHNIQUE

Time Allocation for Procedure

At the authors' center, each client is offered a 30 minute slot to allow for the appropriate preparation, to undergo the actual procedure and to allow for time to feedback to parents, carers, and visiting professionals.

The other challenge for infants is often timing a feed to correlate with the procedure. The hunger drive is often a great asset to the child in encouraging them to accept the modified bolus. Often, parents/carers will reorganize feeding times and delay feeds to provide the optimum setting to encourage oral intake.

Positioning/Seating

Fluoroscopic imaging is often one of the greatest challenges facing any clinician presented with a pediatric client base that could span an age gap of preterm to 19 years of age. Premature infants and full-term babies are often able to be placed side-lying in a cradle attached to the x-ray table. Infants can be seated in their own car seat or small Tumbleform chair where appropriate. The chair base can rest on the floor or upon the step of the fluoroscopy table. The use of the medium-sized Tumbleform chair can also be used alongside positioning with their own buggy. One's own seating is always recommended but a further challenge is often avoiding imaging the integral metal rods that run parallel to the x-ray image of the pharynx and larynx. Ensuring adequate postural support, while gaining a good image is an immense challenge for the clinician. As a last resort, it is at times necessary for a child to be held by a parent. The parent is fully protected using a lead rubber apron and thyroid protector, with the child seated on their knee facing forwards. This practice is generally not promoted due to radiation safety but also the fact that the child is not always well positioned and not fed by a parent. It is essential to ascertain whether a female parent or carer is pregnant, and if so they should be encouraged to bring another carer with them for the procedure.

Radiographic Contrast Products

The most common product used at the authors' center is a preparation of barium sulfate, however access to other water-soluble products is available, including Gastromiro and Omnipaque. The choice of product will normally be led by a consultant radiologist depending on a number of clinical indicators in relation to the infants' age, respiratory status, and medical condition.

Feeding Utensils/Equipment

For the majority of the pediatric population the bolus is offered from their own familiar feeding utensil (e.g., bottle, spoon, cup). This familiarity often aids bolus intake initially. The opportunity to trial specialist equipment within this setting is also available.

Consistencies/Textures

The aim of a pediatric VFSS is to replicate as near as possible a mealtime situation. Encouraging infants to take both the bolus and volume presented can be a great challenge. Familiar foods are requested to be brought from home to trial. This enables masking of the barium within a familiar food-type to encourage oral trials. The ability to add barium preparations to most presented items has become a great skill of many pediatric VFSS teams. The contrast agent is added to the foodstuff to be presented by parents. Barium can be masked well within many yogurt products, baby jars, and other well-known juice bottles and cartons. An approximate aim of 40% barium sulfate to total bolus volume is desired; however, attention must be paid to noting possible changes to texture classification and diluting further if possible.

Order of Bolus Presentation

Within the pediatric population there is no standardized agreement regarding the order of bolus presentation. When managing a compromised neonate, commencing with a strict hierarchy of dummy dips, followed by measured teat trial, followed by bottle trial where appropriate may be beneficial.

For the infant taking both weaning diet and fluids commencing with a clinical decision is necessary as to the "safest" consistency predicted (i.e., least likely to be aspirated) dependent on their developmental age and co-operation. Hiorns and Ryan (2006) state that at the end of the investigation, having assessed multiple swallows and with a range of textures, it is necessary to provide representative and practical advice for feeding due to the fact that aspiration may not be demonstrated with a single bolus.

Anxiety/Behavior Management

There are times when distraction techniques are required. This can be in the form of toys, DVDs, or music in order to get valuable data.

Introducing young adults and those children who have great anxiety associated with the clinical setting to come and view the x-ray department, meet staff, and hear machine noises may be invaluable to aid achieving relaxation and co-operation. The use of a play therapist has also been invaluable at times.

QUANTIFIABLE DATA/SCORING

As previously stated there is a limited evidence base to draw from in the pediatric VFSS field. The clinician endeavors to quantify as much data collected as possible which includes details regarding behavior and cooperation of the child, positioning, exact volumes of fluids taken, and number of teaspoons of diet consumed. When aspiration is seen to occur, the application of the penetration-aspiration scale (Rosenbek et al., 1996) yields useful information, even though its source is from adult data.

CONCLUSION

The modification of VFSS for the pediatric population has provided objective data that cannot be underestimated in its use in the assessment and management of infants and children. This tool has become invaluable in our management of infants and children with complex eating and drinking difficulties. Further research is necessary into the standardization of this procedure, in understanding the rationale for VFSS, interpreting results and formulating management plans.

It must be noted that there are times when the clinician may not achieve a definitive answer using this procedure, which requires further skill and combined MDT knowledge of the client to formulate an appropriate management plan. Management of the infant alongside managing the expectation(s) of the parent/carer, interpreting objective data and implementing it into a plan is a complex skill achieved by the multidisciplinary team within the radiology setting. The skill of the SLP within the MDT is therefore essential to modify this procedure from the adult field in order to provide objective results.

REFERENCES

American College of Radiology. (2012). *Image gently pause and pulse initiative provides materials to help physicians lower radiation dose in fluoroscopic procedures performed on children.* Retrieved February 20, 2012, from http://www.acr.org/SecondaryMainMenuCategories/NewsPublications/FeaturedCategories/CurrentACRNews/Image-Gently-Pause-Pulse-Initiative-.aspx

Arvedson, J., & Lefton–Greif, M. (1998). *Pediatric videofluoroscopic swallow studies.* San Antonio, TX: Communication Skill Builders.

Bader, C. A., & Niemann, G. (2010). Dysphagia in children with cerebral palsy: Fibreoptic endoscopic findings. *Larynogorhinootologie, 89*(2), 90–94.

Baikie, G., South, M. J., Reddihough, D. S., Cook, D. J., Cameron, D. J. S., Olinsky, A., & Ferguson, E. (2005). Agreement of aspiration tests using barium videofluoroscopy, salivagram, and milk scan in children with cerebral palsy. *Developmental Medicine and Child Neurology, 47*, 86–93.

Chau, C. H., & Kung, C. M. (2009). Patient dose during videofluoroscopy swallowing studies in a Hong Kong public hospital. *Dysphagia, 24*(4), 387–390.

Cohen, M. D. (2009). Can we use pulsed fluoroscopy to decrease the dose during video fluoroscopic feeding studies in children? *Clinical Radiology, 64*(1), 70–73.

DeMatteo, C., Matovich, D., & Hjartarson, A. (2005) Comparison of clinical and videofluoroscopic evaluation of children with feeding and swallowing difficulties. *Developmental Medicine and Child Neurology, 47*(3), 149–157.

Hiorns, M. P., & Ryan, M. M. (2006). Current practice in pediatric videofluoroscopy. *Pediatric Radiology, 36*(9), 911–919.

Logemann, J. (1983). *Evaluation and treatment of swallowing disorders.* San Diego, CA: College-Hill Press.

Logemann, J. (1986). *Manual for the videofluorographic study of swallowing.* Boston, MA: Little, Brown.

Logemann, J. (1993). *Manual for the videofluorographic study of swallowing* (2nd ed.). Austin, TX: Pro-Ed.

McNair, J., & Reilly, S. (2007). *The pros and cons of videofluoroscopic assessment of swallowing in children. Database of Abstracts of Reviews of Effects (DARE) (Centre for Reviews and Dissemination).* Retrieved February 20, 2012, from http://www.crd.york.ac.uk/CRDWeb/ShowRecord.asp?ID=12005005019

Morgan, A. T. (2010). Dysphagia in childhood traumatic brain injury: A reflection on the evidence and its implications for practice. *Developmental Neurorehabilitation, 13*(3), 192–203.

Morris, S. E., & Klein, M. D. (2000). *Pre-feeding skills* (2nd ed.). San Antonio, TX. Therapy Skill Builders.

National Institute of Clinical Excellence (NICE). (2007, September). *Triage, assessment, investigation and early management of Head Injury in infants, children and adults.* NICE Guidelines.

O'Donoghue, S., & Bagnall, A. (1999). Videofluoroscopic evaluation in the assessment of swallowing disorders in pediatric and adult populations. *Folia Phoniatrica et Logopaedica, 51*(4–5), 158–171 .

Otapowicz, D., Sobaniec, W., Okurowska-Zawada, B., Artemowicz, B., Sendrowski, K., Brockowski, L., & Kuzia-Smiqieska, J. (2010). Dysphagia in children with infantile cerebral palsy. *Advances in Medical Science, 55*(2), 222–227.

Rosenbek, J. C., Robbins, J. A., Roecker, E. B., Coyle, J. L., & Wood, J. L. (1996). A penetration-aspiration scale. *Dysphagia, 11*(2), 93–98.

SCoR. Society and College of Radiographers. (2005). *The child and the law: The roles and responsibilities of the radiographer.* London, UK: SCoR.

SCoR. Society and College of Radiographers. (2009). *Practice standards for the imaging of children and young people.* London, UK: SCoR.

Splaingard, M. L., Hutchins, B., Sulton, L. D. & Chaudhuri, G. (1998). Aspiration in rehabilitation patients: Videofluoroscopy vs. bedside clinical assessment. *Archives of Physical Medicine and Rehabilitation, 69*(8), 637–640.

Tuchman, D., & Walter, R. (Eds). (1994). *Disorders of feeding and swallowing in infants and children*. San Diego, CA: Singular.

Weir, K. A., McMahon, S. M., Long, G., Bunch, J. A., Pandeya, N., Coakley, K. S., & Chang, A. B. (2007). Radiation doses to children during modified barium swallow studies. *Pediatric Radiology, 3*, 283–290.

Zammit-Maempel, I., Chapple, C. & Leslie, P. (2007). Radiation dose in videofluoroscopic swallow studies. *Dysphagia, 22*(1), 13–15.

Chapter

12

VIDEOFLUOROSCOPY IN LEARNING DISABILITIES

Tracy Lazenby-Paterson and Hannah Crawford

INTRODUCTION

In the United Kingdom, the collective terms "learning disabilities" (LD) or "intellectual disabilities" (ID), refer to individuals with intellectual impairment (IQ of 70 or below) combined with a reduced ability to understand and process information, learn and develop new skills, and function independently. For a diagnosis of LD to apply, there should be evidence of these disabilities having a consistent and long-term impact on development since birth or early childhood (Department of Health [DoH], 2001; Scottish Executive, 2000).

It is estimated that approximately a million people in the U.K. (2% of the general population) have LD, and that incidence and prevalence of the LD population will continue to rise at the same rates as the general population (Emerson & Hatton, 2008). The causes of LD are numerous and complex, resulting in a heterogeneous population of individuals with a wide range of symptoms and conditions. LD can be caused before birth (e.g., chromosomal conditions, inherited condi-

tions, maternal infections, metabolic disorders), around birth (e.g., hypoxia, perinatal illness), and after birth (e.g., childhood illness, acquired brain injury). Down's syndrome and cerebral palsy are the most common specific causes of LD (NHS Health Scotland, 2004); however, many children and adults are diagnosed with LD for which the cause is unknown. People with LD suffer from a variety of conditions and disorders that impact on their health and quality of life. Dysphagia is a particular concern for health professionals as it is an important risk factor in the development of respiratory illness, which is the leading cause of death among people with LD (Cooper, Melville, & Morrison, 2004; Day, Strauss, Shavelle, & Reynolds, 2005; Langmore et al., 1998; National Patient Safety Agency, 2004)

Hollins, Attard, von Fraunhofer, McGuigan, and Sedgwick (1998) found that out of 2000 individuals with LD, 52% died of respiratory disease, contrasting with 32% of the general population who reportedly die of the same condition. Tyrer and McGrother (2009) also report that one of the most common causes of death in people with LD is respiratory disease, five times more common than in the general population. In addition, 45% of people with LD who died in their study had a diagnosis of Down's syndrome.

Glover and Ayub (2010) report similar findings that people with LD have a shorter life expectancy than the general population, and that respiratory illness including pneumonia and pneumonitis is the principal immediate cause of death in people with LD across all age ranges. Lung damage caused by aspiration of solids, liquids, and other foreign bodies was implicated in 14% of deaths in people with LD in their study, relative to just over 2% in the general population. In 60% of cases where the cause of death was aspiration of solids or liquids, dysphagia was also mentioned. Within the LD group, 22% of people who died from these conditions had cerebral palsy.

PREVALENCE AND PATHOPHYSIOLOGY

Although prevalence rates of dysphagia in adults with LD are unknown, estimates range from 36 to 74% (Field, Garland, & Williams, 2003; Hickman & Jenner, 1997; Rogers et al., 1994) and can reach as high as 99% in specific diagnostic groups such as cerebral palsy (Calis, Veugelers, Sheppard, Tibboel, Evenhuis, & Penning, 2008).

Dysphagia and its life-threatening sequelae, including malnutrition, dehydration, obesity, and upper airway obstruction, are widely considered to be more common in individuals with LD than in the general population (Carter & Jancar, 1983; Chadwick & Joliffe, 2009; Chadwick, Joliffe, & Goldbart, 2003; Martin et al., 1994; Stewart, 2003).

There is no common pathophysiology of dysphagia in people with LD. Functional changes in the eating, drinking, and swallowing mechanism vary widely due to the various

causes of LD and the multiple co-morbidities frequently observed in this population. Nonetheless, the literature reports dysphagia to be associated with certain conditions and developmental disabilities more frequently than others, notably cerebral palsy (CP), and Down's syndrome (DS) given the psychomotor impairments associated with these conditions. These patient groups also often suffer from multiple comorbidities such as cardiopulmonary problems, neurological conditions, for example, delayed and disordered neurological development, seizure disorders, Alzheimer's neuropathology, as well as anatomical anomalies, for example, craniofacial abnormalities, abnormal tone of the oropharyngeal musculature, scoliosis, and kyphosis, that are all associated with a higher prevalence of dysphagia (Field et al., 2003).

People with CP have a significant risk for dysphagia given the extent of their neuromotor dysfunction. Dysphagia occurs in the majority of children with CP and persists throughout adulthood. The most profound oropharyngeal problems are associated with greater severity and type of motor impairment (quadriplegia) and greater degree of intellectual impairment. In addition the higher prevalence of epilepsy in this population impacts significantly on psychomotor development, that is, the acquisition of skills pertaining to mental activities and motor movements (Calis et al., 2008; Otapowicz et al., 2010).

Dysphagia signs frequently observed in CP include problems with sucking, swallowing, chewing, retaining food/drink in the mouth (Figure 12–1), oral hypersensitivity, loss of saliva, coughing, vomiting, and abnormal reflexes that interfere with eating, drinking, and swallowing. A large majority of people with CP are also known to present with chronic gastrointestinal problems such as gastroesophageal reflux disease (GERD), as a consequence of psychomotor dysfunction and dysmotility (Del Giudice et al., 1999). Field

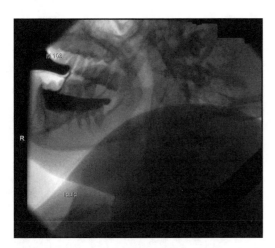

Figure 12–1. *Difficulties highlighted in the oral phase, with poor tongue control and an inability to form a controlled liquid bolus. Liquid is pooling under the tongue.*

et al. (2003) found that GERD was associated with a higher prevalence of dysphagia than in children with other types of gastrointestinal problems.

People with DS are also commonly known to suffer from dysphagia due to the abnormal structure and function of the eating, drinking and swallowing mechanism that are inherent to their syndrome. Their typical craniofacial characteristics (underdeveloped maxilla, protruding mandible, seemingly large tongue relative to the smallness of the oral cavity), combined with systemic low tone frequently lead to tongue protrusion, mouth breathing, upper airway obstruction, malocclusion (poor contact between the upper and lower teeth), and poor coordination of breathing and swallowing (Boston & Rutter, 2003; Lewis & Kritzinger, 2004; Mitchell, Call, & Kelly, 2003; Nargozian, 2004; Oliveira, Paiva, Campos, & Czeresnia, 2008).

Dysphagia problems commonly reported in people with DS include inadequate chewing and subsequent swallowing of food whole (Hennequin, Allison, Faulks, Orliaguet, & Feine, 2005), loss of food and saliva out of the mouth (N'Gom & Woda, 2002), problems coordinating breathing and swallowing (Mitchell et al., 2003), delayed initiation of the pharyngeal swallow (Frazier & Friedman, 1996), and esophageal motor disorders (Wallace, 2007). In addition, many illnesses commonly observed in DS such as congenital heart disease, dental disease, pulmonary conditions, and GERD can also severely impact on the swallowing process (Bittles, Bower, Hussain, & Glasson, 2006; Kerins, Petrovic, Bruder, & Gruman, 2007; Zárate, Mearin, Hidalgo, & Malagelada, 2001). It is also well recognized that aging adults with DS are at increased risk of developing Alzheimer's disease (AD) at an earlier age than the general population (Bush & Beail, 2004; Lott & Head, 2001). Studies have shown early onset of AD in 40% of DS adults by the age of 60, while evidence of the neuropathology in AD can be seen in most people with DS by 40 years of age (Holland, Huppert, Stevens, & Watson, 1998; Malamud, 1964). See Chapter 13, Dementia for a more detailed examination of the impact that dementia has on eating, drinking, and swallowing.

Various studies report that the higher prevalence of *Helicobacter pylori* seropositivity (the bacteria responsible for most ulcers and many cases of chronic gastritis) and GERD in people with LD is linked to the significantly higher rates of gastric cancer and oesophageal cancer observed than in the general population (Duff, Scheepers, Cooper, Hoghton, & Baddeley, 2001; Morad, Merrick, & Nasri, 2002 ; Scheepers, Duff, Baddeley, Cooper, Hoghton, & Harrison, 2000; Wallace, 2007). Maladaptive mealtime behaviors can also interfere with the eating and drinking process. Behaviors such as *cramming* (forcing excessive amounts of food into the mouth at once) and *bolting* (eating extremely quickly) are common in adults with LD and are associated with increased risk of asphyxiation (Samuels & Chadwick, 2006).

Dysphagia is also known to occur as a side effect of many medications. Polypharmacy (the concomitant use of multiple drugs) and the overprescribing of medication in the treatment of adults with LD is a widely reported problem that needs careful monitoring (Royal College of Nursing, 2010). Although many people with LD have multiple conditions for which medication is necessary, the literature also frequently reports the inappropriate prescribing of certain medications such as antipsychotics for the treatment of challenging behavior, despite an absence of any indicating mental health problem (Robertson, Emerson, Gregory, Hatton, Kessissoglou, & Hallam, 2000). The side effects of many of the these medications include dry mouth (xerostomia), compromised immunity, reduced voluntary muscle control for chewing and swallowing, oral hygiene problems, movement disorders, and irritation and injury to the esophageal mucosa (Al-Shehri, 2002; Gallagher & Naidoo, 2009). The use of neuroleptic medication (drugs with a sedative effect, used to treat psychotic conditions) has been associated with over 50% increased risk of pneumonia particularly in the elderly population (Knol, van Marum, Jansen, Souverein, Schobben, & Egberts, 2008)

As the life expectancy of people with LD continues to improve, individuals are likely to experience many of the same age-related conditions associated with dysphagia and changes in the structure, strength, coordination and sensitivity of the swallowing mechanism as members of the general elderly population (Achem & DeVault 2005; Fucile, Wright, Chan, Yee, Langlais, & Gisel, 1998; Jaradeh, 1994; Schindler & Kelly, 2002; see Chapter 7, The Normal Aging Swallow). Aging per se has little functional impact on eating, drinking, and swallowing, as typically healthy adults can compensate effectively for any age-related changes by increasing functional output. Nonetheless, swallowing problems in older persons are common due to a higher prevalence of concomitant illnesses and chronic conditions in the elderly (Kawashima, Motohashi, & Fujishima, 2004). Adults with learning disabilities are already likely to suffer from a range of co-morbid conditions that impact on eating, drinking, and swallowing from an early age. Therefore, their risk of developing swallowing problems with age is likely to be far higher than in healthy aging adults, as they will experience diminished functional reserve and age-related conditions in the same way as the rest of the elderly population, but in addition to their already presenting difficulties.

CLINICAL PRESENTATION

The clinical presentation of dysphagia in this client group is similar to that in other client groups, with signs and symptoms observed at oral, pharyngeal, and esophageal levels. Common signs and symptoms tend to be coughing, choking, and oral stage problems such as anterior food and fluid loss from the mouth (Figure 12–2), pocketing food in the cheeks,

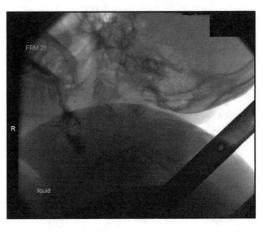

Figure 12–2. *Delayed triggering of the swallow with the bolus filling the pyriform fossae prior to swallow onset.*

and inability to chew food efficiently (NPSA, 2007). Other presentations include behavioral complications at mealtimes such as bolting or cramming food, which is a frequent observation in patients with a history of institutionalized care that increases risk of asphyxiation (Samuels & Chadwick, 2006). What may differ in LD adults relative to the members of the general population is the multitude and higher frequency of co-occurring signs and symptoms associated with dysphagia. Moreover, as with other conditions, dysphagia is at risk of going underreported or misdiagnosed in the ALD population, in part due to complications associated with the self-reporting of symptoms due to communication problems, and the reliance on caregivers who may not know the patient well enough to provide essential information (DoH, 2001).

For the adult with learning disabilities, dysphagia is rarely a "new" presentation. Difficulties tend to be chronic, and request for support may be for a variety of reasons, such as a new member of staff joining the team and being concerned about dysphagic symptoms, a significant choking event, or a recent change or deterioration in skills. When considering dysphagia in this population it is important to recognize that the patient's baseline skills are not likely be the same as those of the general population, and that he or she may always have had some level of dysphagia but has coped well with compensatory strategies and little to no adverse consequences. For this reason, a thorough case history and clinical swallowing examination (see Chapter 2, Alternative Investigations) are essential in the first instance to identify whether dysphagia is actually causing significant problems. Chronic dysphagia alone is insufficient to indicate a videofluoroscopy; it should not be performed exclusively to identify aspiration if there are no reported chest infections, no concerns about weight loss or malnutrition, no dehydration, and no reported or observed distress in the patient. The following case study illustrates that the identification of aspiration alone provides only limited information about pathology and prognosis, and frequently no information about the functional impact on the health and quality of life of the patient, something that should be at the forefront of patient-centered care.

Case Study 1

Mr. A is an adult with learning disabilities and an undiagnosed progressive neurological condition. He coughs frequently during mealtimes, sometimes severe bouts of coughing regardless of the texture of food or drink. Although the SLP suspected that airway penetration was the cause, Mr. A suffered no distress from the coughing, has suffered no periods of ill health, has a healthy and stable weight, and is content with his current diet supported by his staff group. Referral to videofluoroscopy was to confirm SLP suspicions of airway penetration as the cause, and to provide objective feedback for support staff who continued to believe that Mr. A's coughing was a consequence of his intentional and manipulative behavior. The VFSS findings confirmed airway penetration; however, the clinicians who conducted the VFSS had very little experience or background information on Mr. A, and therefore additionally recommended that he would likely require gastrostomy feeding in the near future. This overcautious and inappropriate recommendation was a direct result of a lack of sufficient baseline information about Mr. A, and the purposes for VFSS. Several years later, Mr. A continues to enjoy a full oral diet and is supported by a staff group with a better understanding of his symptoms and his needs.

Dysphagic presentation in learning disabilities is also frequently complicated by poor oral health and hygiene (Cumella, Ransford, Lyons, & Burnham, 2000; Tiller, Wilson, & Gallagher, 2001). This can include decayed or missing teeth, infected gums, or oral thrush

(Royal College of Surgeons of England, 2003). Langmore et al. (1998) report that dysphagia alone is insufficient to predict aspiration pneumonia, whereas the key predictors for aspiration pneumonia were poor oral hygiene, dependency on other people for oral care and having a number of decayed teeth. Subsequent studies confirm the association between poor oral hygiene, harmful bacteria, and the development of aspiration pneumonia (Abe, Ishihara, Adachi, & Okuda, 2008). Therefore, poor oral health in adults with LD generally leads to a higher risk of developing aspiration pneumonia than the general healthy population.

THE ROLE OF VFSS IN THE IDENTIFICATION AND MANAGEMENT OF DYSPHAGIA IN ALD

Videofluoroscopy should be a theory driven adjunct to dysphagia assessment, prior to which a comprehensive case history including breadth and depth of noninstrumental clinical assessment data is essential. Assessment should not focus exclusively on clinical presentation or pathophysiology of the swallow, given that many patients with learning disabilities may present with what appears to be a disordered or abnormal swallow on videofluoroscopy but one that is functional and may cause no serious difficulties. An individual with LD may even display chronic aspiration or silent aspiration on videofluoroscopy, but at the same time not show any negative symptoms or distress. Their clinical history might suggest few to no episodes of chest illness. This may occur because the patient with LD often learns to compensate for their atypical anatomy and physiology and adapt to their dysphagia through postures, positions, and techniques that might appear unusual or even dangerous to the general pop-

ulation. In addition, oral health, positioning, and safe feeding techniques may be supported by experienced and familiar caregivers, which would reduce the risk of chest infections. The clinician's main concerns should center on the ultimate and most serious consequences of the dysphagia, that being respiratory illness. Other considerations following this should include inadequate hydration and nutrition, and distress to the patient.

In order for videofluoroscopy to be useful, the assessing clinician should have a hypothesis and a clear rationale for examination, with the aim of VFSS providing additional information to influence future management. If the hypothesis is to determine whether an individual aspirates on fluids due to coughing at every mealtime, but the patient is not able to follow instructions to modify his/her position and the family and patient will not consider texture modification as a treatment option, the SLP must consider carefully whether a videofluoroscopy is still indicated. In addition, if the assessing clinician does not know the client well, any treatment options in relation to the VFSS findings should be determined and discussed with the client, family and/or carers as well as the community/treating SLP.

Case Study 2

Miss B is 25 years old, with a very low weight and history of chest infections since childhood. She presents with both oral and pharyngeal dysphagia on clinical assessment. She has difficulty with lip closure, chewing, and losing food and fluid from her mouth. She presents with tongue protrusion on presentation of a food bolus and appears to have a delayed swallow trigger, tending to cough on all consistencies. The SLP suggests that videofluoroscopy may show reduced tongue elevation and lateral movement, reduced tongue base movement, reduced pharyngeal wall con-

traction, and reduced laryngeal elevation and closure. She hypothesizes that this will result in food and fluid loss from the mouth, residue in the oral cavity, reduced bolus movement in the oral cavity, residue in the valleculae at the laryngeal inlet, aspiration during swallow, and residue on the pharyngeal walls. Within a multidisciplinary meeting the SLP discusses concerns with the team (care staff, occupational therapist, physiotherapist, dietitian, physician, nurse, and psychologist) and family as her advocate, that Miss B's swallowing difficulties prevent her from safely taking on board adequate food and fluid. Treatment options and prognosis are discussed. Miss B's family report that they feel eating and drinking is very distressing for her, that she takes no pleasure in eating and drinking and they would like the team to consider gastrostomy support for her if this is confirmed by the videofluoroscopy. Under these circumstances the SLP agrees to make the referral and the x-ray goes ahead (Figure 12–3).

Ensuring the best outcome from videofluoroscopy is about putting assessment observations into a context of a whole person rather than simply using the x-ray snapshot to inform future management. As such it is particularly relevant for the treating SLP to be present at the examination if they are not

the SLP directing the exam. In such cases, collaboration between both SLPs is essential to discuss the theory that has been developed through clinical assessment, and plan how the exam will be conducted.

Case Study 3

Ms. S is 32 and has complex physical and learning disabilities. She lives at home with her mother. Ms. S has been prescribed thickener to attempt to reduce coughing on thin liquids in the past but her mother does not believe she likes it and therefore rarely uses it. Ms. S suffers from recurrent chest infections and more recently has suffered from pneumonia. The treating SLP is concerned because Ms. S coughs on normal fluids, and displays signs of distress such as crying and eye watering. She observes that Ms. S has significantly impaired tongue function which means she is not able to control normal fluids in her oral cavity, likely resulting in aspiration before the swallow is triggered. The treating SLP refers Ms. S for videofluoroscopy but does not attend the exam. It is performed by the SLP and the radiologist based in the hospital, both of whom had never previously met Ms. S or her mother. On videofluoroscopy Ms. S displays limited oral control of fluids however a swallow is triggered at the level of the pyriform sinuses and no aspiration occurs. With little knowledge of Ms. S's clinical history, the radiologist and hospital SLP assess that she is safe to continue drinking normal fluids and tell mother that thickener is no longer needed.

Although Ms. S's presentation on videofluoroscopy matches the treating SLP's observations, on the occasion of the assessment, she did not aspirate. Had the treating SLP been present she would have been able to discuss Ms. S's habitual presentation. Recommendations and repeat assessments may have been made more appropriately, incorporating the potential risk relative to her presenting symptoms. In this particular case

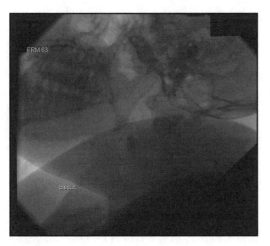

Figure 12–3. Pre-swallow laryngeal penetration.

Ms. S continued to display coughing and distress on fluids, requiring repeat videofluoroscopy assessment 6 months later.

The rationale for videofluoroscopy may also be to support family or carers with implementing recommendations (Royal College of Speech and Language Therapists, 2006). Videofluoroscopy findings can prove to be a useful tool to provide comprehensive and objective visual feedback. The SLP may be very clear as to the nature and consequence of dysphagia, and recommended intervention, but family or carers may find the information difficult to follow, or there may be a great deal of conflict about the appropriate intervention. Used in this way, it can help facilitate discussion about the exact nature of a patient's dysphagia, the potential health risks and appropriate intervention.

In a very few cases, where the clinical picture is unclear, videofluoroscopy may be used to rule out dysphagia in lieu of other conditions, for example, reflux, or mechanical disorders such as achalasia:

Case Study 4

Mr. P is a 55-year-old man with moderate learning disabilities. He is not able to describe his condition in relation to his eating and drinking and has been assessed as not having capacity to consent to assessment and treatment of his eating and drinking. Mr. P is reported to suffer from recurrent chest infections, and he experiences severe choking episodes that require first aid intervention. He sometimes coughs on food and drink. Mr. P's support staff are very concerned that he has severe dysphagia, and as a result have restricted Mr. P to pureed foods in an attempt to prevent choking, also requesting thickener for fluids. On clinical assessment Mr. P appears to have an unimpaired swallow. However, he was referred for a videofluoroscopy to rule out oropharyngeal dysphagia and assess for any signs of

possible esophageal dysphagia. Videofluoroscopy confirmed that Mr. P did not have any form of oral or pharyngeal dysphagia but he displayed marked esophageal dysmotility and gross spontaneous reflux. Further tests following VFSS also revealed a large ulcerated hiatus hernia and Barrett's esophagus.

ETHICAL DILEMMAS

As with the treatment of any other patient group, the rationale for x-ray examination must provide new information and future benefit to the management of the patient in order to justify exposure to radiation (DoH, 2000). The assessing clinician has additional factors to consider for the patient with learning disabilities who is likely to have difficulties fully understanding and consenting to treatment. A thorough preassessment of the patient's needs and challenges should be conducted beforehand to maximize the patient's understanding and compliance and reduce potential distress (Scottish Parliament, 2000; U.K. Parliament, 2005) However, many adults with learning disabilities will still be unable to understand the purpose and implications of assessment, therefore the decision to proceed or not proceed with videofluoroscopy must have a sound rationale backed by an evidence-based model (Sacket et al, 1996), and with the patient's best interests in mind (see Chapter 3).

It is also important to note that people with LD frequently suffer discrimination in the health care setting and as a consequence are excluded from essential treatment or assessment. Issues such as diagnostic overshadowing and assumed noncompliance due to behaviors perceived as challenging are factors that continue to prevent many people with LD from accessing health services (DoH, 2008; Mencap, 2007; NHS Health Scotland, 2004). It is important to avoid the presumption that people with LD will not cope with the assessment environment simply because they have a diagnosis of learning disabilities or challenging behaviors. Many individuals have no difficulty complying with instrumental assessment if the right adaptations are put in place to account for their needs. If videofluoroscopy is clinically indicated, then there must be a clear and evidenced rationale for why it might not be offered to the LD patient.

MODIFICATIONS OF TECHNIQUE

Once videofluoroscopy is chosen as an appropriate assessment for a patient with LD, several considerations must be taken into account in order to ensure the maximum amount of useful clinical information will be gathered with the minimum amount of exposure to radiation. Clinicians must be prepared to be flexible in their approaches according to the needs of each individual. Many adults with LD have structural and postural conditions that prevent the use of conventional seating, therefore mobile units must be used to accommodate for a person's own wheelchair or specialized seating. At the same time, specialized head rests and neck supports may obscure a lateral view on x-ray, as will structural abnormalities and conditions affecting the patient such as kyphosis and scoliosis. Some patients may be unable to sit still, and may rock or move about unintentionally during assessment. LD clients are frequently very sensitive to changes in their routine and environment, and as a result they may become distractible or distressed in clinical environments. This, in turn, may impact on their swallowing performance under examination. It may be necessary to provide a slightly longer time slot to allow for familiarization with the x-ray suite,

or for positioning in the equipment when an individual has a wheelchair that is difficult to place (Mencap, 2004). A preplanned visit to the suite in conjunction with photos of the environment and radiography staff can help the person with LD predict and adapt to the strange environment more readily. In addition, the vast majority of people with LD suffer from difficulties with expression and comprehension (Enderby & Davis, 1989), impacting on their ability to follow and comply with instructions and self-report symptoms. It is essential that the VFSS clinician has thorough and advance background knowledge of a patient's communication system and that he or she carefully weighs performance on videofluoroscopy against baseline information about eating, drinking, and swallowing function provided by caregivers, families, and health professionals who know the patient very well.

People with LD require structure, routine and predictability in their environments in order to maximize understanding and minimize distress. These can be improved for the videofluoroscopy exam by providing the patient with the first clinic appointment of the day or at times where a delay is unlikely, thus avoiding a prolonged and unpredictable stay in the waiting room. Clinicians can help adults with LD better understand their environment and predict what will happen next by employing what is familiar to them, for example, using their own food, specialized utensils, prompts, and seating, and inviting family members or carers with whom the patient is familiar and comfortable to feed and provide information and support. An approach that is familiar to the patient with LD is likely to reduce anxiety and distress and in turn allow for the most representative account possible. For the many people with LD who have hypersensitivities, sound and lighting levels must also be taken into account. Being informed of a patient's needs prior to videofluoroscopy can allow for the clinician to prepare the environment and clinical approach to the best of their ability and thus maximize the chance of a successful and representative assessment. One way of achieving this is through robust communication between hospital and community services, often through a LD hospital liaison nurse who can facilitate communication among staff and caregivers, and ensure that all information is provided to clinicians in advance of assessment.

Frequently, there is a limit to the type and number of environmental alterations that can be realistically achieved in the videofluoroscopy clinic; however, clinicians should still endeavor to achieve as suitable an environment whenever possible. Although videofluoroscopy does not yet follow a universally standardized protocol, it should aim to be systematic and repeatable, even if a modified approach is frequently the best we can do under presenting circumstances.

CONCLUSION

It is important to consider that LD is a label that describes a complex heterogeneous group, where there is no clear pattern of dysphagia or its underlying causes. In addition, multiple health conditions and co-morbidities are common. Dysphagia and its secondary impact, such as respiratory illness, malnutrition, dehydration, distress, and ultimately death, are significant issues in this group. It is often necessary to work within a framework of 'best interests' where a patient has limited capacity to make their own decisions. The clinician should ensure they adhere to statutory mental capacity guidance and work closely with the patient, their family and the multidisciplinary team. The clinician must always be sure that there is a clear clinical rationale for conducting VFSS, but where the impact of dysphagia is

apparent, a VFSS clearly would be indicated. In developing a rationale for VFSS, the clinician must ensure a detailed, extensive case history and clinical assessment are performed, in order to carry out a theory driven systematic examination with clear and functional outcomes and inform future patient management. Under these circumstances the VFSS with adults with learning disabilities is a valuable clinical tool which has considerable utility in evidence-based, individualized patient management.

REFERENCES

Abe, S., Ishihara, K., Adachi, M., & Okuda, K. (2008) Tongue-coating as risk indicator for aspiration pneumonia in edentate elderly. *Archives of Gerontology and Geriatrics, 47*, 267–275.

Achem, S., & DeVault, K. (2005) Dysphagia in aging. *Journal of Clinical Gastroenterology 39*(5), 357–371.

Al-Shehri, & Ali Maeed (2002) Dysphagia as a drug side effect. *Internet Journal of Otorhinolaryngology, 1*(2). Retrieved June 15, 2011, from http://www.ispub.com/journal/the_internet _journal_of_otorhinolaryngology/volume1_ number_2_47/article_printable/dysphagia_as _a_drug_side_effect.html

Bittles, A. H., Bower, C., Hussain, R., & Glasson, E. J. (2006) The four ages of Down syndrome. *European Journal of Public Health, 17*(2), 221–225.

Boston, M., & Rutter, M. (2003) Current airway management in craniofacial anomalies. *Current Opinions in Otolaryngology-Head Neck Surgery, 11*, 428–432.

Bush, A., & Beail, N. (2004) Risk factors for dementia in people with Down syndrome: Issues in assessment and diagnosis. *American Journal on Mental Retardation, 109*(2), 83–97.

Calis, E. A., Veugelers, R., Sheppard, J. J., Tibboel, D., Evenhuis, H. M. & Penning, C.(2008) Dysphagia in children with severe generalized cerebral palsy and intellectual disability. *Developmental Medicine and Child Neurology, 50(8), 625–630.

Carter, G., & Jancar, J. (1983) Mortality in the mentally handicapped: A 50 year survey at the Stoke Park group of hospitals (1930–1980). *Journal of Mental Deficiency Research, 27,* 143–156.

Chadwick, D., & Joliffe, J. (2009) A descriptive investigation of dysphagia in adults with intellectual disabilities. *Journal of Intellectual Disability Research, 53*(1), 29–43.

Chadwick, D., Joliffe, J., & Goldbart, J. (2003) Adherence to eating and drinking guidelines for adults with intellectual disabilities and dysphagia. *American Journal on Mental Retardation, 108*(3), 202–211.

Cooper, S. A., Melville, C., & Morrison, J. (2004) People with intellectual disabilities — their health needs differ and need to be recognised and met. *British Medical Journal, 329,* 414–415.

Cumella, S., Ransford, N., Lyons, J., & Burnham, H. (2000) Needs for oral care among people with intellectual disability not in contact with Community Dental Services. *Journal of Intellectual Disability Research, 44*(1), 45–52.

Day, S., Strauss, D. J., Shavelle, R. M., & Reynolds, R. J. (2005) Mortality and causes of death in persons with Down syndrome in California. *Developmental Medicine and Child Neurology, 47,* 171–176.

Del Giudice, E., Staiano, A., Capano, G., Romano, A., Florimonte, L., Miele, E., . . . Crisanti, A. F. (1999) Gastrointestinal manifestations in children with cerebral palsy. *Brain Development, 21*(5), 307–311.

Department of Health. (2000). *The Ionising Radiation (Medical Exposure) Regulations.* London, UK: Department of Health.

Department of Health. (2001). *Valuing People. A new strategy for learning disability for the 21st Century.* London, UK: Department of Health.

Department of Health. (2008). *Healthcare for all: Report of the independent inquiry into access to healthcare for people with learning disabilities.* London, UK: Department of Health.

Duff, M., Scheepers, M., Cooper, M., Hoghton, M., & Baddeley, P. (2001) Helicobacter pylori: Has the killer escaped from the institution? A possible cause of increased stomach cancer in a population with intellectual disability. *Journal of Intellectual Disability Research, 45*(3), 219–225.

Emerson, E., & Hatton, C. (2008). *People with learning disabilities in England.* Centre for Disability Research Report. Lancaster, UK: Lancaster University.

Enderby, P., & Davies, P. (1989). Communication disorders: Planning a service to meet the needs. *British Journal of Disorders of Communication, 24,* 301–331.

Field, D., Garland, M., & Williams, K. (2003). Correlates of specific childhood feeding problems. *Journal of Paediatrics and Child Health, 39,* 299–304.

Frazier, J., & Friedman, B. (1996). Swallow function in children with Down syndrome: A retrospective study. *Developmental Medicine and Child Neurology, 38,* 695–703.

Fucile, S., Wright, P. M., Chan, I., Yee, S., Langlais, M. E., & Gisel, E. G. (1998). Functional oral-motor skills: Do they change with age? *Dysphagia, 13,* 195–201.

Gallagher, L., & Naidoo, P (2009). Prescription drugs and their effects on swallowing. *Dysphagia, 24,* 159–166.

Glover, G., & Ayub, M. (2010). *How people with learning disabilities die.* Improving Health and Lives, Learning Disability Observatory: Department of Health.

Hennequin, M., Allison, P. J., Faulks, D., Orliaguet, T., & Feine, J. (2005) Chewing indicators between adults with Down syndrome and controls. *Journal of Dental Research, 84*(11), 1057–1061.

Hickman, J., & Jenner, L. (1997, Autumn). Adults with learning disabilities and dysphagia: Issues and practice. *Speech and Language Therapy in Practice,* pp. 8–11.

Holland, A. J., Huppert, F., Stevens, F., & Watson, P. (1998). Population-based study of the prevalence and presentation of dementia in adults with Down's syndrome. *British Journal of Psychiatry, 172,* 493–498.

Hollins, S., Attard, M. T., von Fraunhofer, N., McGuigan, S., & Sedgwick, P. (1998) Mortality in people with learning disability: Risks, causes, and death certification findings in London. *Developmental Medicine and Child Neurology, 40*(1), 50–56.

Jaradeh, S. (1994). Neurolophysiology of swallowing in the aged. *Dysphagia, 9*(4), 218–220.

Kawashima, K., Motohashi, Y., & Fujishima, I. (2004) Prevalence of dysphagia among community-dwelling elderly individuals as estimated using a questionnaire for dysphagia screening. *Dysphagia, 19*, 266–271.

Kerins, G., Petrovic, K., Bruder, M. B., & Gruman, C. (2007). Medical conditions and medication use in adults with Down syndrome: A descriptive analysis. *Downs Syndrome Research and Practice, 12*(2), 1–7.

Knol, W., van Marum, R. J., Jansen, P. A. F., Souverein, P. C., Schobben, A. F. A. M., & Egberts, A. C. G. (2008). Antipsychotic drug use and risk of pneumonia in elderly people. *Journal of the American Geriatric Society, 56*, 661–666.

Langmore, S. E., Terpenning, M. S., Schork, A., Chen, Y., Murray, J. T., Lopatin, D., & Loesche, W. J. (1998). Predictors of aspiration pneumonia: How important is dysphagia? *Dysphagia, 13*(2), 69–81.

Lewis, E., & Kritzinger, A. (2004). Parental experiences of feeding problems in their infants with Down syndrome. *Downs Syndrome Research and Practice, 9*(2), 45–52.

Lott, I., & Head, E. (2001). Down syndrome and Alzheimer's dementia: A link between development and aging. *Mental Retardation and Developmental Disabilities Research Reviews, 7*, 172–178.

Malamud, N. (1964). Neuropathology. In H. Stevens & R. Herber (Eds.), *Mental retardation: A review of research* (pp. 429–452). Chicago, IL: University of Chicago Press.

Martin, B., Corlew, M., Wood, H., Olson, D., Golopol, L., Wingo, M., & Kirmani, N. (1994). The association of swallowing dysfunction and aspiration pneumonia. *Dysphagia, 9*(1), 1–6.

Mencap. (2004). *Treat me right! Better healthcare for people with a learning disability.* London, UK: Mencap.

Mencap. (2007). *Death by indifference. Following up the Treat me right! report.* London: Mencap.

Mitchell, R. B., Call, M. S., & Kelly, J. (2003). Ear, nose and throat disorders in children with Down syndrome. *Laryngoscope, 113*, 259–263.

Morad, M., Merrick, J., & Nasri, Y. (2002). Prevalence of Helicobacter pylori in people with intellectual disability in a residential care center in Israel. *Journal of Intellectual Disability Research, 46*(2), 141–143.

N'Gom, P. I., & Woda, A. (2002). Influence of impaired mastication on nutrition. *Journal of Prosthetic Dentistry, 87*, 667–673.

Nargozian, C. (2004) The airway in patients with craniofacial abnormalities. *Pediatric Anesthesia, 14*, 53–59.

National Patient Safety Agency. (2004). *Understanding the patient safety issues for people with learning disabilities.* London, UK: NPSA.

National Patient Safety Agency. (2007). *Problems swallowing? Ensuring safer practice for adults with learning disabilities who have dysphagia.* London, UK: NPSA.

NHS Health Scotland. (2004). *Health needs assessment report. People with learning disabilities in Scotland.* Edinburgh, UK: NHS.

Oliveira, A. C., Paiva, S. M., Campos, M. R., & Czeresnia, D. (2008). Factors associated with malocclusions in children and adolescents with Down syndrome. (Online only). *American Journal of Orthodontics and Dentofacial Orthopedics, 489*, e1–e8. Retrieved June, 15, 2011.

Otapowicz, D., Sobaniec, W., Okurowska-Zawada, B., Artemowicz, B., Sendrowski, K., Kulak, W., Bockowski, L., & Kuzia-Smigielska, J. (2010). Dysphagia in children with infantile cerebral palsy. *Advances in Medical Sciences, 55*(2), 222–227.

Royal College of Nursing. (2010). *Mental health nursing of adults with learning disability.* London, UK: RCN.

Royal College of Speech and Language Therapists. (2006). *Communicating Quality 3.* London, UK: RCSLT.

Royal College of Surgeons of England's Joint Advisory Committee for Special Care Dentistry. (2003). *A case of need. Proposal for a speciality in special care dentistry.* http://www.bsdh.org.uk/misc/ACase4Need.pdf

Robertson, J., Emerson, E., Gregory, N., Hatton, C., Kessissoglou, S., & Hallam, A. (2000). Receipt of psychotropic medication by people with intellectual disability in residential settings. *Journal of Intellectual Disability Research, 44*(6), 666–676.

Rogers, B., Stratton, P., Msall, M., Andres, M., Champlain, M. K., Koerner, P., & Piazza, J.

(1994). Long-term morbidity and management strategies of tracheal aspiration in adults with severe developmental disabilities. *American Journal on Mental Retardation, 4*, 490–498.

Sacket, D. L., Rosenberg, W. M. C., & Gray, J. A. M. (1996). Evidence-based medicine: what it is and what it isn't. *British Medical Journal, 312*, 71–72.

Samuels, R., & Chadwick, D. (2006) Predictors of asphyxiation risk in adults with intellectual disabilities and dysphagia. *Journal of Intellectual Disability Research, 50*(5), 362–370.

Scheepers, M., Duff, M., Baddeley, P., Cooper, M., Hoghton, M., & Harrison J. (2000). Helicobacter pylori and the learning disabled. *British Journal of General Practice, 50*, 813–814.

Schindler, J., & Kelly, J. (2002). Swallowing disorders in the elderly. *Laryngoscope, 112*, 589–602.

Scottish Executive. (2000). *The same as you? A review of services for people with learning disabilities.* Edinburgh, UK: Scottish Executive.

Scottish Parliament. *Adults with Incapacity (Scotland) Act 2000*, asp 4.

Stewart, L. (2003). Development of the Nutrition and Swallowing Checklist, a screening tool for nutrition and swallowing risk in people with intellectual disability. *Journal of Intellectual and Developmental Disability, 28*, 171–187.

Tiller, S., Wilson, K. I., & Gallagher, J. E. (2001). Oral health status and dental service use of adults with learning disabilities living in residential institutions and in the community. *Community Dental Health, 18*(3), 167–171.

Tyrer, F., & McGrother, C. (2009) Cause-specific mortality and death certificate reporting in adults with moderate to profound intellectual disability. *Journal of Intellectual Disability Research, 53*(11), 898–904.

U. K. Parliament. *Mental capacity act 2005* (c.9).

Wallace, R. A. (2007). Clinical audit of gastrointestinal conditions occurring among adults with Down syndrome attending a specialist clinic. *Journal of Intellectual and Developmental Disability, 32*, 45–50.

Zárate, N., Mearin, F., Hidalgo, A., & Malagelada, J. R. (2001). Prospective evaluation of esophageal motor dysfunction in Down's syndrome. *American Journal of Gastroenterology, 96*(6), 1718–1724.

Chapter

13

DEMENTIA

Pamela A. Smith and Paula Leslie

INTRODUCTION

Dementia is not a medical diagnosis but a clinical syndrome made up of constellations of symptoms. The syndrome is caused by a number of medical diagnoses. How the swallow function and/or nutritional status is affected depends on the specific pathophysiology of a case. Determination of the underlying medical condition is an important piece of the decision making process in managing dysphagia in patients with dementia. Symptoms of dementia include memory impairment plus at least one of the following disturbances in cognitive functioning: **agnosia** (difficulty with recognition of previously familiar items or objects), **aphasia** (language disturbance), **apraxia** (impairment in motor programming affecting execution of learned motor movements), or **reduction in executive functioning** (higher-level problem solving, and planning and organizational skills) (Mazzoni, Pearson, Rowland, & Merritt, 2006). These deficits must be severe enough to cause impairments in functioning either at home or at work and they must represent a decline from previous levels of functioning (American Psychiatric Association, 2000). The condition is progressive and impairs both intellect and behavior to the point where activities of daily living are affected (Mesulam, 2003). Delirium and depression often mimic dementia, but the course of the conditions differ; hence the need for an accurate medical diagnosis.

Delirium is differentiated from dementia by its identifiable onset date, as compared to the more insidious onset seen in dementia (Adelman & Daly, 2005). Delirium is characterized by reduced levels of alertness/consciousness, and extreme fatigue or reduced arousability can be likely markers for delirium. Cognitive and attention issues may interfere with feeding and possibly swallowing function if alertness is affected to such an extent as to impair motor function. Delirium may be caused by multiple factors, including medication reaction, infections, dehydration and metabolic disturbances. The symptoms decrease when the underlying cause of delirium is identified and controlled (Schuurmans, Duursma, & Shortridge-Baggett, 2001).

Depression can be mistaken for dementia in older individuals because it often leads to vague cognitive loss and disorientation. Affect is typically flatter and responses are more likely to be, "I don't know." Reduced appetite and subsequent nutritional deficits can also be seen. For many institutionalized geriatric patients, eating may become a less pleasurable activity. When dysphagia is also present social isolation is more pronounced and accompanied by lower self-esteem and decreased life satisfaction (Ekberg, Hamdy, Woisard, Wuttge-Hannig, & Ortega, 2002). Depression is under diagnosed in the elderly, particularly the institutionalized elderly, where appropriate management of depression can lead to improvement in symptoms (Fessman & Lester, 2000).

Dementia may be caused by a number of diseases, the most common of which is the irreversible condition of Alzheimer's disease. Some dementias are reversible if the underlying cause of the cognitive loss can be identified and managed. The physician makes the diagnosis of Alzheimer's disease through a sequential process of elimination (Adelman & Daly, 2005) with a firm diagnosis only possible on autopsy.

INCIDENCE

Dementia is a collection of symptoms and not a medical diagnosis, which makes incidence numbers difficult to determine. Individuals living in the community may begin to exhibit signs of cognitive decline without having been diagnosed with any specific disease. Diseases that cause dementia are more common in older people and increased life expectancy worldwide will result in a greater incidence of the diseases and conditions that can lead to dementia. Incidence approaches 10% of adults who are age 65 and older, and up to 50% of those who are older than 90 years of age (Adelman & Daly, 2005). Hopper (2007) reports that up to 5 million people in the United States

have clinically diagnosed Alzheimer's disease, which is the most common cause of dementia. In Canada 8% of the population over the age of 65 are estimated to have either Alzheimer's disease or some other related dementing condition. According to the World Alzheimer's Report (2011) 35.6 million people lived with dementia throughout the world in 2010, and this is expected to increase to 65.7 million by 2030 and 115.4 million by 2050 (Alzheimer's Disease International, 2010). Risk increases with advancing age and a positive family history of the disease and lessens with higher educational levels (Holsinger, Deveau, Boustani, & Williams, 2007; Santacruz & Swagerty, 2001). More frequent identification of even preclinical Alzheimer's disease is expected due to expanded diagnostic criteria including the use of biomarkers in addition to traditional clinical criteria (Jeffrey, 2011).

PATHOPHYSIOLOGY

The pathophysiology of the disease may be different depending on the cause of the dementia. This is important for the clinician's decision-making process as the specific impairments and their expected progression are likely to affect motor/perceptual/cognitive function differently.

Alzheimer's Disease

The pathophysiology of Alzheimer's disease has been described as abnormal growths of proteins within (amyloid plaques) and between (neurofibrillary tangles) neurons. These plaques and tangles lead to a reduction in the production of acetylcholine, leading to reduced neurotransmission and global cognitive deficits (Bayles, 2001; Mann & Yates,

1986). Reduced neurotransmission leads to cell death and the cerebral atrophy commonly seen with advanced Alzheimer's disease. Medications such as cholinesterase inhibitors act to reduce the metabolism of acetylcholine which leads to greater availability of necessary chemicals for neurotransmission (Hogan et al., 2008). Improved neurotransmission over time can lead to slower progression of the disease as "functional disuse" is reduced. Medications do not cure the disease. The symptoms seen with Alzheimer's disease will continue to progress even if trials of medications such as Aricept (Donepezil) appear initially successful.

Vascular Dementia/Multi-Infarct

Multiple small (lacunar) infarctions may lead to a global deterioration of cognitive functioning. Multi-infarct dementia, vascular dementia or vascular cognitive impairment, progresses in a more stepwise manner than Alzheimer's disease (Hachinski et al., 2006). This is due to the relationship of symptom progression to the size of the lesion for each new neurological event. Patients with multi-infarct dementia typically exhibit an underlying medical background consistent with risk for stroke such as hypertension, cardiac conditions, diabetes, and so forth (Duron & Hanon, 2008). Medical management of these patients is largely focused on reducing the risk of additional cerebrovascular events (Hachinski et al., 2006).

Other Diseases

A number of disease processes may lead to progressive cognitive loss. The pattern, rate and progression of such loss is dependent on the individual disease process and motor symptoms may often precede the cognitive

symptoms. Diseases such as multiple sclerosis, Parkinson's disease, and other progressive neurological conditions may lead to a frontal lobe syndrome characterized by declining reasoning and reduced higher level problem solving. Other diseases such as Pick's disease, Huntington's disease, and so forth, also cause dementia, and differential diagnosis by the medical professional is important in understanding the specific disease progression (Adelman & Daly, 2005; Santacruz & Swagerty, 2001).

Sequelae: General

On cursory examination many patients with dementia exhibit similar symptoms ("the patient is confused") but there are similarities and differences across underlying causes.

Cognitive/Behavioral

Patients with a diagnosis of dementia may exhibit a wide variety of cognitive/behavior characteristics, including agitation, apathy, memory loss, and attention problems (Bayles, 2001; Fernandez, Gobartt, & Balana, 2010; Forstl & Kurz, 1999; Mega, Cummings, Fiorello, & Gornbein, 1996). Behavioral disturbances may relate to sensory issues and to motor disturbances that may be misinterpreted by carers. For example, restlessness may be misinterpreted as agitation in patients whose medical diagnosis leads to more motor based responses (Kurlan, Richard, Papka, & Marshall, 2000). Problematic behaviors usually first occur in the moderate stages of Alzheimer's disease (Hopper, 2007). These behavioral impairments do not appear to be a direct result of the neuropathological changes associated with the disease process. Such multifactorial causes complicate the effectiveness of management strategies by carers.

Physiological: Motor

Dementing conditions affect global cortical tissue by different mechanisms so the degree of motor involvement varies by condition. Diagnoses with extrapyramidal symptoms such as Parkinson's disease, dementia with Lewy bodies, and multi-infarct/vascular dementia may be more likely to manifest themselves by motor involvement. Such impairments may affect gross as well as finer motor abilities and may impact functional independence for activities of daily living as well as ambulation (Kurlan et al., 2000).

Physiological: Sensory

The same global cell damage can affect sensory function to varying degrees and depends on which specific cortical cells are involved. For example, patients with dementia exhibit sensory disturbances such as visual perceptual impairments (Binetti et al., 1998) and visual hallucinations are more common in dementia with Lewy bodies (Shinagawa et al., 2009). Patients may have difficulty with perception of objects, particularly against complex backgrounds, and they may be easily distracted by both visual and auditory information.

Metabolic

A growing literature on the impact of metabolic dysfunction on the progression and appropriate care of the patient with dementia has led to discussions about the use of enteral feeding with this population. Central nervous system changes leading to impairments in metabolic function have been identified (Hoffer, 2006). The calorific demands far exceed any that could be supplied. Enteral support was originally designed to be a mechanism of short term nutritional support for patients with a temporary dysphagic condition. The ineffectiveness of using enteral tube feeding for all in order to maintain weight, nutritional status, and skin integrity has been demonstrated repeatedly (Brody, 2000; Finucane, Christmas, & Travis, 1999; Murphy & Lipman, 2003; Post, 2001). Using this information often requires family members to make painful decisions that may be at odds with their cultural beliefs. Families need to understand that the nature of the disease leads to reduced absorption of calories by the body's metabolic system. These disease-related changes mean that no matter which route of nutrition it will eventually not be possible to provide adequate calories to sustain weight. Therefore, the use of tube feeding in this population does not aid in maintaining weight or other nutritional markers.

CLINICAL PRESENTATION

The patient with dementia who also exhibits dysphagia is immediately at higher risk than the typical older institutionalized patient for dehydration, malnutrition, weight loss, and aspiration pneumonia due to the cognitive, sensory, and behavioral sequelae of dementia (Easterling & Robbins, 2008). There are no conclusive data about the prevalence of dysphagia among individuals with dementia because there are many different etiologies that may manifest themselves with varying degrees of functional impairments. Such problems already occur in the older population with their own set of comorbidities. Horner et al. (1994) estimated that 45% of institutionalized patients with dementia have some type of dysphagia (Horner, Alberts, Dawson, & Cook, 1994). Easterling and Robbins (2008) suggest that higher incidences of dysphagia in patients with dementia may be a result of several factors: normal aging and the related physiological changes as well as the various disease processes that occur more frequently in older people and may lead to the dementia itself (Easterling & Robbins, 2008).

Impact on Swallow: Cognitive/Behavioral

Cognitive and behavioral factors can affect willingness and ability to self-feed particularly in later stages of the disease (Correia Sde, Morillo, Jacob Filho, & Mansur, 2010). Patients who are dependent on others for feeding are at higher risk of development of pulmonary complications secondary to aspiration as well as having a reduced immune system response due to malnutrition and dehydration (Langmore et al., 1998). This is particularly true in an institutional setting where carer/resident ratios can reduce the available time for feeding, reducing safety and potentially reducing amount of intake. The resistive or agitated resident may be quite difficult to feed, leading to greater risks of malnutrition and dehydration with simultaneous increase in caloric requirements secondary to increased activity (Easterling & Robbins, 2008). Medications that might be used in the management of behavior have potentially multiple side effects including reduced alertness and responsiveness, xerostomia (dry mouth) leading to difficulty with oral manipulation, pharyngeal transit, and esophageal motility (Hogan et al., 2008).

Impact on Swallow: Motor

Symptoms of dysphagia appear as the dementing medical conditions progress but cortical changes related to swallowing in early stages of Alzheimer's disease have been identified before overt symptoms were noted (Humbert et al., 2010). Patients in the advanced stages of disease may develop difficulty with the process of chewing, leading to the need to manipulate diet consistency and the acceptance of risks that are often associated with sensory changes to the diet (Easterling & Robbins, 2008). In the final stages of the disease, patients have greater levels of physical dependence, increasing the risk for poorer oral hygiene. In the final disease stages reduced activity levels further increase the risk for development of pulmonary complications in the event of aspiration (Easterling & Robbins, 2008).

Patients with Alzheimer's disease show longer oral stage swallow function, delayed pharyngeal response, and inefficient pharyngeal clearance as compared to normal controls (Chouinard, 2000). These behaviors are also seen in the swallows of individuals aging normally but in patients with Alzheimer's disease the swallow abnormalities increase proportionally with dementia severity (Horner et al., 1994).

Patients with Parkinson's disease, which often leads to a frontal lobe dementia syndrome, exhibit a characteristic motor pattern of lingual tremors both at rest and during volitional movement. As the disease progresses these patients often develop other symptoms related to impaired motor functioning, such as reduced hyolaryngeal excursion, reduced upper esophageal opening, and reduced pharyngeal clearance (Easterling & Robbins, 2008). Patients with frontotemporal dementia show a higher occurrence of abnormal oral behaviors affecting bite size and chewing as compared to patients with Alzheimer's disease (Ikeda, Brown, Holland, Fukuhara, & Hodges, 2002). Extrapyramidal signs are also commonly seen in dementia with Lewy bodies which is characterized by visual hallucinations, cognitive fluctuations, and noted sensitivity to, or intolerance of, psychotropic medications (Shinagawa et al., 2009). These patients often exhibit motor based feeding and swallowing problems, such as coughing, choking, delayed initiation, and difficulty managing saliva, to a greater degree than patients with Alzheimer's disease (Shinagawa et al., 2009).

Vascular dementia leads to fewer delays in swallow initiation than in patients with Alzheimer's disease (Suh, Kim, & Na, 2009). Patients with vascular dementia are more likely to exhibit reduced hyolaryngeal excursion, reduced epiglottic inversion and silent aspiration. Patients with vascular dementia may exhibit more motor-based dysfunction whereas patients with Alzheimer's disease exhibit more sensory-based dysfunction (Suh et al., 2009).

Poor positioning often affects feeding and swallowing in people with dementias particularly in the later stages. There can be a loss of integrity of dentition affecting mastication as well as general oral cavity health. Primitive oral reflexes may reappear that interfere with feeding or be misinterpreted as feeding refusal in the case of the tonic bite reflex where sustained jaw closure and increased abnormal tone in the jaw muscles occurs in response to stimulation of the teeth or gums (Correia Sde et al., 2010).

Impact on Swallow: Sensory

In Alzheimer's disease the sense of smell characteristically is impaired due to the proximity of the olfactory system to the medial temporal lobes which are often an early site for reduction in cortical function. Reduction in olfaction typically influences the sense of taste and thus patients in the early stages of dementia often complain that foods no longer taste good or taste different than they are used to. Reduced sensory satisfaction related to smell and taste remove some of the reinforcing factors related to eating and drinking in later stages of the disease. Patients may benefit from flavor enhancing substances such as condiments and appropriate sweeteners. Changes in sensitivity to texture may also affect oral acceptance of foods (Correia Sde et al., 2010).

Patients with semantic dementia and frontotemporal dementia are more likely than those with Alzheimer's disease to develop increased appetite, particularly for sweet foods (Ikeda et al., 2002). Patients with semantic dementia are more likely than were patients with other dementias to attempt to eat nonfoods.

Visual impairment has been reported in the middle stages of dementia which is likely to affect the ability to attend to the task of eating and maintain attention to and appropriate use of the objects required for independent feeding (Correia Sde et al., 2010). In later stages of dementia distraction by utensils is often noted, and the need for either finger foods or assistance in feeding may be required. Clinically, patients with sensory disturbances may have difficulty locating a plate on a table, especially if it is the same color, or have difficulty self-feeding due to visual disturbances. Oral sensory impairments can lead to either reduced or heightened sensation for textures, which affects the patient's willingness to orally manipulate foods.

Impact on Swallow: Metabolic

Chouinard, Lavigne, and Villeneuve (1998) describe a pattern of decline in patients with dementia whereby marked weight loss and dysphagia lead to death from pneumonia. They describe observations that suggest a general reduction in homeostatic mechanisms: the patients developed increased episodes of skin breakdown and protein malabsorption regardless of the use of enteral feeding. Catabolic processes that lead to muscle wasting as a direct result of the disease process potentially limit the benefit of nutritional supplementation (Royal College of Physicians and British Society of Gastroenterology, 2010).

ROLE OF VFSS IN THE MANAGEMENT OF THIS PATIENT GROUP

Management of Dysphagia: Influences on Assessment

For a patient with dysphagia secondary to a dementing condition, an understanding of the components of a practical management plan helps to drive an appropriate evaluation procedure. Management for patients with progressive diseases differs markedly from plans of care for patients with diagnoses in which there is potential for recovery. Given what is known about motor, sensory, cognitive, and metabolic changes associated with dementing diseases, it is generally not in the patient's best interest to undergo artificial nutrition and hydration as a long term method of nutritional intake. Best outcomes for management of these patients typically involve the continued use of oral feeding (Gillick, 2000). Motor, sensory, and cognitive impairments can be managed through environmental manipulations, such as reducing distractions while eating, providing 1:1 assistance, frequent redirection and reassurance, and through establishment of patient-specific feeding techniques, thereby preserving the use of hand feeding as the primary means of nutritional intake. Nasogastric and surgically placed feeding tubes involve greater risk than potential benefit for patients with dementia advanced to the point where dysphagia is problematic (Finucane et al., 1999; Royal College of Physicians and British Society of Gastroenterology, 2010).

Appropriate assessment techniques must be considered with regard to the potential management plans and focus on gathering relevant information. Given these management principles the use of videofluoroscopy must be carefully considered for the evaluation of a patient with advanced dementia. This should not be construed as an abandonment of these patients nor a disregard for their very real problems. The goal of an assessment is to establish the highest level of functioning which the patient with dementia might be capable of achieving (ASHA, 2005a, 2005b).

Professional guidelines for the use of instrumental assessment state that assessment is only appropriate where it is likely to result in a change in the management plan for a particular patient. It is not likely that a patient with advanced dementia will be able to make use of independent postures, maneuvers, or swallow strategies. Determination of aspiration itself is never the main objective of a videofluoroscopic swallow study. Outcome data for patients with advanced dementia do not support the routine placement of tubes for feeding so this consideration needs careful justification (Finucane et al., 1999; Gillick, 2000; Murphy & Lipman, 2003).

Intervention for patients with dementia is likely to vary by stage and by underlying medical cause. For most patients with an acute onset of an illness the goal of treatment is recovery. This generally is not a reasonable objective for the patient with an irreversible, progressive medical condition. In such cases compensation and/or palliation are often more appropriate avenues of treatment. Patients in the early stages of a disease leading to dementia are not likely to exhibit overt symptoms of dysphagia but as the underlying disease progresses, symptoms of swallowing difficulty are likely to increase. As disease progresses, end stage patients are more likely to exhibit behavioral symptoms and are less likely to cooperate. For these reasons later stage patients are less likely to benefit from information that is obtained from videofluoroscopy.

There is little evidence supporting intensive direct rehabilitative efforts for recovery of swallowing function in patients with advanced dementia. The care provided by rehabilitation services for these patients is largely supportive in nature and includes such factors as diet modifications, environmental manipulation, modifications of methods of food/liquid presentation, types of communicative interactions/verbal cues, and family and staff training. The most effective intervention for feeding/swallowing issues with patients with dementia routinely involves carer training. This includes training in general swallowing physiology and in communication/cognitive strategies to facilitate maximal functioning in the environment where the patient resides (ASHA, 2005a, 2005b). Hopper (2007) expands this concept of a more holistic intervention program to consider life participation as a meaningful outcome for these patients (Hopper, 2007). Such carer plans are less anatomically/physiologically driven and are not likely to be directly developed from x-ray data.

In order to devise a supportive plan the clinician must assess the patient's cognitive, sensory/perceptual, and motor behaviors in the context of their effects on feeding/swallowing. The level of knowledge and sensitivity of the carer must be assessed. In most cases careful hand feeding has been shown to get the best outcomes in terms of maintaining weight, skin integrity and general health during the inevitable decline associated with dementia. Realistic goal planning must reflect all aspects of the patient's status and must not be determined solely by oral/motor or pharyngeal responses during a swallow.

As the global nature of the decline associated with progressive dementing conditions becomes more pronounced, the type of information that is most useful in the development of a supportive care plan is rarely found through instrumental assessment. General supportive care typically includes positioning, thorough oral hygiene, careful hand feeding, timing of meals/snacks, and reasonable protection against reflux and its complications.

Careful hand feeding may include the use of finger foods, adaptive feeding equipment, specific behavioral cues such as verbal reminders to chew, swallow, and/or clear the mouth, assistance with presentation of foods/drinks, and pacing of meals to reduce impulsiveness and/or to continue intake despite inattention (Royal College of Physicians and British Society of Gastroenterology, 2010). Further components of a feeding program might include 1:1 carer attention versus group dining, provision of favorite foods, augmenting foods with condiments to promote intake, and so forth.

Prandial aspiration of small amounts of food or drink become lesser issues in the larger context of a patient who may not have the sustained attention for the eating task, the recollection of the need to chew, the recollection of the need to hydrate, and the understanding of the need for nutritionally balanced intake. The task of assuring these basic motivations for initiating and continuing oral intake typically fall more on the carer as the disease progresses.

MANAGEMENT OF DYSPHAGIA: INSTRUMENTAL ASSESSMENT

The evaluation of swallowing function may be performed with or without instrumentation but should always begin with the clinical swallowing assessment, the components of which are discussed elsewhere (ASHA, 2002; CASLPA, 2007; RCSLT, 2005). Assessment for all patients should begin with a careful review of the medical record and include an assessment of cognitive/sensory/behavioral factors that influence the ability to successfully feed. In many cases, such an assessment is sufficient to plan supportive care. In the rare instances where it might be practical to complete a videofluoroscopic swallowing study on a patient with advanced dementia, it is important for the clinician to recognize the limitations due to the dementing condition. Instrumental assessments are performed when additional information beyond the clinical exam is required to make treatment decisions (ASHA, 2002; CASLPA, 2007; RCSLT, 2005).

Modifications to the Technique

During an instrumental assessment a number of cognitive/behavioral factors may influence successful completion of the study. Attention must be considered as the patient may be easily distracted by the visual complexity of the radiology suite and the auditory distractions of a busy radiology department. Bells/buzzers and the associated ambient sounds of a busy diagnostic department are likely to be very distracting. Maintaining as quiet an environment as practical will help to maintain the patient's ability to attend to the task for the study. Given the long-term nutritional issues for these patients, with weight loss and muscle wasting, they are often cold, and blankets should be used to keep the patient as comfortable as possible.

Simple explanations and a more conversational approach are likely to be much more effective at facilitating cooperation during the study than a structured clinical progression of tasks. This patient group is often able to interact verbally despite lack of understanding of situational content. The skilled clinician may be able to use the social conversational pragmatics to encourage cooperation. Eye contact, smiling, judicious use of touch, and verbal praise are often effective at encouraging cooperation. Verbalizations to the patient should be directed in a calm, soothing manner, to help offset the clinical setting of a radiology suite and the unnatural act of eating in such a setting. The inclusion of a familiar person (family member, etc.) may be helpful for some patients.

Any videofluoroscopic study is designed to obtain the necessary information in a controlled amount of time, minimizing radiation exposure. Typically, such a study has a standard protocol designed to sample multiple consistencies in multiple controlled quantities. For the cognitively intact and cooperative patient this structure is time efficient and permits the acquisition of a great deal of information in a minimal period of time. For the patient with advanced dementia this level of structure is impractical. Cognitive and behavioral factors typical of patients with dementia may reduce the efficiency of a study due to the patient's need for encouragement, reinforcement, and redirection. This often leads to the need for greater use of clinical analysis skills that require inductive reasoning.

It is unlikely that the full protocol of a standard videofluoroscopic evaluation will be possible. As with any patient the clinician must have specific questions in mind and design the procedure in such a way as to obtain the necessary information in a timely manner. For example, the physician may wish to determine if there is a structural abnormality contributing to the patient's difficulty managing foods/drinks, or it may be important to determine if vegetative oral movements occur in response to specific residue in the pharynx. Perhaps there is concern of bolus retropulsion or a possible obstruction. The presence of penetration or aspiration of the bolus will be less important than obtaining the specific information that might be sought for the purpose of planning an individualized program of care.

CONCLUSIONS

Videofluoroscopic assessment is not appropriate for routine use with patients with advanced dementia. The information needed to devise the management plan can usually be obtained through careful clinical assessment of swallowing coupled with cognitive/behavioral evaluation. Discussions with the care team about a particular patient's behavioral triggers and preferences are very important in developing a care plan. This is particularly true, as these patients are generally not good candidates for complex swallowing rehabilitation programs nor are they generally candidates for alternative routes of nutrition. This is not to say that patients with dementia should be less of a priority for x-ray examination, when the situation requires it. When it is necessary for a videofluoroscopy to be conducted on a patient with dementia, the suggestions that are presented may help in obtaining the information that is needed to plan an appropriate program of care. Given the progressive nature of this disease, the family and care team need to consider frequent reassessments and case reviews so that over time the most appropriate decisions will be made to assure optimal quality of life for their family member.

REFERENCES

Adelman, A. M., & Daly, M. P. (2005). Initial evaluation of the patient with suspected dementia. *American Family Physician, 71*(9), 1745–1750.

Alzheimer's Disease International. (2010). *World Alzheimer's report 2010: The global economic impact of dementia*. London, UK: Author.

American Psychiatric Association. (2000). *Diagnostic and statistical manual of mental disorders* (4th ed., text rev.). Washington DC: Author.

ASHA. (2002). *The roles of speech-language pathologists in swallowing and feeding disorders: Technical report*. Rockville, MD: Author.

ASHA (2005a). *The roles of speech-language pathologists working with individuals with dementia-based communication disorders: Position statement*. Rockville, MD: Author.

ASHA. (2005b). *The roles of speech-language pathologists working with individuals with dementia-based communication disorders: Technical report*. Rockville, MD: Author.

Bayles, K. A. (2001). Understanding the neuropsychological syndrome of dementia. *Seminars in Speech and Language, 22*(4), 251–259; quiz 260.

Binetti, G., Cappa, S. F., Magni, E., Padovani, A., Bianchetti, A., & Trabucchi, M. (1998). Visual and spatial perception in the early phase of Alzheimer's disease. *Neuropsychology, 12*(1), 29–33.

Brody, H. (2000). Evidence-based medicine, nutritional support, and terminal suffering. *American Journal of Medicine, 109*(9), 740–741.

CASLPA. (2007). *Position paper on dysphagia in adults*. Ottawa, ON: Canadian Association of Speech-Language Pathologists and Audiologists.

Chouinard, J. (2000). Dysphagia in Alzheimer disease: A review. *Journal of Nutrition, Health, and Aging, 4*(4), 214–217.

Chouinard, J., Lavigne, E., & Villeneuve, C. (1998). Weight loss, dysphagia, and outcome in advanced dementia. *Dysphagia, 13*(3), 151–155.

Correia Sde, M., Morillo, L. S., Jacob Filho, W., & Mansur, L. L. (2010). Swallowing in moderate and severe phases of Alzheimer's disease. *Arquivos de Neuro-Psiquiatria, 68*(6), 855–861.

Duron, E., & Hanon, O. (2008). Vascular risk factors, cognitive decline, and dementia. *Journal of Vascular Health and Risk Management, 4*(2), 363–381.

Easterling, C. S., & Robbins, E. (2008). Dementia and dysphagia. *Geriatric Nursing, 29*(4), 275–285.

Ekberg, O., Hamdy, S., Woisard, V., Wuttge-Hannig, A., & Ortega, P. (2002). Social and psychological burden of dysphagia: Its impact on diagnosis and treatment. *Dysphagia, 17*(2), 139–146.

Fernandez, M., Gobartt, A. L., & Balana, M. (2010). Behavioural symptoms in patients with Alzheimer's disease and their association with cognitive impairment. *BioMedCentral Neurology, 10,* 87.

Fessman, N., & Lester, D. (2000). Loneliness and depression among elderly nursing home patients. *International Journal of Aging and Human Development, 51*(2), 137–141.

Finucane, T. E., Christmas, C., & Travis, K. (1999). Tube feeding in patients with advanced dementia: A review of the evidence. *Journal of the American Medical Association, 282*(14), 1365–1370.

Forstl, H., & Kurz, A. (1999). Clinical features of Alzheimer's disease. *European Archives of Psychiatry and Clinical Neuroscience, 249*(6), 288–290.

Gillick, M. R. (2000). Rethinking the role of tube feeding in patients with advanced dementia. *New England Journal of Medicine, 342*(3), 206–210.

Hachinski, V., Iadecola, C., Petersen, R. C., Breteler, M. M., Nyenhuis, D. L., Black, S. E., . . . Leblanc, G. G. (2006). National Institute of Neurological Disorders and Stroke-Canadian Stroke Network vascular cognitive impairment harmonization standards. *Stroke, 37*(9), 2220–2241.

Hoffer, L. J. (2006). Tube feeding in advanced dementia: The metabolic perspective. *British Medical Journal, 333*(7580), 1214–1215.

Hogan, D. B., Bailey, P., Black, S., Carswell, A., Chertkow, H., Clarke, B., . . . Thorpe, L. (2008). Diagnosis and treatment of dementia: 5. Nonpharmacologic and pharmacologic therapy for mild to moderate dementia. *Canadian Medical Association Journal, 179*(10), 1019–1026.

Holsinger, T., Deveau, J., Boustani, M., & Williams, J. W., Jr. (2007). Does this patient have dementia? *Journal of the American Medical Association, 297*(21), 2391–2404.

Hopper, T. (2007). The ICF and dementia. *Seminars in Speech and Language, 28*(4), 273–282.

Horner, J., Alberts, M. J., Dawson, D. V., & Cook, G. M. (1994). Swallowing in Alzheimer's disease. *Alzheimer Disease and Associated Disorders, 8*(3), 177–189.

Humbert, I. A., McLaren, D. G., Kosmatka, K., Fitzgerald, M., Johnson, S., Porcaro, E., . . . Robbins, J. (2010). Early deficits in cortical control of swallowing in Alzheimer's disease. *Journal of Alzheimer's Disease, 19*(4), 1185–1197.

Ikeda, M., Brown, J., Holland, A. J., Fukuhara, R., & Hodges, J. R. (2002). Changes in appetite, food preference, and eating habits in frontotemporal dementia and Alzheimer's disease. *Journal of Neurology, Neurosurgery, and Psychiatry, 73*(4), 371–376.

Jeffrey, S. (2011, April 19). New diagnostic criteria for Alzheimer's published. Retrieved April 19, 2011, from http://www.medscape.com/viewarticle/741101

Kurlan, R., Richard, I. H., Papka, M., & Marshall, F. (2000). Movement disorders in Alzheimer's disease: more rigidity of definitions is needed. *Movement Disorders, 15*(1), 24–29.

Langmore, S. E., Terpenning, M. S., Schork, A., Chen, Y., Murray, J. T., Lopatin, D., . . . Loesch, W. J. (1998). Predictors of aspiration pneumonia: How important is dysphagia? *Dysphagia, 13*(2), 69–81.

Mann, D. M., & Yates, P. O. (1986). Neurotransmitter deficits in Alzheimer's disease and in other dementing disorders. *Human Neurobiology, 5*(3), 147–158.

Mazzoni, P., Pearson, T., & Rowland, L. P. (2006). *Merritt's neurology handbook* (2nd ed.). New York, NY: Lippincott, Williams & Wilkins.

Mega, M. S., Cummings, J. L., Fiorello, T., & Gornbein, J. (1996) The spectrum of behavioral changes in Alzheimer's disease. *Neurology, 46*(1), 130–135.

Mesulam, M. M. (2003). Primary progressive aphasia—a language-based dementia. *New England Journal of Medicine, 349*(16), 1535–1542.

Murphy, L. M., & Lipman, T. O. (2003) Percutaneous endoscopic gastrostomy does not prolong survival in patients with dementia. *Archives of Internal Medicine, 163*(11), 1351–1353.

Post, S. G. (2001). Tube feeding and advanced progressive dementia. *Hastings Center Report, 31*(1), 36–42.

RCSLT. (2005). *Clinical guidelines.* Bicester, UK: Speechmark Publishing.

Royal College of Physicians and British Society of Gastroenterology. (2010). *Oral feeding difficulties and dilemmas: A guide to practical care, particularly towards the end of life.* London, UK: Royal College of Physicians.

Santacruz, K. S., & Swagerty, D. (2001). Early diagnosis of dementia. *American Family Physician, 63*(4), 703–713, 717–708.

Schuurmans, M. J., Duursma, S. A., & Shortridge-Baggett, L. M. (2001). Early recognition of delirium: Review of the literature. *Journal of Clinical Nursing, 10*(6), 721–729.

Shinagawa, S., Adachi, H., Toyota, Y., Mori, T., Matsumoto, I., Fukuhara, R., . . . Ikeda, M. (2009). Characteristics of eating and swallowing problems in patients who have dementia with Lewy bodies. *International Psychogeriatrics, 21*(3), 520–525.

Suh, M. K., Kim, H., & Na, D. L. (2009). Dysphagia in patients with dementia: Alzheimer versus vascular. *Alzheimer Disease and Associated Disorders, 23*(2), 178–184.

Chapter

14

HEAD AND NECK CANCERS

Jo Patterson and Margaret Coffey

INTRODUCTION

Head and neck cancer (HNC) constitutes a diverse group of diseases arising from the oral cavity, pharynx and larynx and other less common sites such as the salivary glands, nose and sinuses. Approximately 7,500 new patients are diagnosed in the United Kingdom per year with over 550,000 cases worldwide. The most common sites are the larynx and oral cavity, with the vast majority being squamous cell carcinomas. Males are affected more than females with a ratio ranging from 2:1 to 4:1. There are three main types of treatment; surgery, radiotherapy, and chemoradiotherapy. Early disease is likely to be treated using single modality treatment (i.e., surgery or radiotherapy) whereas advanced tumors usually require a combination of treatments (e.g., surgery with adjuvant radiotherapy or chemoradiotherapy). Dysphagia, both at presentation and following treatment is usually complex and multifactorial, involving both anatomical and physiological changes. This chapter aims to give a broad overview of videofluoroscopy in the assessment and management of HNC dysphagia and postlaryngectomy voice.

PRE-TREATMENT DYSPHAGIA

Symptoms of HNC are variable and much will depend on which structures are involved. At presentation, most patients have a functional swallow (Pauloski et al., 2000). Videofluoroscopy studies have shown those with advanced disease commonly have pharyngeal residue, longer swallow transit times and are at greater risk of aspiration (Frowen, Cotton, Corry, & Perry, 2009; Pauloski et al., 2000; van der Molen et al., 2009). The incidence of aspiration appears to vary according to the site of the tumor, for instance, patients with oral disease rarely aspirate (Brown, Rieger, Harris, & Selkaly, 2010) compared to reports of 11% for oropharyngeal disease (Feng et al., 2010). However, laryngeal penetration may also occur in approximately one half of patients with early stage glottic cancer despite other biomechanical measurements being within normal range (Ford, Gollins, Hobson, & Vyas, 2009). Therefore, evidence suggests that aspiration is a relatively uncommon event in pretreatment HNC patients, but those with large pharyngeal cancers are at greater risk than those in other tumor groups.

(Chemo-)Radiotherapy

External radiotherapy delivers high energy x-rays to destroy cancer cells. Radiotherapy is combined with chemotherapy (CRT) as an intervention for some advanced HNC tumors. Patients can experience a number of functional impairments months and even years following treatment, dysphagia being the most common side effect (Hanna et al., 2004). In the acute phase, oral mucositis can be severe and painful, making eating and drinking very difficult. Mucosal adhesions at the postcricoid level can develop, sometimes completely obliterating the upper esophageal lumen i.e. total stricture. Xerostomia (dry mouth) due to salivary gland damage, compromises patient comfort and creates difficulties for food bolus formation. Unfortunately, for CRT patients, there are limited improvements to swallowing pathophysiology over time (Logemann et al., 2008). Tissues can become fibrotic, atrophic, or remain edematous, significantly affecting the movement and co-ordination of swallowing (Figure 14–1). Some may experience an unremitting course of fibrotic changes and a small percentage may be left with a nonfunctioning larynx.

The true incidence of dysphagia is difficult to ascertain as most studies have small subject numbers or have selected patients on the basis of a suspected dysphagia. Our own cohort identified that 28% of patients aspirated at 1 year post-CRT compared to just 5% of those receiving radiotherapy alone (Patterson, 2011). Common problems contributing to swallowing safety, severity, and inefficiency are as follows:

- Reduced pharyngeal contractile wave (Chang et al., 2003; Eisbruch, 2004; Kotz, Abraham, Beitler, Wadler, & Smith, 1999; Smith, Kotz, Beitler, & Wadler, 2000)
- Reduced base of tongue retraction (Eisbruch, 2004; Graner et al., 2003; Hutcheson et al., 2008; Logemann et al., 2008)

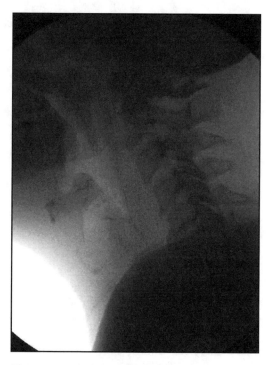

Figure 14–1. *Lateral view with the image displaying gross edema of the epiglottis, pharyngeal walls, and arytenoids in a patient 12 months postchemoradiotherapy.*

- Incomplete or delayed laryngeal closure (Eisbruch, 2004; Hutcheson et al., 2008; Logemann et al., 2008)
- Impaired hyolaryngeal elevation (Eisbruch, 2004; Hutcheson, et al., 2008; Logemann et al., 2008)
- Impaired epiglottic inversion (Eisbruch, 2004; Hutcheson et al., 2008; Smith, et al., 2000)
- Abnormal upper esophageal opening or stricture (Eisbruch, 2004; Hutcheson et al., 2008; Logemann et al., 2005)

Different chemotherapy protocols have shown minimal differences in dysphagic features (Eisbruch et al., 2004; Logemann et al., 2008). Higher radiation doses and bilateral treatment to the neck result in worse swallowing function (Frowen et al., 2009; Patterson, 2011). Preliminary results on intensity modulated radiotherapy (IMRT), where surrounding healthy tissues receive less radiation, suggest a reduction in dysphagia symptoms (Feng et al., 2010; Roe et al., 2010). A dose-effect relationship has been found between the involvement of specific structures and swallowing outcomes (pharyngeal constrictors, glottis, supraglottis, and upper esophagus). The reported incidence of an upper esophageal stricture (Figure 14–2) ranges from 13 to 37% (Caglar et al., 2008; Nguyen et al., 2008), which may be treated with a surgical or radiological dilatation. Strictures are likely to co-occur with oropharyngeal dysphagia and, therefore, dilatation alone is unlikely to fully rehabilitate the swallow and patients should be counseled accordingly.

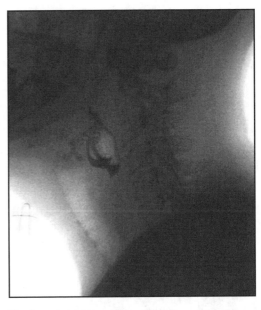

Figure 14–2. *Lateral view of total upper esophageal stricture in a patient 2 months postchemoradiotherapy.*

Surgery for Oral/Oropharyngeal Tumors

Surgery aims to completely excise the tumor, alongside a margin of healthy tissue, giving the best chance of microscopic clearance. Primary closure, that is, where the remaining tissues are left to heal, appears to result in better swallowing function (McConnel et al., 1998). However, larger resections will require some form of "flap" reconstruction, usually with a local or free tissue transfer, harvested from elsewhere in the body such as the forearm. In the absence of nerve grafting, free flap reconstruction will be insensate and adynamic. Flaps need to have sufficient bulk for function, but this needs to be balanced against being too bulky, which could restrict movement and airflow for breathing. Swallowing impairment can change over time, with edema being more prevalent in the early postoperative period and atrophy or scarring being more common in the long term (Figure 14–3). Furthermore, surgery can result in temporary or permanent nerve damage. Many patients will go on to have adjuvant

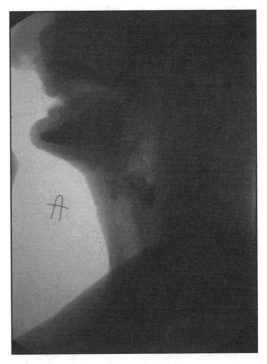

Figure 14–3. *Lateral view showing atrophy of the base of tongue in a patient 25 years following an oropharyngeal resection and reconstruction.*

radiotherapy, or will have had primary radiotherapy followed by salvage surgery, adding to the detrimental effect on swallowing (Mittal et al., 2003).

A small resection in the oral cavity usually has minimal effects on swallowing, secondary to edema, reduced sensation, and pain, often settling within a matter of weeks. A large tumor in this area may require a composite resection, that is, removal of a portion of more than one structure such as the floor of the mouth combined with a mandibulectomy (removal/resection of the lower jaw). Removal of all or some teeth is often required. Where indicated, a neck dissection (removal of the lymph glands) is also performed, usually unilaterally on the same side as the tumor. Swallowing will be significantly impaired in these patients, and a period of tube feeding is usually required. Clearly, there will be difficulties at the oral and oral preparatory stage of swallowing. Depending on the site of the surgery, this can include difficulties with lip seal, jaw opening (trismus), chewing, bolus preparation, control, and propulsion (Pauloski, Logemann, & Rademaker, 1993). There may be a degree of tongue tethering, affecting the pharyngeal stage. Where the muscles of the floor of the mouth are detached, this reduces the capacity for hyolaryngeal elevation (Pauloski et al., 1993). Even a neck dissection alone can have a detrimental impact, potentially increasing scarring and sensory changes (Lango et al., 2010). Aspiration can remain a problem in the long term (Pauloski, Logemann, & Rademaker, 1993; Tei et al., 2007). Removal of a maxillary tumor will require either a palatal obdurator (a prosthetic device) or flap repair, to restore the division between the oral and nasal cavity. Nasal penetration can occur where a repair is not entirely effective. If the patient is undergoing adjuvant radiotherapy, then it is often advisable that obdurators are temporarily removed, limiting both speech and swallowing function.

Tumors of the oropharynx include critical swallowing sites such as the base of tongue, tonsil, soft palate and pharyngeal wall. Early cancers may be treated with laser or transoral robotic surgery, affording a minimally invasive approach. Swallowing outcomes appear promising (Haughey et al., 2011; Iseli et al., 2009; Sinclair et al., 2011), although little has been published using instrumental swallowing assessment. Generally, the larger volume resected, the poorer the outcome, with the most important predictor being the extent of tongue base resected (Fujimoto, Hasegawa, Yamada, Ando, & Nakashima, 2007; Pauloski et al., 2004; Smith et al., 2008). For instance, a total glossectomy will result in problems at all stages of the swallow (Figure 14–4). Many patients with advanced disease have a composite resection, resulting in a multifaceted dysphagia. Problems can include premature bolus spillage, nasal backflow, impaired pharyngeal

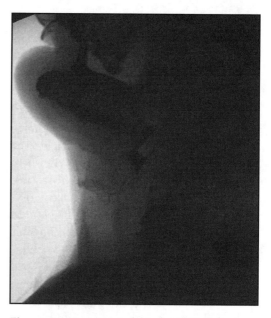

Figure 14–4. *Lateral view of a total glossectomy and mandibulectomy, reconstructed with a radial forearm free flap and mandibular plate. A backward head thrust is required to propel the bolus posteriorly.*

contraction, reduced airway closure, and increased oral and pharyngeal transit times (Borggreven et al., 2007; McConnel et al., 1998; Rieger et al., 2007). The incidence of aspiration varies, with reports ranging from 7 to 50% (Borggreven et al., 2007; Rieger et al., 2007; Tei et al., 2007).

A small number of studies have reported on surgical techniques to try to improve swallowing outcomes, such as laryngeal suspension where the larynx is raised and secured to the mandible, thus placing it in a more protective position. Retaining soft palate function is particularly problematic and there are some successful reports of using pharyngeal flaps and tendons to act as a sling to maintain elevation (McCombe, Lyons, Winkler, & Morrison, 2005; Seikaly et al., 2008). Strategies to retain the bulk of tongue base flaps have been described for the purpose of improved swallowing (Seikaly et al., 2009).

Modification to the Videofluoroscopy Technique

For the majority of cases, a videofluoroscopy may be carried out according to the procedures outlined in previous chapters. However, interpretation can be challenging as the usual anatomical landmarks explained in Chapters 4 and 6 may be absent or altered and reconstruction materials such as a mandibular plate may be visible (see Figure 14–4). Asymmetry from a unilateral defect, tethered structures, edema, flap shape, or neurological impairment may require an anterior-posterior radiographic view. Patients with an extended neck dissection may have some degree of shoulder droop requiring an oblique position. Swallowing techniques may be introduced during the procedure. The "dump and swallow" technique, often used in patients with a total glossectomy, requires a head thrust backwards, so positioning needs to be planned (see Figure

14–4). The availability of equipment such as modified spoons or a syringe may be useful for patients with oral preparatory problems.

LARYNGECTOMY

Total laryngectomy involves the removal of the entire larynx, resulting in the separation of swallowing and respiratory functions. As a consequence, patients breathe through a permanent open neck stoma, lose the ability to produce voice in a conventional manner and experience significant changes in ability to smell, taste, and swallow. An appreciation of the normal swallow facilitates understanding of the specific anatomical changes described in this chapter that occur after laryngectomy. Chapter 4 provides a full description of the anatomy and physiology of the normal swallow, with Chapter 6 outlining the biomechanics of the normal swallow in detail. Prelaryngectomy anatomy is illustrated in Figure 14–5.

A standard total laryngectomy typically involves an initial separation and "skeletonization" of the larynx from the jugular and carotid vessels on either side of the neck (Figure 14–6). The larynx is usually dissected from above the hyoid bone to below the cricoid cartilage. The suprahyoid muscles are then dissected off the hyoid bone. The thyropharyngeus is shaved off the thyroid cartilage and the cricopharyngeus is removed from the cricoid cartilage. All of these muscles are preserved and later reconstructed to form the pharyngoesophageal segment (PES) which allows for optimum voice and swallow function.

Once the larynx is removed, the open trachea and pharynx remain. The exposed upper part of the trachea is secured to an opening in the neck to form a stoma, through which the patient will breathe. A surgical puncture can be performed between the trachea and

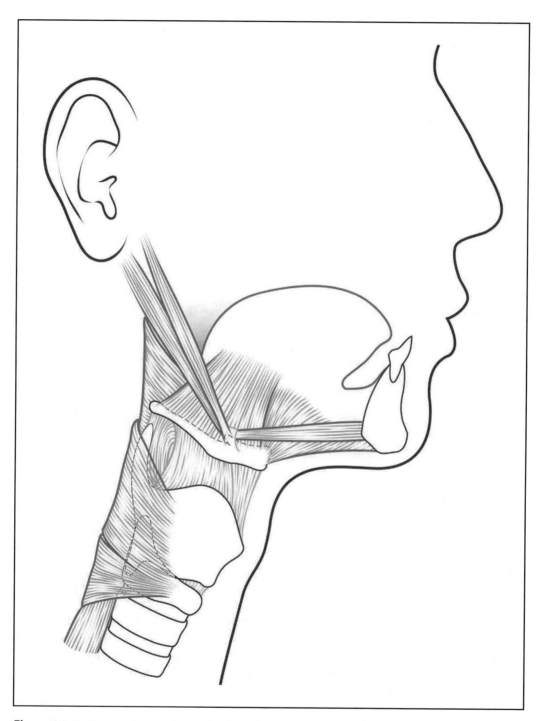

Figure 14–5. Preoperative anatomy. The thyropharyngeus and cricopharyngeus muscles lie posteriorly and are attached laterally to the thyroid and cricoid cartilages. Copyright © Y. Edels & P. Clarke (2005). Used with permission.

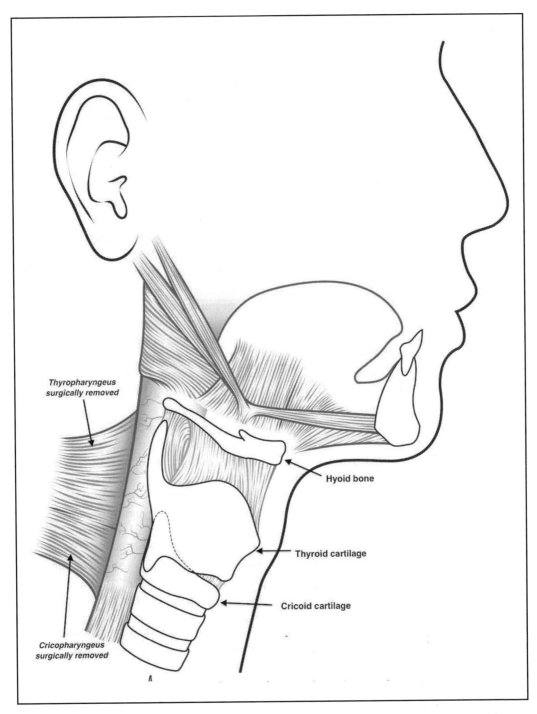

Thyropharyngeus
surgically removed

Hyoid bone

Thyroid cartilage

Cricoid cartilage

Cricopharyngeus
surgically removed

Figure 14–6. *Skeletonization of the larynx during laryngectomy surgery. Copyright © Y. Edels & P. Clarke (2005). Used with permission.*

esophagus to permit voice prosthesis placement and facilitate restoration of voice. This usually takes place at the time of laryngectomy surgery (primary puncture) but may also take place at a later date (secondary puncture).

The open pharynx is then closed. Provided enough thyropharyngeal and cricopharyngeal muscle remains, these are used as a second level of closure over the repaired pharynx. This second layer of closure inwardly compresses the repaired pharyngeal tissue. At rest this is seen on videofluoroscopy as a closed narrow area and is referred to as the pharyngoesophageal (PE) or reconstructed segment. The amount, constriction, and muscle tone of the thyropharyngeus and cricopharyngeus muscle used for this second level of repair will influence voice quality postsurgery. The ability of the PES to dilate, coupled with power created at the base of tongue and the length of time the PES remains open dictates the patient's ease to swallow a variety of food consistencies.

Reconstruction of the suprahyoids by suturing them onto the superior margin of the repaired thyropharyngeus (Perry, McIvor, & Chalton, 1987) provides a third level of closure over the repaired pharynx, which importantly is believed to prevent the formation of a pseudodiverticulum. During swallow, it is thought that the reconstructed suprahyoids maintain ability to contract and in doing so, pull the repaired thyropharyngeus forward and facilitate opening of the upper esophagus for swallowing. Figure 14–7 illustrates complete reconstruction of the pharynx after laryngectomy. The reconstructed pharynx after laryngectomy is sometimes referred to as a neopharynx.

A surgical procedure called a myotomy is recommended during surgery to improve both voice and swallow functions (Bayles & Deschler, 2004; Blom & Singer, 1981; Scott, Bleach, Perry, & Cheesman, 1993). A myotomy involves cutting individual muscle fibers. A "short" myotomy involves dividing the muscle fibers running from the lower third of the reconstructed PES to below the tracheoesophageal puncture, approximately parallel with the lower stomal lip as in Figure 14–8. Before laryngectomy, the force of the upper esophageal wave prevents the bolus from refluxing back into the pharynx as discussed in Chapters 4 and 6. Postlaryngectomy myotomy has the effect of reducing the upper oesophageal peristaltic wave force. Furthermore, this procedure creates an air reservoir at the top of the esophagus for voicing and increases the width of the esophageal lumen for swallowing, helping to prevent prosthesis fouling. An alternative procedure is the pharyngeal plexus neurectomy, which involves surgical denervation of middle constrictor muscle and partial denervation of thyropharyngeus and cricopharyngeus muscles. Three to five nerve branches of the pharyngeal plexus are divided, cauterized with a segment removed as part of this procedure (Bayles & Deschler, 2004; Blom, Singer, & Hamaker, 1986). Neurectomy provides surgical outcomes similar to a myotomy.

Patients whose cancer has extended beyond the boundaries defined for total laryngectomy to areas such as the hypopharynx, postcricoid region, and cervical esophagus may require a partial or total pharyngectomy or partial or total esophagectomy in addition to removal of the larynx. All usually involve tissue transfer from other parts of the body such as radial forearm, anterior lateral thigh, pectoralis major, jejunum, and, in some cases, stomach, or colon. The decision on the type of surgery that the patient will have will be influenced by the extent and location of disease.

Voicing After Laryngectomy

After laryngectomy, the larynx, including vocal folds, is removed and the patient has no means to produce normal voice. The patient now breathes by taking air in through a stoma in

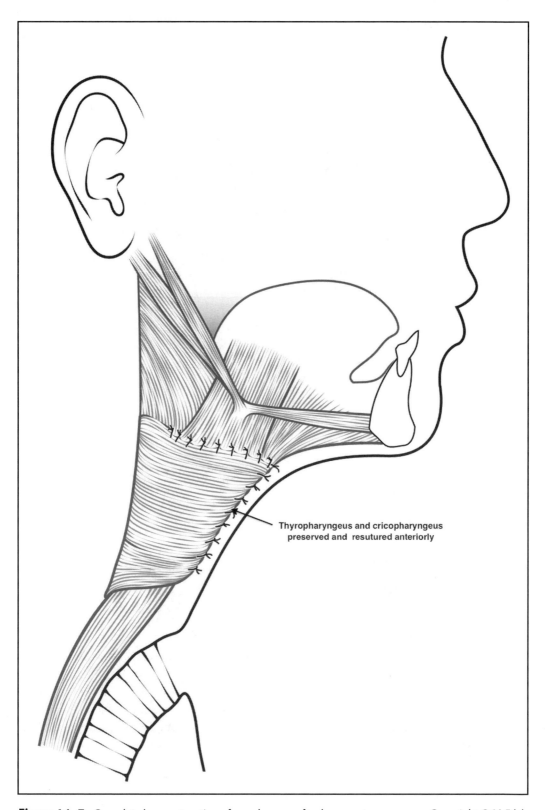

Thyropharyngeus and cricopharyngeus
preserved and resutured anteriorly

Figure 14–7. *Completed reconstruction of neopharynx after laryngectomy surgery. Copyright © Y. Edels & P. Clarke (2005). Used with permission.*

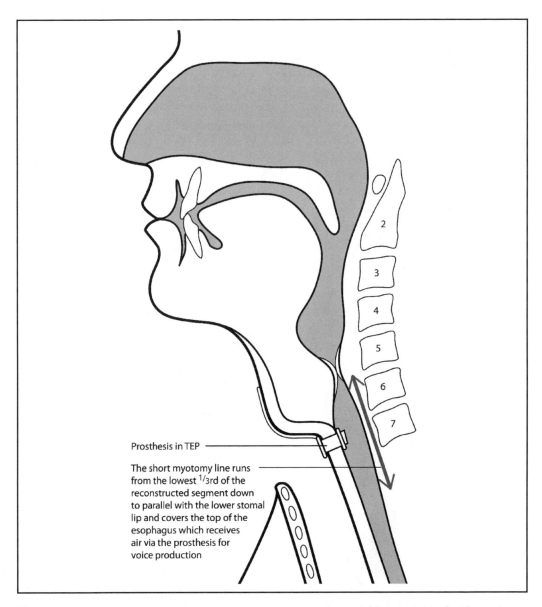

Prosthesis in TEP

The short myotomy line runs from the lowest ¹/₃rd of the reconstructed segment down to parallel with the lower stomal lip and covers the top of the esophagus which receives air via the prosthesis for voice production

Figure 14–8. *Short myotomy in a laryngectomy patient. Copyright © Y.Edels (2012). Used with permission.*

the neck rather than through the mouth and nose. In order to communicate, a new vibratory source is required to replace the vocal folds.

Esophageal speech involves injecting or inhaling air so that it enters the esophagus. This air is forced back out of the esophagus and into the PES where a vibration is produced. Alternatively, an *electrolarynx* communication aid may be used. This is a handheld vibratory device that can be placed against muscle tissue in the neck or cheek. It provides the vibration which supplies sound as the patient articulates allowing communication.

In 1979, Dr. Eric Blom and Dr. Mark Singer (Blom & Singer, 1979) introduced a silicone voice prosthesis, which was placed in the puncture site between the trachea and esophagus. The prosthesis itself does not produce voice; rather this one-way valve allows inspired air to be shunted from the lungs into the esophagus and then via the PES which vibrates to produce voice. This device rapidly became the intervention of choice for voice restoration after laryngectomy and has largely replaced previous rehabilitation methods.

Swallowing After Laryngectomy

Laryngectomy patients appear to experience dysphagic symptoms that affect quality of life, such as taking a longer time than others to eat, or an over-reliance on modified diets. A seminal Australian study (Ward, Frisby, & Stephens, 2002) highlighted the significance of this problem with the suggestion that the incidence of dysphagia may be as high as 48% for total laryngectomy and 50% for pharyngo-laryngectomy three years postsurgery. A more recent study (Maclean, Cotton, & Perry, 2009), found an even higher incidence, with 72% of laryngectomy patients in this study self-reporting symptoms of dysphagia.

It is now acknowledged that dysphagia is not only a real and common problem after total laryngectomy but one that appears to be under reported (Landera, Lundy, & Sullivan, 2010). It is understood that dysphagia may arise because of anatomical changes postsurgery, sensory impairments to taste and smell, and side effects of radiotherapy and/or chemotherapy. Table 14–1 compares swallowing for laryngeal and alaryngeal patients from oral to esophageal stages.

Modification to Videofluoroscopy Technique

Videofluoroscopic examination in laryngectomy patients requires a number of modifications to the standard technique. Some important modifications are now described.

Placement of Stoma Marker

Before commencing videofluoroscopic examination of the laryngectomy patient, a metal marker should be placed to the patient's right hand side of the stoma (Figure 14–9). Care should be taken to avoid obscuring the voice prosthesis during imaging. This marker will indicate stoma level during videofluoroscopic examination and assists with identification and examination of the voice prosthesis.

Positioning the Patient

Positioning the patient to achieve the best view of anatomical structures and swallowing physiology is crucial for the laryngectomy patient. Placing the patient in a lateral oblique position, as in Figure 14–9, facilitates observation of the voice prosthesis, hypopharyngeal area, and upper esophagus. This prevents the patient's shoulders from obscuring these structures in the videofluoroscopic image.

Examination of Voicing Function

A microphone should be attached to the patient to enable voice recording, see Figure 14–9. It may be appropriate for some patients without a voice prosthesis to undergo an air insufflation test (Blom, Singer, & Hamaker, 1985) to assess suitability for future surgical voice restoration with placement of a voice prosthesis. The radiological technique used to assess voicing potential of the reconstructed pharynx of postlaryngectomy patients using air insufflation has been previously described (McIvor, Evans, Perry, & Cheesman, 1990; Sloane, Griffin, & O'Dwyer, 1991).

Magnification

During the videofluoroscopic examination, magnification of the voice prosthesis can be requested to enhance ability to observe the

Table 14–1. *Comparison of Laryngeal and Alaryngeal Swallow*

	Oral	Pharyngeal	Laryngeal	Proximal Esophagus	Esophagus
Laryngeal Swallow	Lips seal, teeth, tongue, hard and soft palate form bolus and pass it to the back of the mouth	Soft palate elevates to close the nasal port. Base of tongue and posterior pharyngeal wall close together. Stripping action propels the bolus onward. Swallow sequence fires.	Suprahyoids contract elevating and tilting the larynx forward under the tongue. Epiglottis seals tracheal entrance and laryngeal sphincters close to protect the airway. Cricopharyngeal muscles relax permitting entrance of esophagus to open. Bolus can pass.	Esophageal entrance opens. Bolus enters.	Gravity and sequential peristaltic wave carry bolus to stomach. Lower esophageal sphincter relaxes and opens to allow bolus to pass.
Alaryngeal Swallow	Lips seal, teeth, tongue, hard and soft palate form bolus and pass it to the back of the mouth	Soft palate elevates. Tongue base approximates posterior pharyngeal wall. Partial / reduced stripping action of posterior pharyngeal wall due to surgery and denervation. Bolus transits pharynx under power created here. Swallow sequence follows.	Reattached suprahyoids contract, pull on reconstructed segment, helping to lift the pharynx which in turn helps to relax reconstructed thyropharyngeus (and possibly cricopharyngeus) opening entrance to esophagus. Bolus under reduced pressure from tongue base and pharyngeal wall contraction exerts pressure from above. This (plus gravity) moves the bolus onward.	Esophageal entrance opens. Bolus enters.	Gravity and sequential peristaltic wave carry bolus to stomach. Lower esophageal sphincter relaxes and opens to allow bolus to pass.

Source: Copyright © Edels (2011). Used with permission.

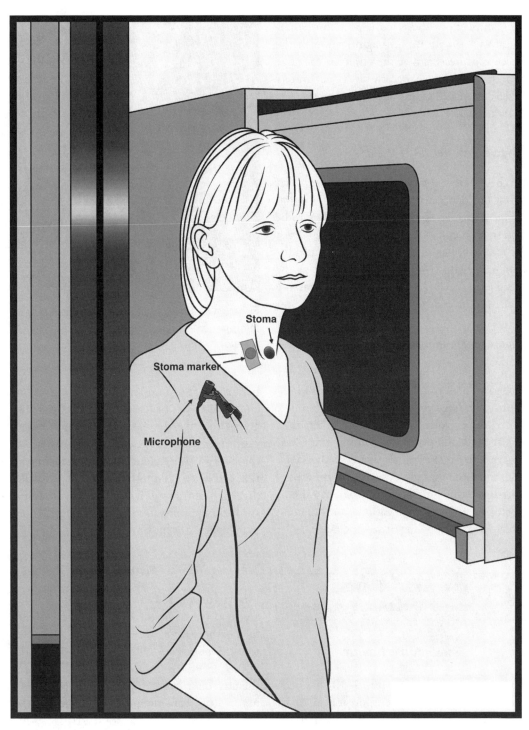

Figure 14–9. *Positioning a laryngectomy patient for videofluoroscopy with stoma marker and microphone in place. Copyright © Y. Edels (2012). Used with permission.*

proximity of prosthesis to the posterior esophageal wall. In addition, magnification of the voice prosthesis allows the clinician to judge whether the voice prosthesis is accurately sized and placed within the tracheoesophageal puncture.

Anteroposterior (AP) View

In the AP view, following the bolus as it passes from the neopharynx through the cricopharyngeus enables the esophageal swallow to be screened in collaboration with the radiologist or radiographer, and other relevant multidisciplinary team (MDT) members such as the head and neck surgeon, specialist nursing staff, and physiotherapist(s).

Fluoroscopic Images

It may be appropriate to request that x-ray images of anatomical features such as pseudodiverticulum (see next section for full definition), stricture, or voice prosthesis are taken during the videofluoroscopic examination. These images can later be made available to the MDT to facilitate any surgical, medical, or behavioral management. Fluoroscopic images may also be useful in providing education to the patient about their swallowing or voicing issues.

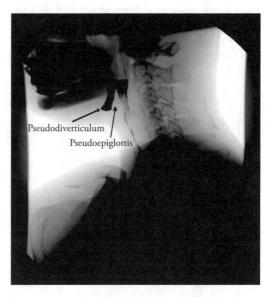

Figure 14–10. *Lateral view of a postlaryngectomy patient with a pseudodiverticulum and a pseudoepiglottis.*

because of the appearance on barium swallow and other types of imaging. It has been suggested that the use of the suprahyoid repair, previously described, can reinforce the area at the base of tongue and help prevent formation of a diverticulum (Edels, 2011). A smaller diverticulum may not impact on functional swallowing ability but a larger diverticulum may obstruct bolus flow.

Fistula

Pharyngocutaneous fistulae (Figure 14–11) are reported to be the most common nonfatal postoperative complication of laryngectomy (Galli et al., 2009; Sullivan & Hartig, 2001). Previous radiotherapy and chemotherapy have been implicated as predisposing factors causing post-operative fistulae (Klozar, Cada, & Koslabova, 2012) with a greater risk in those patients having concurrent chemotherapy rather than radiotherapy alone (Driven, Swinson, Gao, & Clark, 2009). Larger tumors (T3, T4) requiring salvage lar-

---

CLASSIC FINDINGS AND IMAGES

Pseudodiverticulum

Pseudodiverticulum (Figure 14–10) has been described as a mucosalized pouch at the base of the tongue, separated from the remaining pharynx by a posterior tissue band (Deschler, Blevins, & Ellison, 1996). The diverticulum has been alternatively called a *pseudovallecula* and the posterior tissue band a *pseudoepiglottis*

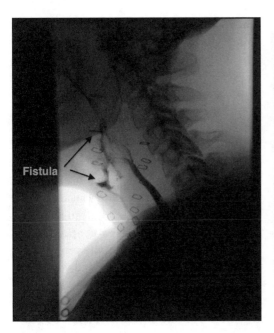

Figure 14–11. *Lateral view of a postlaryngec-tomy patient with area of fistualization.*

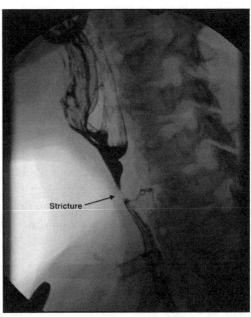

Figure 14–12. *Lateral view of a postlaryngectomy patient with a stricture within the neopharynx.*

yngectomy are thought to pose a greater risk for fistula formation (Aarts, Rovers, Grau, Grolman, & Vanderheijden, 2011). Other studies (Cavalot et al., 2000; Boscolo-Rizzo, De Cillis, Marchioni, Carpenè, & Da Mosto, 2008) have identified factors such as diabetes, liver disease and anemia as predictors of fistualization. Generally, patients with suspected fistualization are referred for alternative imaging procedures such as a gastrografin contrast swallow. However, should a fistula be observed during a videofluoroscopic study, multidisciplinary discussion should be initiated to ascertain whether it is appropriate to continue and whether alternative diagnostic procedures and contrast agents need to be considered.

Stricture

Strictures (Figure 14–12) within the neopharynx in a laryngectomy patient may be observed on videofluoroscopy as an area of limited dila-tion and abnormal tightness. Stricture may occur at one point within the neopharynx or along the entire length and generally impedes bolus flow particularly on more solid consistencies. Stricture is often a result of scar tissue, fibrosis, or recurrent disease. Some authors have suggested that strictures are more likely to occur in patients with a history of previous radiotherapy or chemoradiation treatment (Silverman & Deschler, 2008).

Reduced Propulsion in Neopharynx

In the normal swallow, the tongue base retracts and the posterior pharyngeal wall contracts causing pharyngeal pressure to build. As both structures make contact, the pharyngeal wall contraction continues progressively down the pharynx (Logemann, 1998). This contraction ensures efficient bolus transit with minimal or no residue. In laryngectomy patients, neo-pharyngeal contraction is significantly altered by surgical repair of this area. A recent study, using a combination of videofluoroscopy and manometry, concluded that not only are pharyngeal propulsive forces impaired but there is also resistance to bolus flow across the pharyngoesophageal segment (Maclean, Szczesniak, Cotton, & Perry, 2011). In many laryngectomy patients, bolus transit is achieved primarily by gravity, rather than by propulsive forces within the neopharynx. As a result, it is not uncommon to observe reduced pharyngeal bolus clearance and sometimes, significant residue (Figure 14–13) on videofluoroscopy examination.

Aspiration

Placement of a voice prosthesis is now considered the gold standard for communication rehabilitation after laryngectomy (Elmiyeh et al., 2010). The voice prosthesis is placed in a surgical puncture between the trachea and the esophagus. The one-way valve, which opens

when the patient produces voice but stays closed during swallowing, can trigger specific difficulties. Certain situations may cause the voice prosthesis to leak either around the prosthesis or through the center of the prosthesis, including an inaccurately sized voice prosthesis. Similarly, voice prosthesis leakage may occur when it is approaching the natural end of its lifespan or because it has been colonized by a fungal infection such as candidiasis (thrush). Leakage, if present, can usually be observed under radiological imaging magnification of the area where the voice prosthesis is located. Figure 14–14 illustrates central voice prosthesis leakage. The stoma and voice prosthesis should also be observed for evidence of contrast medium resulting from voice prosthesis leakage and measures should be taken to limit any aspiration. As a consequence, the

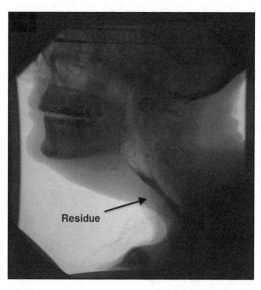

Figure 14–13. *Lateral view of a postlaryngectomy patient with residue within the neopharynx.*

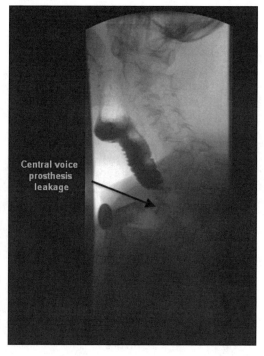

Figure 14–14. *Lateral view of central voice prosthesis leakage in a postlaryngopharyngectomy patient with jejunal reconstruction.*

videofluoroscopic examination may need to be temporarily suspended until voice prosthesis issues are resolved.

Reflux

Anecdotal evidence suggests that some laryngectomy patients experience a degree of esophageal stage swallowing disorder including delayed esophageal transit. Laryngectomy patients appear to experience reduced amplitude and duration of contractions in the proximal esophagus (Dantas, Aguiar-Ricz, Gielow, & Mello-Filho, 2005). A high incidence of gastropharyngeal reflux has also been found in a study of a small number of laryngectomy patients (Smit et al., 1998).

LARYNGEAL CONSERVATION SURGERY

Laryngeal conservation surgery is the treatment of choice for a select group of patients with laryngeal cancer. The appropriateness of this intervention will depend on the position of the disease and the patient's rehabilitation potential. Treatment involves removing a portion of larynx while maintaining speech, swallowing, and respiratory function. A spectrum of procedures is reported in the literature, including general categories of cordectomy (resection of the vocal folds, ranging from subepithelial cordectomy to an extended procedure, including the laryngeal ventricle), and partial or extended partial laryngectomy (including supraglottic and vertical laryngectomy). Describing all the different types of reconstruction is beyond the scope of this chapter. Again, the incidence and severity of dysphagia will much depend on the nature and extent of the resection. The oral stage is

usually left intact, but multiple breakdowns are possible at the pharyngeal stage, such as pharyngeal paresis or weakness and decreased laryngeal elevation (Figure 14–15). Airway protection is a major issue, with aspiration being possible before, during and after the swallow. A poorer outcome is predicted when the arytenoids are included in the resection. The procedure may be combined with a temporary tracheostomy which may further compromise swallowing. Aspiration has been reported in up to a third of patients following cordectomy (Bernal-Sprekelsen, Vilaseca-Gonzalez, & Blanch-Alejandro, 2004), which may be transient until healing is complete. For more extended resections, reports of aspiration ranges from a third to up to 94% (Kreuzer et al., 2000; Lewin et al., 2008; Simonelli et al., 2010).

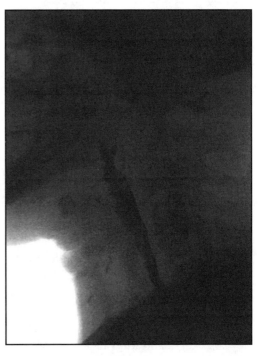

Figure 14–15. *Lateral view of a patient following a supraglottic partial laryngectomy, with reduced hyolaryngeal elevation.*

ROLE OF VIDEOFLUOROSCOPY IN HEAD AND NECK CANCER

A "bedside" examination of swallowing provides important clinical information, and for the laryngectomy patient, additional information on voice prosthesis function and ability to achieve surgical voice restoration. However, given that HNC patients often present with major anatomical changes, complex pathophysiology, and comorbidities, a full picture cannot be determined by clinical assessment alone. Instrumental swallowing evaluations including endoscopy, manometry, and videofluoroscopy provide a more comprehensive, objective evaluation (see Chapter 2). Videofluoroscopy is the most commonly reported instrumental assessment in the HNC literature, although protocols for its use in laryngectomy care are yet to be definitively researched.

Instrumental assessments form a valuable part of clinical management and swallowing rehabilitation. Information on safety and efficiency are important for decisions regarding potential impact on respiratory function and/or ability to maintain sufficient oral intake. Assessments can provide visual feedback to educate patients on the problem and intervention aims. They aid treatment decision-making such as assessing candidacy for laryngeal conservation surgery or method of voice rehabilitation. Conducting a baseline videofluoroscopy prior to therapy results in more targeted, individually tailored interventions (Logemann et al., 1992). For example, aspiration can be eliminated or reduced by specific swallowing postures and/or maneuvers (Lazarus, 1993; Logemann, Pauloski, Rademaker, & Colangelo, 1997; Nguyen et al., 2007; Zuydam, Rogers, Brown, Vaughan, & Magennis, 2000). A videofluoroscopy can help determine the patient's readiness for oral intake and timing of removal or placement of a feeding tube (Lazarus, Logemann, & Gibbons, 1993).

The information derived can help the clinician to identify and monitor which swallowing exercises are indicated for the presenting dysphagia (Logemann et al., 2009). A videofluoroscopy can confirm whether an upper esophageal stricture is present, guiding the necessary management. Furthermore, it can provide an indication of prognosis for long-term swallowing outcome (Denk, Swoboda, Schima, & Eibenberger, 1997).

A choice of HNC treatments may be offered (surgery or radiotherapy), where survival outcomes for interventions are in equipoise. Unfortunately, clinical trials comparing treatments have infrequently included swallowing endpoints, or have used surrogate measures such as the presence of a feeding tube. Patients need to be adequately informed about the consequences for their function and given realistic expectations. The use of videofluoroscopy in HNC research has helped to profile the characteristics of dysphagia associated with different treatments.

CLINICAL DILEMMAS

Some of the clinical dilemmas presented here are equally applicable to other populations. Frequent assessment is usually part of ongoing dysphagia management and therefore, radiation exposure needs to be a consideration (Aviv et al., 2001). The nature of the dysphagia can change over time, so selecting an appropriate time point for a videofluoroscopy is an important consideration. Furthermore, radiation exposure sets a time limit on the assessment period when vital information such as aspiration of residue may be lost. A full understanding of the anatomical changes can be difficult to ascertain on VFSS alone. A clear distinction between healthy tissue, disease, flap reconstruction, or edema can be difficult to decipher during VFSS.

The risk of pneumonia secondary to aspiration can pose a management dilemma, due to conflicting reports in the literature. One study reported a 9% mortality rate in patients known to aspirate, and therefore it was suggested that oral feeding should only be reinstated once aspiration has been ruled out (Nguyen et al., 2006; Nguyen et al., 2009). Elsewhere, only half of patients with chronic aspiration had a history of pneumonia (Lundy et al., 1999). As with other dysphagic populations, additional factors may need to be present for pneumonia to develop, such as neutropenia, that is, abnormal decrease in white blood cells, cachexia, poor oral hygiene, history of smoking, high metabolic rate, and fatigue (Nguyen et al., 2004; Purkey, Levine, Prendes, Norman, & Mirza, 2009). Prolonged aspiration and chronic chest infections have been associated with pulmonary fibrosis, a condition that HNC patients may be susceptible to, especially as swallowing can deteriorate in the long-term. Anecdotally, it is not uncommon for patients to be re-referred with persistent chest problems secondary to aspiration, several years after their initial treatment. Experts in the field agree that patients need to be regularly monitored to identify any deterioration (Logemann et al., 2008; Nguyen et al., 2005; Rosenthal, Lewin, & Eisbruch, 2006). Management of swallowing safety in the palliative care patient requires special attention. Patients may present with aspiration, but still desire to eat and drink. An instrumental assessment may be beneficial in facilitating patient participation in decision-making over feeding route and devising strategies that may minimize risk and/or increase efficiency.

Another consideration is that swallowing disorders observed on instrumental assessments do not appear to have a strong relationship with how HNC patients perceive their dysphagia (Gillespie et al., 2005; Patterson, 2011; Thomas et al., 2008). A complete understanding of the impact of a swallowing problem cannot be assessed by instrumentation alone. Collecting information on the impairment and the patient's perspective is necessary for a comprehensive evaluation of the problem.

CONCLUSION

This chapter has introduced some of the highly diverse anatomical and physiological changes in swallow and communication function arising from a diagnosis of HNC. The location and extent of disease in this population together with the type of treatment modality can influence the nature of dysphagia encountered. Although modifications to standard techniques are sometimes required, the use of videofluoroscopy and other instrumental swallow evaluation tools allows dysphagia to be investigated and rehabilitated in a comprehensive manner. Dysphagia in this population is unlikely to be static and instrumental evaluation allows swallowing baselines to be established as well as monitoring progress over time. Videofluoroscopy also plays a valuable role in giving patients a greater understanding and appreciation of the rationale for swallowing therapy. Crucially, the multidisciplinary management of clinical issues such as chronic aspiration and palliative care is enhanced by the judicious use of instrumental swallow evaluation tools including videofluoroscopy.

REFERENCES

Aarts, M., Rovers, M., Grau, C., Grolman, W., & Vanderheijden, G. (2011). Salvage laryngectomy after primary radiotherapy: What are prognostic factors for the development of pharyngocutaneous fistulae? *Otolaryngology-Head and Neck Surgery, 144*(1), 5–9.

Aviv, J. E., Sataloff, R. T., Cohen, M., Spitzer, J., Ma, G., Bhayani, R., & Close, L. G. (2001).

Cost-effectiveness of two types of dysphagia care in head and neck cancer: A preliminary report. *Ear, Nose, and Throat Journal, 80*(8), 553–556.

Bayles, S., & Deschler, D. (2004). Operative prevention and management of voice limiting pharyngoesophageal spasm. *Otolaryngologic Clinics of North America, 37*(3), 547–558.

Bernal-Sprekelsen, M., Vilaseca-Gonzalez, I., & Blanch-Alejandro, J. L. (2004). Predictive values for aspiration after endoscopic laser resections of malignant tumors of the hypopharynx and larynx. *Head and Neck, 26*(2), 103–110.

Blom, E., & Singer, M. (1979). Surgical-prosthetic approaches for post-laryngectomy voice restoration. *Laryngectomy Rehabilitation*. Houston, TX: College-Hill Press.

Blom, E., & Singer, M. (1981). Selective Myotomy for voice restoration after total laryngectomy. *Archives of Otolaryngology, 107*, 670–673.

Blom, E., Singer, M., & Hamaker, R. (1985). An improved esophageal insufflation test. *Archives of Otolaryngology-Head and Neck Surgery, 111*, 211–212.

Blom, E., Singer, M., & Hamaker, R. (1986). Pharyngeal plexus neurectomy for alrayngeal speech rehabilitation. *Laryngoscope, 96*, 50–53.

Borggreven, P. A., Verdonck-de Leeuw, I., Rinkel, R. N., Langendijk, J. A., Roos, J. C., David, E. F. L., de Bree, R., & Leemans, C. R. (2007). Swallowing after major surgery of the oral cavity or oropharynx: A prospective and longitudinal assessment of patients treated by microvascular soft tissue reconstruction. *Head and Neck Journal for the Sciences and Specialties of the Head and Neck, 29*(7), 638–647.

Boscolo-Rizzo, P., DeCillis, G., Marchioni, C., Carpenè, S., & Da Mosto, M. (2008). Multivariate analysis of risk factors for pharyngocutaneous fistula after total laryngectomy. *European Archives of Otorhinolaryngology, 265*(8), 929–936.

Brown, L., Rieger, J., Harris, J., & Selkaly, H. (2010). A longitudinal study of functional outcomes after surgical resection and microvascular reconstruction for oral cancer: Tongue mobility and swallowing function. *Journal of Oral and Maxillofacial Surgery, 68*(11), 2690–2700.

Caglar, H. B., Tishler, R. B., Othus, M., Burke, E., Li, Y., Goguen, L., . . . Allen, A. M. (2008).

Dose to larynx predicts for swallowing complications after intensity-modulated radiotherapy. *International Journal of Radiation Oncology, Biology, Physics, 72*(4), 1110–1118.

Cavalot, A., Gervasio, C., Nazionale, G., Albera, R., Bussi, M., Staffieri, A., . . . Cortesina, G. (2000). Pharyngocutaneous fistula as a complication of total laryngectomy: Review of the literature and analysis of case records. *Otolaryngology-Head and Neck Surgery, 123*(5), 587–592.

Chang, Y. C., Chen, S. Y., Lui, L. T., Wang, T. G., Wang, T. C., Hsiao, T. Y., . . . Lien, I. N. (2003). Dysphagia in patients with nasopharyngeal cancer after radiation therapy: A videofluoroscopic swallowing study. *Dysphagia, 18*(2), 135–143.

Dantas, R., Aguiar-Ricz, L., Gielow, I., & Mello-Filho, F. (2005). Proximal esophageal contractions in laryngectomised patients. *Dysphagia, 20*(2), 101–104.

Denk, D. M., Swoboda, H., Schima, W., & Eibenberger, K. (1997). Prognostic factors for swallowing rehabilitation following head and neck cancer surgery. *Acta Oto-Laryngologica, 117*(5), 769–774.

Deschler, D., Blevins, N., & Ellison, D. (1996). Post laryngectomy dysphagia caused by an anterior neopharyngeal diverticulum. *Otolaryngology-Head and Neck Surgery, 115*, 167–169.

Driven, R., Swinson, R., Gao, K., & Clark, S. (2009). The assessment of pharyngocutaneous fistula rate in patients treated primarily with definitive radiotherapy followed by salvage surgery of the larynx and hypopharynx. *Laryngoscope, 119*(9), 1691–1695.

Edels, Y. (2011). *Anatomy, physiology and complications of the post laryngectomy swallow.* Paper presented at the Advanced Surgical Voice Restoration Course, Imperial College, London.

Eisbruch, A. (2004). Dysphagia and aspiration following chemo-irradiation of head and neck cancer: Major obstacles to intensification of therapy. *Annals of Oncology, 15*(3), 363–364.

Eisbruch, A., Schwartz, M., Rasch, C., Vineberg, K., Damen, E., Van As, C. J., et al. (2004). Dysphagia and aspiration after chemoradiotherapy for head-and-neck cancer: Which anatomic structures are affected and can they be spared by IMRT? *International Journal of Radiation Oncology, Biology, Physics, 60*(5), 1425–1439.

Elmiyeh, B., Dwivedi, R., Jallall, N., Chisholm, E., Kazi, R., Clarke, P., . . . RhysEvans, P. (2010). Surgical voice restoration after laryngectomy: An overview. *Indian Journal of Cancer, 47*(3).

Feng, F. Y., Kim, H. M., Lyden, T. H., Haxer, M. J., Worden, F. P., Feng, M., . . . Eisbruch, A. (2010). Intensity-modulated chemoradiotherapy aiming to reduce dysphagia in patients with oropharyngeal cancer: Clinical and functional results. *Journal of Clinical Oncology, 28*(16), 2732–2738.

Ford, S., Gollins, S., Hobson, P., & Vyas, S. (2009). Structural displacements during the swallow in patients with early laryngeal cancers and other early primary cancers of the head and neck. *Dysphagia, 24*(2), 127–136.

Frowen, J., Cotton, S., Corry, J., & Perry, A. (2009). Impact of demographics, tumor characteristics, and treatment factors on swallowing after (chemo)radiotherapy for head and neck cancer. *Head and Neck, 32*(3).

Fujimoto, Y., Hasegawa, Y., Yamada, H., Ando, A., & Nakashima, T. (2007). Swallowing function following extensive resection of oral or oropharyngeal cancer with laryngeal suspension and cricopharyngeal myotomy. *Laryngoscope, 117*(8), 1343–1348.

Galli, J., Valenza, V., Parillo, C., Galla, J., Marchese, M., Castaldi, P., . . . Paludetti, G. (2009). Pharyngocutaneous fistula onset after total laryngectomy: Scintigraphic analysis. *Acta Oto-Rhinolaryngologica Italia, 29*(5), 242–244.

Gillespie, M. B., Brodsky, M. B., Day, T. A., Sharma, A. K., Lee, F. S., & Martin-Harris, B. (2005). Laryngeal penetration and aspiration during swallowing after the treatment of advanced oropharyngeal cancer. *Archives of Otolaryngology-Head and Neck Surgery, 131*(7), 615–619.

Graner, D. E., Foote, R. L., Kasperbauer, J. L., Stoeckel, R. E., Okuno, S. H., Olsen, K. D., . . . Strome, S. E. (2003). Swallow function in patients before and after intra-arterial chemoradiation. *Laryngoscope, 113*(3), 573–579.

Hanna, E., Alexiou, M., Morgan, J., Badley, J., Maddox, A. M., Penagaricano, J., . . . Suen, J. (2004). Intensive chemoradiotherapy as a primary treatment for organ preservation in patients with advanced cancer of the head and neck: efficacy, toxic effects, and limitations. *Archives of Otolaryngology-Head and Neck Surgery, 130*(7), 861–867.

Haughey, B. H., Hinni, M. L., Salassa, J. R., Hayden, R. E., Grant, D. G., Rich, J. T., . . . Krishna, M. (2011). Transoral laser microsurgery as primary treatment for advanced-stage oropharyngeal cancer: A United States multicenter study. *Head and Neck-Journal for the Sciences and Specialties of the Head and Neck, 33*(12), 1683–1694.

Hutcheson, K. A., Barringer, D. A., Rosenthal, D. I., May, A. H., Roberts, D. B., & Lewin, J. S. (2008). Swallowing outcomes after radiotherapy for laryngeal carcinoma. *Archives of Otolaryngology-Head and Neck Surgery, 134*(2), 178–183.

Iseli, T. A., Kulbersh, B. D., Iseli, C. E., Carroll, W. R., Rosenthal, E. L., & Magnuson, J. S. (2009). Functional outcomes after transoral robotic surgery for head and neck cancer. *Otolaryngology-Head and Neck Surgery, 141*(2), 166–171.

Klozar, J., Cada, Z., & Koslabova, E. (2012). Complications of total laryngectomy in the era of chemoradiation. *European Archives of Otorhinolaryngology, 269*(1), 1691–1695.

Kotz, T., Abraham, S., Beitler, J. J., Wadler, S., & Smith, R. V. (1999). Pharyngeal transport dysfunction consequent to an organ-sparing protocol. *Archives of Otolaryngology-Head and Neck Surgery, 125*(4), 410–413.

Kreuzer, S. H., Schima, W., Schober, E., Pokieser, P., Kofler, G., Lechner, G., . . . Denk, D. M. (2000). Complications after laryngeal surgery: Videofluoroscopic evaluation of 120 patients. *Clinical Radiology, 55*(10), 775–781.

Landera, M., Lundy, D., & Sullivan, P. (2010). Dysphagia after total laryngectomy. *Perspectives on Swallowing and Swallowing Disorders, 19*(2).

Lango, M. N., Egleston, B., Ende, K., Feigenberg, S., D'Ambrosio, D. J., Cohen, R. B., . . . Ridge, J. A. (2010). Impact of neck dissection on long-term feeding tube dependence in patients with primary radiation or chemoradiation. *Head and Neck-Journal for the Sciences and Specialties of the Head and Neck, 32*(3), 341–347.

Lazarus, C., Logemann, J. A., & Gibbons, P. (1993). Effects of maneuvers on swallowing function in a dysphagic oral-cancer patient. [Article]. *Head* and *Neck-Journal for the Sciences and Specialties of the Head and Neck, 15*(5), 419–424.

Lazarus, C. L. (1993). Effects of radiation therapy and voluntary maneuvers on swallow functioning in head and neck cancer patients. *Clinics in Communication Disorders, 3*(4), 11–20.

Lewin, J. S., Hutcheson, K. A., Barringer, D. A., May, A. H., Roberts, D. B., Holsinger, C., & Diaz, E. M. (2008). Functional analysis of swallowing outcomes after supracricoid partial laryngectomy. *Head and Neck-Journal for the Sciences and Specialties of the Head and Neck, 30*(5), 559–566.

Logemann, J. (1998). *Evaluation and treatment of swallowing disorders* (2nd ed.). Austin, TX: Pro-Ed.

Logemann, J. A., Pauloski, B. R., Rademaker, A. W., & Colangelo, L. A. (1997). Super-supraglottic swallow in irradiated head and neck cancer patients. *Head and Neck, 19*(6), 535–540.

Logemann J. A., Pauloski B. R., Rademaker A. W., Lazarus, C., Gaziano, J., Stachowiak, L., . . . Mittal, B. (2008). Swallowing disorders in the first year after radiation and chemoradiation. *Head and Neck, 30*(2), 148–158.

Logemann, J. A., Rademaker, A., Pauloski, B. R., Kelly, A., Stangl-McBreen, C., Antinoja, J., . . . Shaker, R. (2009). A randomized study comparing the shaker exercise with traditional therapy: A preliminary study. *Dysphagia, 24*(4), 403–411.

Logemann, J. A., Rademaker, A., Pauloski, B. R., Lazarus, C., Mittal, B. B., Brockstein, B., . . . Liu, D. (2005). Site of disease and treatment protocol as correlates of swallowing function in patients with head and neck cancer treated with chemoradiation. *Head and Neck, 28*, 64–73.

Logemann, J. A., Roa Pauloski, B., Rademaker, A., Cook, B., Graner, D., Milianti, F., . . . Lazarus, C. (1992). Impact of the diagnostic procedure on outcome measures of swallowing rehabilitation in head and neck cancer patients. *Dysphagia, 7*(4), 179–186.

Lundy, D. S., Smith, C., Colangelo, L., Sullivan, P. A., Logemann, J. A., Lazarus, C. L., . . . Gaziano, J. (1999). Aspiration: Cause and implications. *Otolaryngology-Head and Neck Surgery, 120*(4), 474–478.

Maclean, J., Cotton, S., & Perry, A. (2009). Post laryngectomy: It's hard to swallow. An Australian study of prevalence and self reports of swallow function after total laryngectomy. *Dysphagia, 24*(2).

Maclean, J., Szczesniak, M., Cotton, S., & Perry, A. (2011). Impact of a laryngectomy and surgical closure technique on swallow biomechanics and dysphagia severity. *Otolaryngology-Head and Neck Surgery, 144*(1), 21–28.

McCombe, D., Lyons, B., Winkler, R., & Morrison, W. (2005). Speech and swallowing following radial forearm flap reconstruction of major soft palate defects. *British Journal of Plastic Surgery, 58*(3), 306–311.

McConnel, F. M., Pauloski, B. R., Logemann, J. A., Rademaker, A. W., Colangelo, L., Shedd, D., . . . Johnson, J. (1998). Functional results of primary closure vs flaps in oropharyngeal reconstruction: A prospective study of speech and swallowing. *Archives of Otolaryngology-Head and Neck Surgery, 124*(6), 625–630.

McIvor, J., Evans, P., Perry, A., & Cheesman, A. (1990). Radiological assessment of post laryngectomy speech. *Clinical Radiology, 41*(5), 312–316.

Mittal, B. B., Pauloski, B. R., Haraf, D. J., Pelzer, H. J., Argiris, A., Vokes, E. E., . . . Logemann, J. A. (2003). Swallowing dysfunction-preventative and rehabilitation strategies in patients with head-and-neck cancers treated with surgery, radiotherapy, and chemotherapy: A critical review. *International Journal of Radiation Oncology, Biology, Physics, 57*(5), 1219–1230.

Nguyen, N. P., Frank, C., Moltz, C. C., Vos, P., Smith, H. J., Bhamidipati, P. V., . . . Sallah, S. (2006). Aspiration rate following chemoradiation for head and neck cancer: An underreported occurrence. *Radiotherapy and Oncology, 80*(3), 302–306.

Nguyen, N. P., Frank, C., Moltz, C. C., Vos, P., Smith, H. J., Nguyen, P. D., . . . Sallah, S. (2009). Analysis of factors influencing aspiration risk following chemoradiation for oropharyngeal cancer. *British Journal of Radiology, 82*, 675–680.

Nguyen, N. P., Moltz, C. C., Frank, C., Karlsson, U., Smith, H. J., Nguyen, P. D., . . . Sallah, S. (2005). Severity and duration of chronic dysphagia following treatment for head and neck cancer. *Anticancer Research*, *25*(4), 2929–2934.

Nguyen, N. P., Moltz, C. C., Frank, C., Vos, P., Smith, H. J., Karlsson, U., . . . Sallah, S. (2004). Dysphagia following chemoradiation for locally advanced head and neck cancer. *Annals of Oncology*, *15*(3), 383–388.

Nguyen, N. P., Moltz, C. C., Frank, C., Vos, P., Smith, H. J., Nguyen, P. D., . . . Sallah, S. (2007). Impact of swallowing therapy on aspiration rate following treatment for locally advanced head and neck cancer. *Oral Oncology*, *43*(4), 352–357.

Nguyen, N. P., Smith, H. J., Moltz, C. C., Frank, C., Millar, C., Dutta, S., . . . Sallah S. (2008). Prevalence of pharyngeal and esophageal stenosis following radiation for head and neck cancer. *Journal of Otolaryngology-Head and Neck Surgery*, *37*(2), 219–224.

Patterson, J. (2011). *Swallowing in head and neck cancer patients treated with (chemo)radiotherapy.* Unpublished thesis, Newcastle University.

Pauloski, B. R., Logemann, J. A., & Rademaker, A. (1993). Speech and swallowing function after anterior tongue and floor of mouth resection with distal flap reconstruction. *Journal of Speech Language and Hearing Research*, *36*, 267–276.

Pauloski, B. R., Logemann, J. A., Rademaker, A. WMcConnel, F.M.S., Stein, D,. Beery, Q., . . . Baker, T. (1993). Speech and swallowing function after anterior tongue and floor of mouth resection with distal flap reconstruction. *Journal of Speech and Hearing Research*, *36*(2), 267–276.

Pauloski, B. R., Rademaker, A. W., Logemann, J. A., McConnel, F. M., Heiser, M. A., Cardinale, S., . . . Beery, Q. (2004). Surgical variables affecting swallowing in patients treated for oral/oropharyngeal cancer. *Head and Neck*, *26*(7), 625–636.

Pauloski, B. R., Rademaker, A. W., Logemann, J. A., Stein, D., Beery, Q., Newman, L., . . . MacCracken, E. (2000). Pretreatment swallowing function in patients with head and neck cancer. *Head and Neck*, *22*(5), 474–482.

Perry, A., AD, C., McIvor, J., & Chalton, R. (1987). A British experience of surgical voice restoration techniques as a secondary procedure following total laryngectomy. *Journal of Laryngology and Otology*, *101*(2), 155–163.

Purkey, M. T., Levine, M. S., Prendes, B., Norman, M. F., & Mirza, N. (2009). Predictors of aspiration pneumonia following radiotherapy for head and neck cancer. *Annals of Otology Rhinology and Laryngology*, *118*(11), 811–816.

Rieger, J. M., Zalmanowitz, J. G., Li, S. Y. Y., Sytsanko, A., Harris, J., Williams, D. . . . Seikaly H. (2007). Functional outcomes after surgical reconstruction of the base of tongue using the radial forearm free flap in patients with oropharyngeal carcinoma. *Head and Neck-Journal for the Sciences and Specialties of the Head and Neck*, *29*(11), 1024–1032.

Roe, J. W. G., Carding, P. N., Dwivedi, R. C., Kazi, R. A., Rhys-Evans, P. H., Harrington, K. J., . . . Nutting, C. M. (2010). Swallowing outcomes following intensity modulated radiation therapy (IMRT) for head and neck cancer—A systematic review. *Oral Oncology*, *46*(10), 727–733.

Rosenthal, D. I., Lewin, J. S., & Eisbruch, A. (2006). Prevention and treatment of dysphagia and aspiration after chemoradiation for head and neck cancer. *Journal of Clinical Oncology*, *24*(17), 2636–2643.

Scott, P., Bleach, N., Perry, A., & Cheesman, A. (1993). Complications of pharyngeal myotomy for alrayngeal voice rehabilitation. *Journal of Laryngology and Otology*, *107*, 403–433.

Seikaly, H., Rieger, J., O'Connell, D., Ansari, K., AlQahtani, K., & Harris, J. (2009). Beavertail modification of the radial forearm free flap in base of tongue reconstruction: Technique and functional outcomes. *Head and Neck-Journal for the Sciences and Specialties of the Head and Neck*, *31*(2), 213–219.

Seikaly, H., Rieger, J., Zalmanowitz, J., Tang, J. L., Alkahtani, K., Ansari, K., . . . Harris, J. R. (2008). Functional soft palate reconstruction: a comprehensive surgical approach. *Head and Neck-Journal for the Sciences and Specialties of the Head and Neck*, *30*(12), 1615–1623.

Silverman, J., & Deschler, D. (2008). A novel approach for dilation of neopharyngeal stricture following total laryngectomy using the tracheosophageal puncture site. *Laryngoscope*, *118*, 2011–2013.

Simonelli, M., Ruoppolo, G., de Vincentiis, M., Di Mario, M., Calcagno, P., Vitiello, C., . . . Gallo, A. (2010). Swallowing ability and chronic aspiration after supracricoid partial laryngectomy. *Otolaryngology-Head and Neck Surgery, 142*(6), 873–878.

Sinclair, C. F., McColloch, N. L., Carroll, W. R., Rosenthal, E. L., Desmond, R. A., & Magnuson, J. S. (2011). Patient-perceived and objective functional outcomes following transoral robotic surgery for early oropharyngeal carcinoma. *Archives of Otolaryngology-Head and Neck Surgery, 137*(11), 1112–1116.

Sloane, P., Griffin, J., & ODwyer, T. (1991). Esophageal insufflation and videofluoroscopy for evaluation of esophageal soeech in laryngecatomy patients: Clinical implications. *Radiology, 181*(2), 433–437.

Smit, C., Tan, J., Mathus-Vliegen, L., Devriese, P., Brandsen, M., Grolman, W., . . . Schouwenberg, P. (1998). High incidence of gastropharyngeal and gastroesophageal reflux after total laryngectomy. *Head and Neck, 20*(7), 619–622.

Smith, J. E., Suh, J. D., Erman, A., Nabili, V., Chhetri, D. K., & Blackwell, K. E. (2008). Risk factors predicting aspiration after free flap reconstruction of oral cavity and oropharyngeal defects. *Archives of Otolaryngology-Head and Neck Surgery, 134*(11), 1205–1208.

Smith, R. V., Kotz, T., Beitler, J. J., & Wadler, S. (2000). Long-term swallowing problems after organ preservation therapy with concomitant radiation therapy and intravenous hydroxyurea: Initial results. *Archives of Otolaryngology-Head and Neck Surgery, 126*(3), 384–389.

Sullivan, P., & Hartig, G. (2001). Dysphagia after total laryngectomy. *Current Opinion in Otolaryngology-Head and Neck Surgery, 9*, 139–146.

Tei, K., Maekawa, K., Kitada, H., Ohiro, Y., Yamazaki, Y., & Totsuka, Y. (2007). Recovery from postsurgical swallowing dysfunction in patients with oral cancer. *Journal of Oral and Maxillofacial Surgery, 65*(6), 1077–1083.

Thomas, L., Jones, T. M., Tandon, S., Katre, C., Lowe, D., & Rogers, S. N. (2008). An evaluation of the University of Washington Quality of Life swallowing domain following oropharyngeal cancer. *European Archives of Oto-Rhino-Laryngology, 265*, S29–S37.

van der Molen, L., van Rossum, M. A., Ackerstaff, A. H., Smeele, L. E., Rasch, C. R. N., & Hilgers, F. J. M. (2009). Pretreatment organ function in patients with advanced head and neck cancer: Clinical outcome measures and patients' views. *BioMedCentral Ear, Nose, and Throat Disorders, 9*, 10.

Ward, E., Frisby, J., & Stephens, M. (2002). Swallowing outcomes following laryngectomy and pharyngolaryngectomy. *Archives of Otolaryngology-Head and Neck Surgery, 128*(2).

Zuydam, A. C., Rogers, S. N., Brown, J. S., Vaughan, E. D., & Magennis, P. (2000). Swallowing rehabilitation after oro-pharyngeal resection for squamous cell carcinoma. *British Journal of Oral and Maxillofacial Surgery, 38*(5), 513–518.

Chapter

15

STRUCTURAL CAUSES OF HIGH DYSPHAGIA

Roger D. Newman

INTRODUCTION

Structural causes of high dysphagia, although not normally life-threatening, may prove disabling to the individual and have varying levels of impact upon the swallowing function, both structural and neurological. Videofluoroscopic examinations of swallowing are a key component in highlighting the exact nature of the pathology, plus any secondary deficit. There are a number of causes of pharyngoesophageal dysphagia, and as a result not all can be described in detail in one chapter. The nature and incidence of four different disorders are presented, explaining the pathophysiology, clinical presentation, and the role of videofluoroscopy in the assessment and management of this client group. The disorders to be described in detail are cervical osteophytes, Zenker's diverticulum, cricopharyngeal prominence, and the interesting but rare incidence of a postcricoid web.

CERVICAL OSTEOPHYTES

Incidence

Cervical osteophytes are bony outgrowths of the anterior cervical spine associated with vertebral degenerative disease. Differential diagnosis of the origin of such bony outgrowths is extensive and includes osteoarthritis (OA), spondylosis deformans, acromegaly, hypoparathyroidism, fluorosis, ochronosis, and trauma (Resnick, 1995). However, the most common causes are reported as being diffuse idiopathic skeletal hyperostosis (DISH) (also known as Forestier's disease) and ankylosing spondylitis (AS) (Carlson, Archibald, Graner, & Kasperbauer, 2011).

DISH is a skeletal disease characterized by ossification of the anterolateral side of the spine and various extraspinal ligaments (Kiss, Szilagyi, Paksy, & Poor, 2002). Although patients with DISH may also suffer from OA, it is reported that patients affected by DISH may differ from patients with primary OA in several aspects. Important examples of these are the cause of cervical osteophytes being the anatomic site of primary involvement (i.e., the primary site for DISH to present being the *cervical* spine); the prevalence in the general population; gender distribution; and the size and distribution of osteophytes in the spine (Sarzi-Puttini & Atzeni, 2004).

Ankylosing spondylitis is a chronic inflammatory spinal disease of unknown cause and belongs to a group of diseases which includes reactive arthritis, arthritis/spondylitis associated with inflammatory bowel disease, and psoriatic arthritis/spondylitis (Chen & Liu, 2009).

The vast majority of patients with cervical osteophytes are asymptomatic, but for those patients who are symptomatic, dysphagia (especially to solids) may be the only presenting complaint. In some patients, respiratory compromise may also be present, but this is thought to be rare.

The prevalence of cervical osteophytes secondary to DISH is greater in males than in females (Childs, 2004), with severe radiological changes reported more commonly in males (Bloom, 1984). Research has shown that the prevalence of DISH is greater in Caucasians, Japanese, Pima Indians, African Blacks, and Jews in Jerusalem, but is less common in American Blacks, suggesting a genetic origin of the condition (Weinfeld, Olson, Maki, & Griffiths, 1997). Incidence also increases with age, and in total is predicted to account for approximately 30% of the population (Granville, Musson, Altman, & Silverman, 1998). An association with obesity has been noted since the early description of the condition by Forestier and Rotes-Querol (1950).

Conversely, ankylosing spondylitis is reported to affect approximately 0.1 to 0.5% of the population (Sciuba et al., 2008) and has a worldwide prevalence ranging up to 9% (Braun et al., 1998). Etiology and pathogenesis are not yet fully understood (Sieper et al., 2002). However, immune-mediated mechanisms (abnormal activity of the body's immune system) plus genetic and environmental factors are thought to have key roles (Sieper et al., 2002).

Pathophysiology

Cervical osteophytes may form when the vertebral disk begins to degenerate which in turn compromises spinal stability. Biomechanical analysis of vertebral movement has shown that the intervertebral disk forms a stabilizing medium, and when degeneration of this disk commences, spinal support is reduced (Kumaresan et al., 2001). The increased level of stress this causes precipitates the need for increased stability, hence the formation of increased bone tissue forming an outgrowth (osteophyte) on the anterior surface of the cervical spine.

Similar stress-induced osteophytic growth also has been shown to occur following trauma and certain surgical procedures where the cervical vertebrae have been involved and support to the neck has become reduced (Ortega-Martínez, Cabezudo, Gómez-Perals, & Fernández-Portales, 2005). Metabolic factors have been identified as being associated with DISH which relate to insulin-associated excessive bone growth in Type II diabetes mellitus (Denko & Malemud, 2006). As the population ages, the proportion of metabolically vulnerable people increases secondary to societal weight gain and, with an associated increase in diabetes, the prevalence of DISH is predicted to increase (Ngian & Littlejohn, 2010). It therefore is likely that the occurrence of cervical osteophytes will also increase, though this remains to be seen.

Clinical Presentations

In addition to dysphagia, compression of the upper airway caused by the outgrowth of the cervical spine may lead to shortness of breath, stridor, and cough, all of which may be related to the onset of dysphagia or stand alone as an isolated symptom. Other complications include musculoskeletal symptoms such as fusion of the osteophytes causing a "bamboo"appearance, particularly in AS (Figures 15–1 and 15–2), sleep apnea, and complete airway obstruction. Although quite rare, pain may also be present as a result of advanced osteophytic growth and fusion causing compression of the pharyngeal cavity and irritation of the nerve endings, but the pain may only be present upon moving the head and/or swallowing. Interestingly, although it is acknowledged that there is a higher incidence of DISH and secondary osteophytes in males, pain and tenderness associated with osteophytic growth secondary to DISH in the cervical spine has been shown to be higher in females (Ngian & Littlejohn, 2010).

Large osteophytes, similar to those seen in Figure 15–3, are known to cause oropharyngeal dysphagia through a variety of mechanisms, including: direct compression of the oro- and hypopharynx (Resnick & Niwayama, 1976); disturbances of the level of normal epiglottic tilt over the laryngeal inlet by the

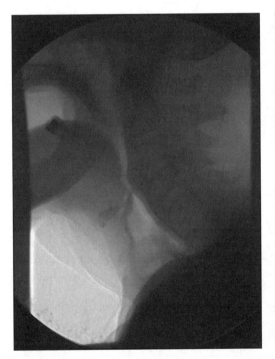

Figure 15–1. *Lateral view of the pharynx and cervical spine clearly demonstrating large osteophytic growth and secondary fusion. The fusion may have extended into the thoracic spine but this is not possible to ascertain due to the patient's shoulder obliterating the view.*

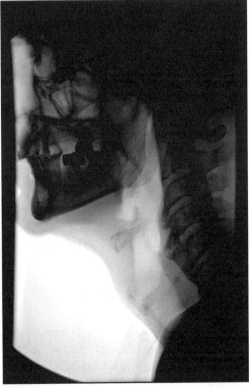

Figure 15–2. *Large cervical osteophytes at C3–C5, with secondary fusion of C5–C7. Neck movement was significantly difficult.*

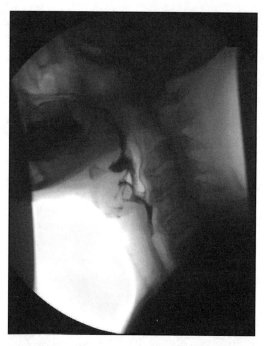

Figure 15-3. *The impact that osteophytic growth has on the posterior pharyngeal wall. Note the contrast coating the pharyngeal mucosa highlighting the abnormal bulges that impact upon the success of the hypopharyngeal pump.*

osteophytes at the level of C3-C4 (Lambert, Tepperman, Jimenez & Newman, 1981; Suzuki, Ishida & Ohmori, 1991); inflammatory reactions in the tissues around the pharynx and esophagus (Akhtar, O'Flynn, Kelly & Valentine, 2000) and cricopharyngeal spasm (Forestier & Rotes-Querol, 1950).

Ethical Dilemmas

Cervical osteophyte-induced dysphagia secondary to AS has been shown to respond to treatment with non-steroidal anti-inflammatory drugs (NSAIDs) that decrease the amount of inflammation of the soft tissue surrounding the bony outgrowth (Ozgocmen, Kiris, Kocakoc, & Ardicoglu, 2002). However, as previously discussed, osteophyte-induced dysphagia may

simply be caused by compression of the pharynx and esophagus (to varying degrees) rather than by an inflammatory process (Unlu et al., 2008). In these instances, surgical resection may be the only option. Surgical resection of the osteophyte is a highly invasive procedure usually involving a left sided neck incision and retraction of the structures and complex nerve fibers and muscle tissue to reveal the cervical vertebrae. Depending on the vertebral level of the osteophytic change, a transoral approach with resection of the posterior pharyngeal wall may be necessary (Ergun & Kahrilas, 1997). Dissection of the osteophytes to the level of the anterior cortices of the vertebral bodies is then completed via the use of a bone cutter and high-speed air drill with diamond burs (Miyamoto et al., 2009).

Although this has been reported to be an effective treatment to remove the bony outgrowth and improve the symptoms including dysphagia, the potential for post-surgical osteophyte recurrence must be considered. Miyamoto et al., (2009) demonstrated that complete relief from dysphagia is successful after surgical resection or "shaving" of the anterior osteophyte compressing into the pharyngeal cavity. However, they went on to show that *all* the patients in their study that underwent the surgical resection later developed recurrence of the cervical osteophytes (demonstrated by radiological examination) 4 years after the original osteophyte resection. The recurrent osteophytes were then shown to continue to grow in thickness.

This demonstrates that while surgical recovery and relief from symptoms including dysphagia can be successful in the short term, longer-term recovery may be compromised by osteophyte regrowth. It must be remembered that the *cause* of the original osteophytic growth will persist, even after the osteophytes have been removed.

Consideration must be given to the patients' need for a repeat VFSS and therefore increased radiation exposure, or simply to repeat bedside oral trials. Close collaboration between the patient and all professionals involved in the examination is necessary to examine the pros and cons of repeating a VFSS.

ZENKER'S DIVERTICULUM

Incidence

The first documented evidence of a Zenker's diverticulum (also known as a pharyngeal pouch) was described by Abraham Ludlow in 1769 who reported an irregular dilation of the posterior pharyngeal wall during a postmortem examination of a patient who had complained of chronic dysphagia (Siddiq, Sood, & Strachan, 2001). However, the pharyngeal pouch became synonymous with Friedrich Albert von Zenker, a German pathologist and physician, following his publication in 1877 describing a series of 34 patients with this acquired diverticulum. Zenker's diverticulum remains the most common form of outpouching of the gastrointestinal tract, and has an estimated annual occurrence of two per 100,000 in the United Kingdom (Laing et al., 1995), yet the etiology remains unclear. In the majority of patients, the cause of Zenker's diverticulum is likely to involve a number of elements or factors. However, recent research suggests a geographical variation in its global occurrence, as the condition has been found to be more prevalent in Northern Europe (Klockars & Mäkitie, 2010), but is rarely seen in Japan or Indonesia (Siddiq, Sood, & Strachan, 2001). It is generally accepted that age plays a role, with pouches being found most commonly in patients age over 70 (Siddiq, Sood, & Strachan, 2001). Rarely, some familial cases of Zenker's diverticulum have been reported (Klockars, Sihvo, & Mäkitie, 2008; Marcus et al., 2005) with approximately 2% of patients presenting with Zenker's diverticulum having a positive family history. Very specific research has demonstrated the rare case of identical twins with Zenker's diverticulum which provides further evidence supporting a genetic predisposition (Klockars & Mäkitie, 2010).

Pathophysiology

A clear understanding of the origin of pharyngeal pouches is not definitively documented within medical literature. Several notions exist regarding the development of such diverticula. These include the irregular function of the cricopharyngeal muscle, and an anatomical predisposition due to a small triangular area on the posterior hypopharyngeal wall between the oblique fibers of the thyropharyngeus muscle and the transverse fibers of the cricopharyngeus muscle. This area is known as Killian's triangle/dehiscence, and has the point of least resistance during swallowing due to its lack of muscle fiber (Figure 15–4). The reduced resistance associated with Killian's dehiscence is due to the reduced density of muscle. Pouch formation is suggested to be triggered by a raised intrabolus pressure exacerbated by the loss of tissue elasticity and reduction in muscle tone, potentially associated with increased age (van Overbeek, 2003).

Clinical Presentation

The area of weakness can enable the mucosa to initially form a pulsion diverticulum that might subsequently develop into a pouch incarcerated through the dehiscence (Figure 15–5). Pouch formation is made more likely if the muscular triangle that forms the dehiscence is large (Siddiq, Sood, & Strachan, 2001). The most common and consistent feature of

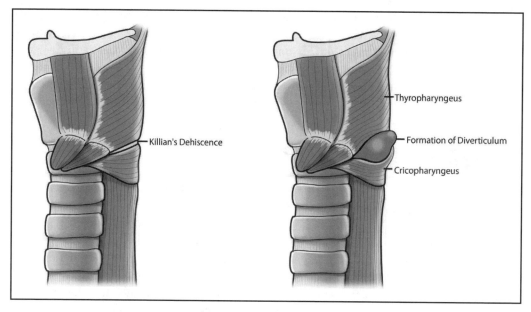

Figure 15–4. *Lateral view of the thyropharyngeus and cricopharyngeus muscles, with the triangular space between the two known as Killian's dehiscence. A Zenker's diverticulum can be seen forming via compression of the posterior pharyngeal wall through the dehiscence, creating the outpouching seen with such diverticula. This image can also be seen in full color in the color insert.*

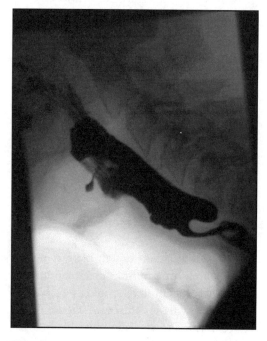

Figure 15–5. *A classic view of a Zenker's diverticulum, with the entrance sitting at the level of C6-C7. Note the diversion of the bolus flowing through the pharynx.*

a Zenker's diverticulum is dysphagia, whereby the patient may complain of *globus pharyngeus*: the constant sensation of a lump in the throat. However, the food or fluids filling the pouch will create this sensation so the perception of a lump in the throat will indeed be real, something that may not be found with "true" globus. In addition, simple successive swallowing may not clear its contents causing increased patient frustration. Other symptoms include regurgitation of undigested food, choking, a "grumbling" sound in the cervical region (the sound that usually occurs in normal circumstances in the lower gastrointestinal tract when hungry or just after eating), chronic cough, throat clearing, halitosis, and weight loss. A less common symptom is hoarseness, potentially caused by the actual regurgitation or overspill into the laryngeal inlet, or constant coughing or throat clearing causing varying degrees of damage to the vocal folds. In more severe cases, aspiration may occur due to overspill of contents from the pouch. The pouch distending with food, liquid, or saliva can compress the esophagus reducing the lumen size to a fraction of normal. In addition the esophagus can deviate anteriorly as it passes over the ballooned pouch. The duration of these symptoms may vary from weeks to several years as patients may ignore the signs and continue as normal, but continued deglutition of all consistencies will cause repeated filling of the pouch and enable it to increase in size (Figure 15–6). As the pouch enlarges, symptoms generally worsen, and large diverticula can result in severe malnutrition (Bowdler, 1997). Dietetic advice is extremely valuable in these cases.

Ethical Dilemmas

As there is no medical remediation for this condition, all patients who have such a diver-ticulum should be considered as potential candidates for surgical treatment (Cassivi et al., 2005). However, many patients may be elderly with comorbidities that must be taken into account. Various surgical techniques exist and depend on the nature and size of the diverticula, but the surgical approach most commonly used is open surgery with *cricopharyngeal myotomy* (Aly, Devitt, & Jamieson, 2004). Other interventions include endoscopic stapling of the entrance to the diverticulum (Sen, Kumar & Bhattacharyya, 2006) and interventional radiological approaches such as balloon dilation of the neck of the pouch. Both of these approaches offer the benefit of reduced hospital stay. A review by Crescenzo et al., (1998) revealed that 94% of patients over the age of 75 who underwent surgical treatment for Zenker's diverticulum demonstrated an improvement, and no intraoperative deaths were reported.

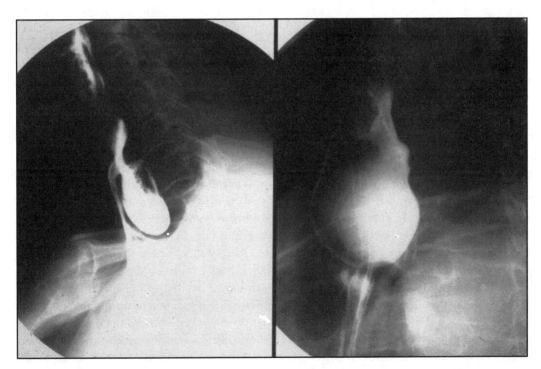

Figure 15–6. *Lateral and anterior-posterior view of a large Zenker's diverticulum filled with contrast extending into the mediastinum. From: Gastrointestinal Tract Imaging: An Evidence-Based Practice Guide (p. 119), by J. M. Nightingale & R. L. Law. Copyright © 2010 Elsevier. All rights reserved. Used with permission.*

However, the patient's comorbidities must be taken into account, and they may not be a suitable candidate for surgical intervention of any kind. The comorbidity may be related to the Zenker's diverticulum with regard to respiratory compromise, or it may be completely unrelated, but whatever the cause, the ethical dilemma remains of whether the patient should risk undergoing surgery. As previously mentioned, other potential treatments include endoscopy and interventional radiology, so these must be considered as viable treatment options for the patient.

POSTCRICOID WEB

Incidence

A web found in the cricopharyngeal region or the postcricoid esophagus can be defined as a thin, membranous tissue covered with squamous epithelium that compromises the cricopharyngeal sphincter or the lumen of the esophagus (Liu & Kahrilas, 2006). Webs can be subdivided into both congenital and acquired. The difference between the two is that congenital webs usually occur in the mid to lower esophagus, and are likely to lie on the full circumference of the esophageal wall and have a central opening and have a "ring" appearance; whereas acquired webs are characteristically thin and translucent, much more prevalent than congenital webs, and are often located only on the anterior surface of the superior esophageal and postcricoid regions. The terms *ring* and *web* often are used interchangeably in the literature, but in the case of an acquired postcricoid web, the term *ring* cannot be used due it not forming a full "ring."

The incidence of acquired postcricoid webs is complex in nature and can be attributed to many things. Literature reports that there is an association between postcricoid dysphagia,

upper esophageal webs, and iron deficiency anemia which is known as *Plummer-Vinson syndrome* in the United States and *Paterson-Kelly syndrome* in the United Kingdom (Liu & Kahrilas, 2006). However, despite the difference in the name, both disorders are identical, and in the early to mid-20th century were found to be more common in females than in males (Odin, 1937).

Pathophysiology

Despite Plummer-Vinson/Paterson-Kelly syndrome now being considered rare, isolated postcricoid webs can occasionally be seen with VFSS. Webs have also been reported to be associated with extracutaneous manifestations of blistering skin disorders such as *epidermolysis bullosa* (Ergun, Lin, Dannenberg, & Carter, 1992) and *bullous pemphigoid*, both chronic or acute autoimmune skin conditions (Foroozan, Enta, Winship, & Trier, 1967). Although the literature for this is now quite old, no updated research into the disorders is available and it is therefore presumed that these underlying conditions are still thought to precede a postcricoid web in some instances. However, more recent data report *gastroesophageal reflux disease* as a precipitating factor for the formation of such a web (Gordon et al., 2001), plus autoimmune conditions such as *rheumatoid arthritis, pernicious anemia, celiac disease*, and *thyroiditis* (Dickey & McConnell, 1999; Elwood, Pitman, Jacobs, & Entwistle, 1964).

In Sweden, where much of the research regarding Plummer-Vinson/Paterson-Kelly syndrome originated, results suggested an increase in presentations during the long winter season, when nutrient rich foods were traditionally less available creating the onset of an iron-deficiency and secondary internal upper gastrointestinal epithelial blistering (Wynder, Hultberg, Jacobsson, & Bross, 1957). It must be stated that in the research, correction of the hematologic abnormality which causes the anemia did not actually improve the symptoms of dysphagia or delay any spread or enlarging of existing esophageal webs (Elwood et al., 1964). This led to the proposal that any web-related dysphagia associated with iron-deficiency anemia may in fact be purely coincidental, especially considering the rarity of the phenomenon, and also when considering the fact that it remains as rare in geographical areas where iron deficiency anemia is widespread, for example, in certain areas of Africa. Despite this, full liaison with a dietician and obtaining blood results may prove beneficial in confirming a diagnosis to aid multidisciplinary treatment.

Clinical Presentation

The principal symptom for patients presenting with a postcricoid web is dysphagia. The severity of the dysphagia is directly related to the size and location of the web, and it is usual to find that the patient has greatest difficulty swallowing solids. Patients may also present with nasopharyngeal reflux as a result of the web causing some degree of regurgitation (potentially secondary to cricopharyngeal spasm), aspiration due to reflux or diversion depending on the size of the web, and spontaneous perforation (Beggs & Morgan, 1989). Another presenting complaint for patients with a web is the acute impaction of solid food that may prompt admission to hospital, and the diagnosis of the web itself.

Pain associated with heartburn and the sensation of food sticking in the throat has been reported with postcricoid webs (Weaver, 1979), and although it cannot be completely ruled out, this data is now old and heartburn-associated pain is thought to be more usually linked with a lower esophageal web. The altered "lump in the throat" sensation associated with *globus pharyngeus* has been reported

with postcricoid webs and confirmed by either barium swallow or videofluoroscopy (Takwoingi, Kale, & Morgan, 2005) (Figure 15–7).

Ethical Dilemmas

Secondary to its rarity, a postcricoid web may go undetected for some time. Though not a direct precursor to malignancy and extremely rare, cancers may form proximally to the web and have been anecdotally reported as arising secondary to chronic irritation (Swami & Ramakrishnan, 2009). This must be borne in mind for the purposes of differential diagnosis, and when forming hypotheses for treatment options. A patient's desire to be informed of

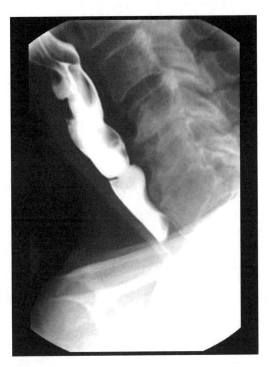

Figure 15–7. *Lateral pharynx with the classic view of an anterior postcricoid web. From: Gastrointestinal Tract Imaging: An Evidence-Based Practice Guide (p. 120), by J. M. Nightingale & R. L. Law. Copyright © 2010 Elsevier. All rights reserved. Used with permission.*

the outcome of a VFSS is likely to be extremely high, but if soft tissue swelling is noted in the region of a web, extreme caution must be executed to allay any unnecessary fears. Referral to other appropriate members of the multidisciplinary team must be implemented to rule out any possibility of malignancy.

In the asymptomatic patient, treatment may not be necessary at all. For patients with mild symptoms, simple lifestyle modifications such as complete bolus preparation, reduced rate of eating, and avoiding certain foods can often eliminate symptoms. This option may indeed be more preferable to the patient, and must be accepted as their choice.

CRICOPHARYNGEAL PROMINENCE

Incidence

The cricopharyngeus, also known as the upper esophageal sphincter (UES), was first described by Valsalva in 1717. It arises from the dorsolateral aspect on one side of the cricoid cartilage then, making a horizontal loop around the esophagus, inserts into the dorsolateral aspect on the opposite side of the cricoid cartilage. A cricopharyngeal prominence may result from persistent spasm of the UES resulting in symptoms of dysphagia. This was described by Asherton in 1950 as cricopharyngeal achalasia (Asherton, 1950) but this is now considered a misnomer. Cricopharyngeal prominence is characterized on barium swallow as an impression on the posterior wall of the pharyngeal esophagus that normally would not be seen (Goyal, 1984).

Dysfunction of the cricopharyngeus is a common cause for dysphagia in the elderly (Leaper, Zhang, & Dawes, 2005). Several factors open the esophageal lumen at the level of the cricopharyngeus: *relaxation; hyolaryngeal elevation; pharyngeal contraction;* and *bolus pressure.* As a result of the combination of the rapid movement of the bolus through the pharynx, the elderly swallow may not be as able to cope with the speed of transition and the cricopharyngeus may not relax as much as is necessary, resulting in a prominent appearance on VFSS.

Pathophysiology

The pathogenesis of esophageal constriction by the cricopharyngeus muscle is uncertain but may be due to neuromuscular activity, spasm, or fibrotic shortening of the muscle band. Five percent of asymptomatic pharyngeal barium swallows will demonstrate prominence of the cricopharyngeus.

The most common symptom is dysphagia, although globus pharyngeus is also common. Disruption to the function of the cricopharyngeus muscle is also considered to be associated with the pathogenesis of Zenker's diverticulum. Medical treatment can include therapy associated with gastroesophageal reflux disease. Injecting the cricopharyngeus muscle with botulinum toxin is said to provide temporary relief of approximately 4 months and has onset around day seven (Moerman, 2006). Although the procedure can be considered to be technically difficult, complication rates are low. Surgically, cricopharyngeal myotomy can be used for longer term symptomatic relief.

Clinical Presentation

A cricopharyngeal prominence can result from spasm, hypertrophy, or pharyngeal weakness. Theoretically, the cricopharyngeus should open completely to allow free passage of the bolus into the proximal esophagus. However, the cricopharyngeus may open late, incompletely or close early, sometimes trapping fluid in the sphincter segment. As previously mentioned, this may be the precursor to a Zenker's diverticulum, being the pressure to force open Killian's dehiscence and form the pouch. In addition, a cricopharyngeal prominence is often seen in those patients who present with a Zenker's diverticulum.

Radiographically, a cricopharyngeal prominence will present as a posterior indentation at approximately the C5–C6 or C6–C7 level during bolus passage, indicating the level of the cricopharyngeus (Figure 15–8).

Ethical Dilemmas

The main problem encountered when a cricopharyngeal prominence is discovered is how to

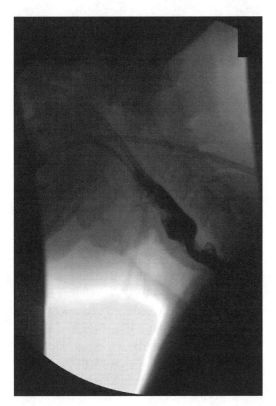

Figure 15–8. *Lateral view of the cricopharyngeal prominence at the level of C5–C6.*

resolve it. As mentioned, botulinim toxin is often used to relax the CP sphincter, but this usually involves a general anesthetic and the patient may not be a suitable candidate. Alternatively, a cricopharyngeal myotomy completed via endoscopy under local anesthetic may be viable, but complications including fistula, wound infection and even procedure-related mortality have been reported (Takes, van den Hoogen, & Marres, 2005). The main questions to ask when completing the VFSS are: "How severe is the deficit?" and "What impact is it having?" Once these questions have been answered and various consistencies have been trialed, the next step to take can then be decided.

ROLE OF VIDEOFLUOROSCOPY IN THE MANAGEMENT OF THIS PATIENT GROUP

It is acknowledged that alternative instrumental examinations such as fiberoptic endoscopic evaluation of swallowing (FEES) have a definite positive role in the examination of the structure of the oro- and hypopharynx (see Chapter 2). The images obtained from FEES will demonstrate the nature of the obstruction from a superior-inferior viewing perspective, but if the partial obstruction is too narrow for the endoscope to pass, then the inferior level to which the obstruction extends cannot be viewed. In many cases the pharyngeal mucosa may be thinner or may have been weakened by the obstruction/diverticulum and the risk of trauma or potential perforation by the endoscope must be considered.

VFSS will demonstrate the nature and extent of the dysphagia, particularly of the lower hypopharynx, and any adverse impacts on swallowing function. Diverticula and lower pharyngeal webs may not be visible upon endoscopic examination, but should be well demonstrated by VFSS. The impact that these obstructions have upon swallowing can be extremely severe.

Conducting the VFSS in the lateral projection will reveal the size, level and nature of cervical osteophytes, plus the extent of any fusion. The lateral projection will demonstrate the location and size of any diverticulum and pharyngeal web. It will also enable the differentiation of a postcricoid web and a cricopharyngeal bar, a web being anterior and a bar typically being posterior and often associated with a Zenker's diverticulum (Cook, 2006). Lateral fluoroscopy will also reveal any functional impact upon the swallow such as the amount and level of contrast collection, plus secondary reflux or spasm caused as a result. Anterior-posterior projections will highlight any laterality of deficit, but will also identify the inferior extent of the pouch (Figure 15–9), something that only a VFSS is able to do.

While the swallowing function (and any subsequent deficit) is traditionally considered to be within the domain of the SLP, examination of the anatomical structures of the pharynx and esophagus and the cervical/thoracic vertebrae is generally considered aligned to the role of the radiographer/radiologist. The multidisciplinary team approach to videofluoroscopic examination therefore has distinct advantages in identifying a definitive diagnosis and appropriate patient management strategies. As mentioned in previous chapters, high density barium is more suited to highlight structure by coating the mucosa, whereas low density contrast is better suited to highlight function. If a structural abnormality or pharyngeal obstruction is revealed during VFSS, the radiographer/radiologist may decide it is in the patient's best interests to change the contrast being used from low density to high density to precisely reveal the nature of the anomaly. Similarly, the option to convert to a conventional barium swallow to more thoroughly examine a possible concurrent esophageal pathology may be considered.

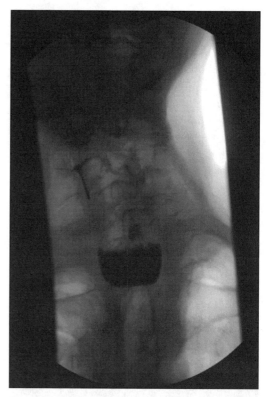

Figure 15–9. *Anterior-posterior view of a large Zenker's diverticulum extending from the inferior pharyngeal cavity into the superior mediastinum with the lower surface of the pouch lying in the midline below the level of the clavicles.*

There are various elements that all clinicians involved in the VFSS should be aware of when an obstruction has been identified. Capturing a control fluoroscopic image prior to commencing oral trials will potentially highlight the size and level of the obstruction. When trials have commenced, the extent of hyolaryngeal excursion should be examined to ascertain if this is reduced as a result of the obstruction. Epiglottic inversion may also be incomplete, particularly in the case of cervical osteophytes where the outgrowth may act as a "shelf like" structure in the hypopharynx, inhibiting epiglottic retroflexion leaving a patent airway for peri- or post-swallow aspiration to occur. Post-swallow residue (plus the level and amount thereof) must also be examined as this offers a potential threat of post swallow aspiration, even if airway closure was complete during the swallow. If the presence of a diverticulum is established, its location is of great importance due to the threat of post swallow aspiration, but also for any surgery or interventional radiology to be successful. Depending on its size and location, a diverticulum typically empties its contents upward into the hypopharynx. A true Zenker's diverticulum may therefore not be evident on initial screening, but the presence of aspirated contrast post swallow without locating an original source indicates regurgitation (Coyle, 2010). Oblique or anterior-posterior positioning is therefore beneficial to expose the diverticulum and the impact the structural abnormality has on the functional swallow.

In the case of a postcricoid web, it is essential that a clear unobstructed view of the upper esophagus is obtained to reveal the size, shape, and extension of the obstruction, plus the nature and extent of any reflux or regurgitation caused by spasm.

MODIFICATIONS TO THE TECHNIQUE

As with all videofluoroscopic examinations, the aim is not only to establish the cause of a dysphagia, but also find the safest method of feeding for patients. This can be through positional modification, altering the consistency of the bolus presented, or both of the above. However, as a significant structural deficit has been identified, the usual techniques outlined in Chapter 1 may not be of benefit to the patient, and in fact may cause more harm.

As previously mentioned, the use of high density contrast to coat the pharyngeal mucosa and subsequently the obstruction will highlight the irregularity in more detail, but it cannot be forgotten that the main purpose of a VFSS is to examine the *functional swallow* and

the *functional deficit*. Two separate examinations may therefore be warranted, one using high density contrast to highlight the nature, location and size of the structural obstruction, and one using low density contrast to examine the impact that the obstruction has on the swallowing function. Close monitoring of radiation exposure must therefore be taken into account (see Chapter 8).

Ascertaining laterality or preferential side of bolus transit is warranted, as this will highlight if positional modification is likely to prove beneficial. In the case of cervical osteophytes, alternating solid and liquid boluses may facilitate pharyngeal clearance (Clark, 2010) though normal aging swallowing and any existing neurologic deficit must be taken into account. This is because vallecular residue may impact upon any fluid boluses subsequently taken, and may influence the safe passage of fluid: the solid bolus may direct the liquid bolus into the airway where under normal circumstances it would remain in the valleculae. In addition, while cervical osteophytes may appear on a lateral image to be symmetric, there may be some degree of unilaterality to the obstruction. As a result, Logemann (1998) reports that tilting the head to the unaffected side or rotating the head to the affected side improve bolus transition for safe passage into the esophagus, hence the need for an A-P viewing plane. This is also beneficial for patients with a diverticulum where laterality of deficit has been identified. Siddiq, Sood, & Strachan (2001) showed that the majority of true Zenker's diverticula deviate slightly left of the midline, although not in all cases, so examination in A-P positioning is vital to ascertain the laterality of deficit and the benefit of positional modification.

When a patient exhibits laryngeal penetration or aspiration, it is usual to attempt a chin tuck to aid laryngeal elevation and epiglottic inversion. However, in patients with cervical osteophytes, this movement may in fact further narrow the oro- and hypopharynx, and reduce the space available for bolus transition already impacted upon, and intensify any pain the patient is suffering. However, Carlson et al. (2011) suggest that not all patients will experience this and it may prove beneficial. However, in Zenker's diverticulum, a chin tuck may not be of benefit due to the fact that the entrance to the diverticulum may be increased in size, allowing greater residue to accumulate and potentially spill out or regurgitate post swallow. However, minimal evidence is available to support this theory and so each case must be analyzed individually. Again, this exemplifies the benefit of VFSS whereby the success of such modifications can be examined.

One technique which is useful for many cases where pharyngeal obstruction is present is a supraglottic swallow (see Chapter 1) to aid airway protection. In all cases described, the use of a supraglottic swallow followed by simple throat clearing and a dry swallow may be sufficient to protect the airway at the primary swallow and clear any residue from the voluntary successive swallow(s).

The main modification to the procedure is to examine the structural anomaly in addition to the functional deficit it has on the patient's swallowing mechanism, plus attempt various techniques to assess safe bolus transition and potential prognosis for improvement. Planning the next steps to be taken for either behavioral or surgical management is also of significant importance.

CONCLUSION

The range of nonmalignant obstructions can be considered as wide as their malignant counterparts. However, the nature of such disorders is very different, and bedside assessment is not enough to form a detailed plan of action. The presentation on VFSS not only proves extremely interesting, but is an essential part of diagnostic decision making. It is important to remember that although positional modifications or swallowing maneuvers may be enough to overcome the problem at the immediate stage, future treatment needs to be considered, and a wide range of multidisciplinary colleagues may need to be involved in the care of the patient. Those professionals outside of the fluoroscopy suite range from dieticians to ENT surgeons, but all have a valuable role in patient care. Given the progressive nature of many of the nonmalignant obstructions described, plus their potentially huge impact on the individual, repeat examinations may be necessary to examine the success of any intervention. The patient's quality of life must always be considered.

Acknowledgments. Many thanks to Robert L. Law, Consultant Gastrointestinal Radiographer from North Bristol NHS Trust for the provision of invaluable direction regarding some of the pharyngoesophageal structural anomalies which may lead to varying degrees of dysphagia.

REFERENCES

Akhtar, S., O'Flynn, P. E., Kelly, A., & Valentine, P. M. W. (2000). The management of dysphagia in skeletal hyperostosis. *Journal of Laryngology and Otology, 114,* 154–157.

Aly, A., Deviit, P. G., & Jamieson, G. G. (2004). Evolution of surgical treatment for pharyngeal pouch. *British Journal of Surgery, 91,* 657–664.

Asherton, N. (1950). Achalasia of the cricopharyngeus sphincter: Record of cases with profile pharyngograms. *Journal of Laryngology and Otology, 64,* 747–758.

Beggs, D., & Morgan, W. E. (1989). Spontaneous perforation of cervical oesophagus associated with oesophageal web. *Journal of Laryngology and Otology, 103*(5), 537–538.

Bloom, R. A. (1984). The prevalence of ankylosing hyperostosis in a Jerusalem population—with description of a method of grading the extent of the disease. *Scandanavian Journal of Rheumatology, 13*, 181–189.

Bowdler, D. A. (1997). Pharyngeal pouches. In A. Kerr (Ed), *Scott Brown's textbook of otorhinolaryngology* (6th ed., pp. 1–21). Oxford, UK: Butterworth-Heinemann.

Braun, J., Bollow, M., Remlinger, G., Eggens, U., Rudwaleit, M., Distler, A., & Sieper, J. (1998). Prevalence of spondylarthropathies in HLA-B27 positive and negative blood donors. *Arthritis and Rheumatism, 41*(1), 58–67.

Carlson, M. L., Archibald, D. J., Graner, D. E., & Kasperbauer, J. L. (2011). Surgical management of dysphagia and airway obstruction in patients with prominent ventral cervical osteophytes. *Dysphagia, 26*, 34–40.

Cassivi, S. D., Deschamps, C., Nichols, F. C., Allen, M. S., & Pairolero, P. C. (2005). Diverticula of the esophagus. *Surgical Clinics of North America, 85*, 495–503.

Chen, J., & Liu, C. (2009). *Sulfasalazine for ankylosing spondylitis.* The Cochrane Collaboration. Retrieved December 22, 2011, from http://onlinelibrary.wiley.com/doi/10.1002/14651858.CD004800.pub2/pdf/standard

Childs, S. G. (2004). Diffuse idiopathic skeletal hyperostosis: Forestier's disease. *Orthopedic Nursing, 23*(6), 375–382.

Clark, H. M. (2010). Cervical osteophytes. In H. N. Jones & J. C. Rosenbek (Eds.), *Dysphagia in rare conditions: An encyclopedia.* San Diego, CA: Plural.

Cook, I. J. (2006). Clinical disorders of the upper esophageal sphincter. *GI Motility Online.* Retrieved November 17, 2011, from http://www.nature.com/gimo/contents/pt1/full/gimo37.html

Coyle, J. L. (2010). Zenker's diverticulum. In H. N. Jones & J. C. Rosenbek (Eds.), *Dysphagia in rare conditions: An encyclopedia.* San Diego, CA: Plural.

Crescenzo, D. G., Trastek, V. F., Allen, M. S., Deschamps, C., & Pairoleret, P.C. (1998). Zenker's diverticulum in the elderly: Is operation justified? *Annals of Thoracic Surgery, 66*(2), 347–349.

Denko, C. W., & Malemud, C. J. (2006). Body mass index and blood glucose: Correlations with serum insulin, growth hormone, and insulin-like growth factor-1 levels in patients with diffuse idiopathic skeletal hyperostosis (DISH). *Rheumatology International, 262*, 292–297.

Dickey, W., & McConnell, B. (1999). Celiac disease presenting as the Paterson-Brown Kelly (Plummer-Vinson) syndrome. *American Journal of Gastroenterology, 94*(2), 527–529.

Elwood, P. C., Pitman, R. G., Jacobs, A., & Entwistle, C. C. (1964) Epidemiology of the Paterson-Kelly syndrome. *Lancet, 2*, 716–720.

Ergun, G. A., & Kahrilas, P. J. (1997). Medical and surgical treatment interventions in deglutitive dysfunction. In A. L. Perlman & K. Schulze-Delrieu (Eds.), *Deglutition and its disorders: Anatomy, physiology, clinical diagnostics and management* (pp. 463–490). San Diego, CA: Singular.

Ergun, G. A., Lin, A. N., Dannenberg, A. J., & Carter, D. M. (1992). Gastrointestinal manifestations of epidermolysis bullosa. A study of 101 patients. *Medicine (Baltimore), 71*(3), 121–127.

Forestier, J., & Rotes-Querol, J. (1950). Senile ankylosing hyperostosis of the spine. *Annals of the Rheumatic Diseases, 9*, 321–330.

Foroozan, P., Enta, T., Winship, D. H., & Trier, J. S. (1967). Loss and regeneration of the esophageal mucosa in pemphigoid. *Gastroenterology, 52*(3), 548–558.

Gordon, A. R., Levine, M. S., Redfern, R. O., Rubesin, S. E., & Laufer, I. (2001). Cervical esophageal webs: Association with gastroesophageal reflux. *Abdomial Imaging, 26*(6), 574–577.

Goyal, R. J. (1984). Disorders of the cricopharyngeus muscle. Symposium on the larynx. *Otolaryngological Clinics of North America, 17*(1), 115–130.

Granville, L., Musson, N., Altman, R., & Silverman, M. (1997). Anterior cervical osteophytes as a cause of pharyngeal stage dysphagia. *Journal of the American Geriatric Society, 46*, 1003–1007.

Kiss, C., Szilagyi, M., Paksy, A., & Poor, G. (2002). Risk factors for diffuse idiopathic skeletal hyperostosis: A case-control study. *Rheumatology, 41*(1), 27.

Klockars, T., & Mäkitie, A. (2010). Case report of Zenker's diverticulum in identical twins: Further evidence for genetic predisposition. *Journal of Laryngology and Otology, 124*, 1129–1131.

Klockars, T., Sihvo, E., & Mäkitie, A. Familial Zenker's diverticulum. *Acta Otolaryngologica, 128*, 1034–1036.

Kumaresan, S., Yoganandan, N., Pintar, F. A., Maiman, D. J., & Goel, V. K. (2001). Contribution of disc degeneration to osteophyte formation in the cervical spine: A biomechanical investigation. *Journal of Orthopaedic Research, 19*, 977–984.

Laing, M. R., Murthy, P., Ah-See, K. W., & Cockburn, J. S. (1995). Surgery for pharyngeal pouch: audit of management with short and long-term follow-up. *Journal of the Royal Colleges of Surgeons of Edinburgh, 40*, 315–318.

Lambert, J. R., Tepperman, P. S., Jimenez, J., & Newman, A.(1981). Cervical spine disease and dysphagia. Four new cases and a review of the literature. *American Journal of Gastroenterology, 76*, 35–40.

Leaper, M., Zhang, M., & Dawes, P. J. D. (2005). An anatomical protrusion exists on the posterior hypopharyngeal wall in some elderly cadavers. *Dysphagia, 20*(1), 8–14.

Liu, J. J., & Kahrilas, P. J. (2006). Pharyngeal and esophageal diverticula, rings, and webs. *GI Motility Online.* doi:10.1038/gimo41. Retrieved November 15, 2011, from http://www.nature.com/gimo/contents/pt1/full/gimo41.html

Logemann, J. A. (1998). *Evaluation and treatment of swallowing disorders* (2nd ed.). Austin, TX: Pro-Ed.

Marcus, K., Harris, P., Thorne, M., & Prince, M. E. (2005). Familial Zenker's diverticulum: Case study and historical perspective. *Journal of Otolaryngology, 34*, 437–439.

Miyamoto, K., Sugiyama, S., Hosoe, H., Iinuma, N., Suzuki, Y., & Shimizu, K. (2009). Postsurgical recurrence of osteophytes causing dysphagia in patients with diffuse idiopathic skeletal hyperostosis. *European Spine Journal, 18*, 1652–1658.

Moerman, M. (2006). Cricopharyngeal Botox injection: indications and technique. *Current Opinion in Otolaryngology-Head and Neck Surgery, 14*(6), 431–436.

Ngian, G. S., & Littlejohn, G. O. (2010). Is DISH painful? *Journal of Rheumatology, 37*(9), 1797–1799.

Odin, M. (1937). Diseases and frequency of diseases in upper Norrland, with special reference to composition of diet. In N. Hellström (Ed.), *An investigation into questions of social hygiene in the countries of Västerbotten and Norrbotten, Sweden, Part 2* (pp. 15–57). Lund, Sweden: Hakan Ohlsson.

Ortega-Martínez, M., Cabezudo, J. M., Gómez-Perals, L. F., & Fernández-Portales, I. (2005). Anterior cervical osteophyte causing dysphagia as a complication of laminectomy. *British Journal of Neurosurgery, 9*(2), 174–178.

Ozgocmen, S., Kiris, A., Kocakoc, E., & Ardicoglu, O. (2002). Osteophyte-induced dysphagia: Report of three cases. *Joint, Bone, and Spine, 69*, 226–229.

Resnick, D. (1995). *Diagnosis of bone and joint disorders* (3rd ed.). Philadelphia, PA: Saunders.

Resnick, D., & Niwayama, G. (1976). Radiographic and pathologic features of spinal involvement in diffuse idiopathic skeletal hyperostosis (DISH). *Radiology, 119*, 559–568.

Sarzi-Puttini, P., & Atzeni, F. (2004). New developments in our understanding of DISH (diffuse idiopathic skeletal hyperostosis). *Current Opinion in Rheumatology, 16*(3), 287–292.

Sciubba, D. M., Nelson, C., Hsieh, P., Gokaslan, Z. L., Ondra, S., & Bydon, A. (2008). Perioperative challenges in the surgical management of ankylosing spondylitis. *Neurosurgical Focus, 24*(1), E10.

Sen, P., Kumar, G., & Bhattacharyya, A. K. (2006). Pharyngeal pouch: Associations and complications. *European Archives of Oto-Rhino-Laryngology, 263*, 463–468.

Siddiq, M. A., Sood, S., & Strachan, D. (2001). Pharyngeal Pouch (Zenker's diverticulum). *Postgraduate Medical Journal, 77*, 506–511.

Sieper, J., Braun, J., Rudwaleit, M., Boonen, A., & Zink, A. (2002). Ankylosing spondylitis: An overview. *Annals of the Rheumatic Diseases, 61*, iii8–iii18.

Suzuki, K., Ishida, Y., & Ohmori, K. (1991). Long-term follow-up of diffuse idiopathic skeletal hyperostosis in the cervical spine. Analysis of progression of ossification. *Neuroradiology*, *33*, 427–431.

Swami, H., & Ramakrishnan, R. (2009). Post cricoid web excision. *Medical Journal of the Armed Forces of India*, *65*, 69–70.

Takes, R. P., van den Hoogen, F. J. A., & Marres, H. A. M. (2005). Endoscopic myotomy of the cricopharyngeal muscle with CO_2 laser surgery. *Head and Neck*, *27*(8),703–709.

Takwoingi, Y. M., Kale, U. S., & Morgan, D. W. (2005). Rigid endoscopy in globus pharyngeus: How valuable is it? *Journal of Laryngology and Otology*, *120*, 42–46.

Unlu, Z., Orguc, S., Eskiizmir, G., Aslan, A., & Tasci, S. (2008). The role of phonophoresis in dysphagia due to cervical osteophytes. *International Journal of General Medicine*, *1*, 11–13.

van Overbeek, J. J. (2003). Pathogenesis and methods of treatment of Zenker's diverticulum.

Annals of Otology, Rhinology, and Laryngology, *112*, 583–593.

Weaver, G. A. (1979). Upper esophageal web due to a ring formed by a squamocolumnar junction with ectopic gastric mucosa (another explanation of the Paterson-Kelly, Plummer-Vinson syndrome). *Digestive Diseases and Sciences*, *24*(12), 959–963.

Weinfeld, R. M., Olson, P. N., Maki, D. D., & Griffiths, H. J. (1997). The prevalence of diffuse idiopathic skeletal hyperostosis (DISH) in two large American Midwest metropolitan hospital populations. *Skeletal Radiology*, *26*(4), 222–225.

Wynder, E. L, Hultberg, S., Jacobsson, F., & Bross, I. J. (1957). Environmental factors in cancer of the upper alimentary tract: A Swedish study with special reference to Plummer-Vinson (Paterson-Kelly) syndrome. *Cancer*, *10*, 470–482.

Chapter
16

STANDARDIZED CLINICAL REPORTING: WRITING FOR THE READER

Martin B. Brodsky

INTRODUCTION

Clinical reporting is the universally accepted, formal, and legal mode by which clinicians relate procedures, findings, interpretations, and recommendations to other clinicians. To this end, clinical reports are often regarded as, "if it was not documented, it did not happen." As a part of becoming more involved in one's own health care, patients are demonstrating greater interest to read their own medical record as a means of gaining greater understanding of their conditions (Fowles et al., 2004). It is, therefore, essential that clinical writing is clear, concise, and logical. Kibbee and Lilly (1988) pointedly summarize the purpose for including this chapter: "Although excellence in documentation certainly does not guarantee good clinical . . . care, it is difficult to minimize the obstacle that poor record-keeping poses for clinical excellence" (p. 6). The focus of this chapter is to address the need for a standardized method of reporting findings from videofluoroscopic swallowing studies (VFSS), offer definitions for physiological function of swallowing that can be used to describe VFSS outcomes, and describe the role that the Penetration-Aspiration Scale (Rosenbek, Robbins, Roecker, Coyle, & Wood, 1996) has in clinical practice. It is not within the purview of this chapter, however, to address content of the clinical report related to regulatory issues, accrediting guidelines, and accounting practices.

Need for Standardization

In a report by the World Health Organization (WHO, 2006), *standardization* refers to the "creation of accepted specifications (e.g., definitions, norms, units, rules) that establishes a common language as a basis for understanding and exchange of information between different parties" (p. 1). The report justifies the use of standardization, when used consistently, as this augments "accuracy, efficiency, reliability, and comparability of health information at local, regional, national, and international levels. . . . [Moreover, it supports] statistical reporting, decision-making, measurement of outcomes and performance, and cost analysis" (p. 1). To some clinicians, standardization immediately suggests constraints and feelings of discomfort, that is, "This is what I *must* do." To other clinicians, standardization offers a format to follow, a "rules-based" paradigm, providing comfort in knowing that as long as the rules are followed, the result will be "correct." Regardless of perspective, standardization leaves little room for interpretation, creating an environment that is properly focused.

Research in swallowing physiology has come a distance in its standardization and measurement. In the 1970s, there was little or no management of oropharyngeal swallowing disorders except by feeding tubes. Since publication of Jeri Logemann's book *Evaluation and Treatment of Swallowing Disorders* in 1983 (Logemann, 1983), there has been a very large leap forward with the amount of research in swallowing physiology. A MEDLINE search using the key words "deglutition," "swallowing," and "dysphagia" revealed 10,213 citations. Since then, there has been a rise in the rate of research in the areas of swallowing and swallowing disorders (Figure 16–1), with over 52,200 citations at the end of 2010. In fact, in the 27 years between 1983 and 2010, the amount of published literature in swallowing and swallowing disorders continues to double approximately every 11 years. Although this collective knowledge has undoubtedly proved to be beneficial for the diagnosis and treatment of swallowing disorders, there are unfortunate side effects, for example the introduction of non-standardized terminology and the use of

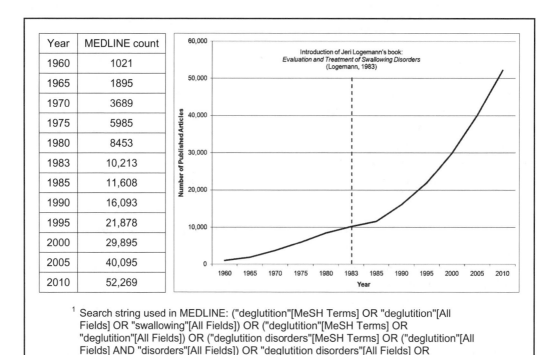

Year	MEDLINE count
1960	1021
1965	1895
1970	3689
1975	5985
1980	8453
1983	10,213
1985	11,608
1990	16,093
1995	21,878
2000	29,895
2005	40,095
2010	52,269

[1] Search string used in MEDLINE: ("deglutition"[MeSH Terms] OR "deglutition"[All Fields] OR "swallowing"[All Fields]) OR ("deglutition"[MeSH Terms] OR "deglutition"[All Fields]) OR ("deglutition disorders"[MeSH Terms] OR ("deglutition"[All Fields] AND "disorders"[All Fields]) OR "deglutition disorders"[All Fields] OR "dysphagia"[All Fields])

Figure 16–1. *MEDLINE citations for swallowing and swallowing disorders.*[1]

non-uniform language in scientific writing and clinical reporting.

The basis for learning clinical reporting appears to be scientific inquiry (i.e., published studies) and is proposed in Figure 16–2. Consumers of the scientific literature will find no surprise in the number of different terms and descriptions associated with any given concept. These differences are largely the result of philosophical or empirically meaningful differences in the literature perceived by different groups of researchers. New studies "tweak" terminology already present in the literature to suit the needs of that research team and its scientific endeavors. Consider the concept of *initiation of the pharyngeal swallow* (and its disordered counterpart "delayed initiation of the pharyngeal swallow") as one example. Among

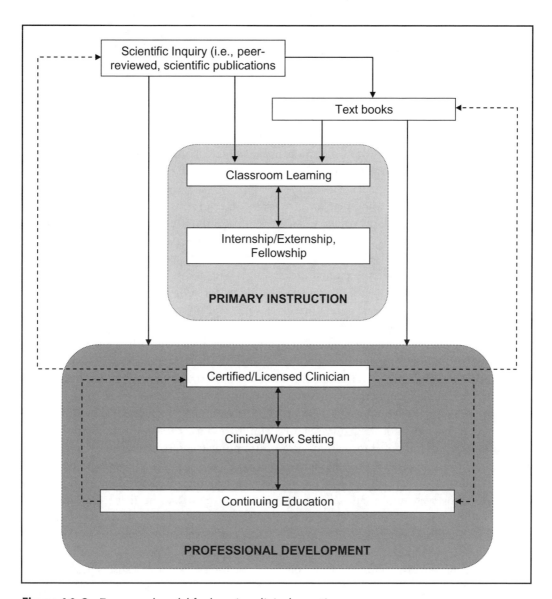

Figure 16–2. *A proposed model for learning clinical reporting.*

the earliest terms used to describe this physiological phenomenon of swallowing in the literature are: initiation of the swallowing reflex (Logemann, 1983), stage transition duration (Robbins, Hamilton, Lof, & Kempster, 1992), and pharyngeal dwell time (Palmer, Rudin, Lara, & Crompton, 1992; Perlman, Booth, & Grayhack, 1994). As each of these titles implies, each research team identifies important nuances as differences in its operational definition. Specific to initiation of the pharyngeal swallow, differences are largely defined by the movement of the bolus and anatomical movements indicating the onset of the pharyngeal swallow. In turn, these differences begin the use of non-uniform language. In fact, it is quite interesting that in the United States alone, the instrumental procedure for viewing oropharyngeal swallowing function using video-recorded, fluoroscopic images can have many different names, such as videofluoroscopy, videofluorography, modified barium swallow study, dynamic swallow study, cookie swallow (study), and cine esophagopharyngogram. If institutions across one country cannot agree on the name of an examination, how will international clinicians ever agree on the content and presentation of standardized reports from the procedure?

In writing textbooks, authors and editors are responsible for amassing and interpreting the scientific literature for a particular subject, which is no small feat. They go to great efforts to create a cohesive understanding of the topics, reviewing published research to synthesize large volumes of information into an efficient, overall message as a chapter or textbook. During this synthesis of scientific information, however, authors and editors are often forced to "choose sides" for which non-standard/non-uniform language will be used, introducing new terminology or perpetuating (or ignoring) previously published terminology. In turn, the combination of scientific

publications and textbooks are the foundation for classroom learning and continuing education, each interpreted with the instructor's own use (i.e., biases) of language. Because the amount of information is economically bundled in the form of textbooks, students may never read all of the original publications that contributed to any given chapter or textbook. At a minimum, the textbook and the instructor's lecture may be the only sources of students' learning, effectively creating a basis for the language the student uses professionally. In professional settings that vary to a great degree throughout the world, whether during student training or working as a licensed and certified clinician, supervisors use their own "locally accepted" language. Finally, as a professional you may experience changes in setting (e.g., school, clinic, hospital, extended care facility) or changes between locations (e.g., cities, states, countries) but maintain the same setting, and the language may change as well. In summary, the roots of clinical reporting are in non-standard and/or non-uniform literature that is, in turn, interpreted with bias, taught with additional bias, and interpreted by students for professional practice with additional (and often increased) levels of bias. It is with this basis that a proposed proforma using peer-reviewed, validated language for the VFSS clinical report is suggested.

The term *pro forma* (Latin: "for form," modern English usage: proforma) suggests function applied to formality. Regarding the clinical report, the proforma is the basic or minimum structure of the report and its contents. Figure 16–3 is an example of a basic report structure used by many clinicians for narrative reports. Note that using this structure offers a great deal of latitude for *how* clinicians communicate findings from the VFSS. That is, narrative reports allow each clinician to use his or her own (non-standard, non-uniform) language to report patient obser-

VIDEOFLUOROSOCOPIC SWALLOWING STUDY

Patient Name: Date of Birth:
Sex:

BACKGROUND/HISTORY
Date of Onset   Evaluation Date:
Primary Medical Diagnosis:
History of Present Illness/Reason for Testing:
Past Medical/Surgical History:
Social History:
Cognitive Status:
Current Diet/Liquids/Medication Route:
Patient's Goals:

SUBJECTIVE
General Observation:

OBJECTIVE
Patient Position (i.e., seating, standing):
Contrast Type (e.g., barium):
View Planes:
        Consistencies Tested:
        Radiologist (if present):
Oral Phase:
Pharyngeal Phase:
Esophageal Phase:

Laryngeal Penetration/Aspiration:

Compensatory Strategies:

Additional Findings/Comments:

ASSESSMENT/IMPRESSION
(Description of swallowing physiology, presence of laryngeal penetration and/or aspiration,
    delivery methods of the bolus, compensatory strategies used, effectiveness of the
    compensatory strategies)

Prognosis

Cultural preferences towards eating/diet (if applicable)

RECOMMENDATIONS
Diet/Liquids:
Medication Route:
Compensatory Strategies:
Short-term/Long-term Goals:
Referrals/Additional Consults:

_____   _____
Clinician Signature: Date:

Figure 16-3. *Example of a proforma videofluoroscopic swallowing study report.*

vations. In doing so, clinicians may not be consistent with the same language from report to report. Even within the same department of an institution, clinicians are not likely to use the same language. More often, as an attempt to simplify (rather than standardize) clinical reporting across all forms of diagnostic and treatment reports, clinicians and institutions depart from the labor-intensive narrative to a more succinct, "check the box" summary of findings. In converting reporting styles, this small (albeit often arduous) change effectively ratifies agreement between clinicians for *how* the clinical report will be constructed and the language used to communicate findings. Thus, standardization is achieved within the department and, consequently, the institution. Of course, this does not imply that all clinicians and all institutions across the world are using the same format and/or language to communicate findings. To date, there is no such standardization for any report, let alone the VFSS report.

Proforma for the VFSS Clinical Report

The American speech-language pathology student and clinician should initially turn to the American Speech-Language-Hearing Association (ASHA) as a reference for what is required to be in the VFSS clinical report. Other countries may have similar licensing and governing bodies that may be used similarly, for example, the United Kingdom's Royal College of Speech and Language Therapists (RCSLT) Policy Statement (RCSLT, 2006). Students and clinicians belonging to other professions involved in the VFSS procedure and reporting thereof (e.g., radiographers/radiologists) should refer to their own governing body's policy. The ASHA policy statement, *Knowledge and Skills Needed by Speech-Language Pathologists Performing Videofluoroscopic Swallowing Studies* (ASHA, 2004) clearly outlines

the minimum requisite contents for the VFSS clinical report. The policy, however, neither standardizes the format nor the language used for this type of clinical report. The first study that standardized the VFSS was published in 2008 (Martin-Harris et al., 2008), 25 years after the publication of Jeri Logemann's textbook (Logemann, 1983). The remainder of this chapter will propose a *language* proforma for the VFSS clinical report, employing the validated terminology from the study (Martin-Harris et al., 2008). This terminology will be used to describe the components of swallowing physiology, effectively creating a *standard language* that may be used by clinicians.

Defining Components of Swallowing Physiology

The following sections describe the components of swallowing physiology validated by expert consensus (Martin-Harris et al., 2008). Each component is listed in Table 16–1 and is bolded in the following text after its description. An outline of the components is presented and is followed by a discussion related to the Penetration-Aspiration Scale (Robbins, Coyle, Rosenbek, Roecker, & Wood, 1999; Rosenbek et al., 1996) and its clinical implications as an adjunct to these components.

Oral Components

The oral preparatory stage of normal swallowing begins as the bolus enters the oral cavity. Upon bolus entry, the mandible closes and the lips seal (**lip closure**) to contain the bolus anteriorly in the oral cavity. Although the tongue is the most mobile element of the oral cavity during the oral preparatory phase, it also plays a major role in bolus containment and airway maintenance with coordination of the soft palate (Palmer et al., 1992; Storey, 1976). This coordination forms a posterior seal of the oral

Table 16–1. *Validated Components of Swallowing Physiology and Corresponding Radiological Plane for Assessment*

Physiological Swallowing Component	Radiological Plane Used for Assessment
Lip closure	Lateral
Tongue control during bolus hold[a]	Lateral
Bolus preparation/mastication	Lateral
Bolus transport/lingual motion	Lateral
Oral residue[b]	Lateral
Initiation of the pharyngeal swallow	Lateral
Soft palate elevation	Lateral
Laryngeal elevation	Lateral
Anterior hyoid excursion[a]	Lateral
Epiglottic movement	Lateral
Laryngeal vestibular closure[a]	Lateral
Pharyngeal stripping wave	Lateral
Pharyngeal contraction	Anterior-Posterior
Pharyngoesophageal segment opening	Lateral
Tongue base retraction	Lateral
Pharyngeal residue[b]	Lateral
Esophageal clearance in the upright position	Anterior-Posterior

[a]Since publication of the study by Martin Harris et al. (2008), the names of these components have been slightly modified to more precisely describe swallowing physiology. The table contains the updated names of the components. Tongue control during bolus hold, anterior hyoid excursion, and laryngeal vestibular closure were updated from hold position/tongue control, anterior hyoid motion, and laryngeal closure, respectively.

[b]Oral and pharyngeal residue are the results of disordered swallowing physiology; they, are not physiological. They are related to and describe bolus flow.

Source: Martin-Harris et al. (2008)

cavity, preventing posterior loss of the bolus **(tongue control during bolus hold)** (Dodds, Logemann, & Stewart, 1990; Dodds, Stewart, & Logemann, 1990). The bolus is manipulated by the tongue and masticated (if appro-priate), during which the ingested material is mixed with saliva and tasted **(bolus preparation/mastication)**, a motion that is integrated into the oral swallowing process (Hiiemae et al., 1996; Hiiemae & Palmer, 1999; Palmer et al., 1992; Storey, 1976). When the bolus is adequately prepared (considering size and consistency), it is re-collected, formed into a cohesive bolus that is placed on the center of the tongue and transported posteriorly toward the pharynx (**bolus transport/lingual motion**) (Cook, Dodds, Dantas, Kern, et al., 1989; Hiiemae et al., 1996; Hiiemae & Palmer, 1999). Portions of the bolus remaining in the oral cavity after the swallow (**oral residue**) may increase a patient's risk for inadequate nutrition, inadequate hydration, and/or possible airway invasion (Perlman et al., 1994). The onset of bolus propulsion is then stimulated by sensory receptors in the posterior oral cavity and oropharynx that begin the pharyngeal swallow (**initiation of the pharyngeal swallow**) (Ardran & Kemp, 1952; Cook, Dodds, Dantas, Kern, et al., 1989; Doty, 1968; Logemann, 1998; Martin-Harris, Brodsky, Michel, Lee, & Walters, 2007; Perlman et al., 1994; Robbins et al., 1992).

Pharyngeal Components

The normal pharyngeal swallow comprises overlapping and well-coordinated mechanical events. In continuing bolus movement posteriorly from the oral cavity, retraction and elevation of the soft palate (**soft palate elevation**) occur to prevent the bolus from entering the nasopharynx (Dantas, Dodds, Massey, Shaker, & Cook, 1990; Dua, Shaker, Ren, Arndorfer, & Hofmann, 1995; Matsuo, Hiiemae, & Palmer, 2005). The larynx is displaced superiorly as the arytenoid cartilages approximate the base of the epiglottis (**laryngeal elevation**) (Ku, Ma, McConnel, & Cerenko, 1990; Logemann et al., 1992; Ohmae, Logemann, Kaiser, Hanson, & Kahrilas, 1995; Shaker, Dodds, Dantas, Hogan, & Arndorfer, 1990) while being pulled anteriorly by displacement of the hyoid bone (**anterior hyoid excursion**) (Cook, Dodds, Dantas, Massey, et al., 1989;

Shaker et al., 1992), moving the airway out of the bolus's path. During hyolaryngeal excursion (anterior and superior movement of the larynx via contractions of muscles attached to the hyoid bone) and tongue base retraction, the epiglottis begins its movement from upright to inverted until it approximates the arytenoid cartilages (**epiglottic movement**) (Ekberg & Nylander, 1982; Ekberg & Sigurjónsson, 1982) and the laryngeal vestibule folds on itself sealing the upper airway from the bolus (**laryngeal vestibular closure**) (Ku et al., 1990; Logemann et al., 1992; Ohmae et al., 1995; Shaker et al., 1990; Shaker et al., 1992).

Observed in the lateral plane, contraction of the pharyngeal constrictors creates a wavelike motion (**pharyngeal stripping wave**) (Kahrilas, Logemann, Lin, & Ergun, 1992; McConnel, 1988) that is believed to assist with bolus clearance from the pharynx. From an anterior-posterior viewing plane, contraction of the pharyngeal constrictors (Castell, Dalton, & Castell, 1990; Kahrilas et al., 1992; McConnel, 1988) is observed to move medially (**pharyngeal contraction**). In addition to airway protection, hyolaryngeal excursion is mechanically and physiologically linked to the opening and duration of distension in the transition area from pharynx to esophagus containing the cricopharyngeus, the pharyngoesophageal segment (Cook, Dodds, Dantas, Massey, et al., 1989; Hiss & Huckabee, 2005; Jacob, Kahrilas, Logemann, Shah, & Ha, 1989; Kahrilas, Dodds, Dent, Logemann, & Shaker, 1988). **Pharyngoesophageal segment [PES] opening** permits entry of the ingested material into the cervical esophagus by placing traction on the cricoid cartilage during hyolaryngeal excursion, thus opening the compliant PES. Movement of the tongue base toward the posterior pharyngeal wall (**tongue base retraction**) in a wavelike motion places a strong pressure on the bolus tail, promoting pharyngeal clearance and prevention of pharyngeal residue (Atkinson, Kramer, Wyman, & Ingelfinger, 1957; Kahrilas et al., 1992; McConnel, Cerenko, & Mendelsohn, 1988; Sokol, Heitmann, Wolf, & Cohen, 1966). Finally, portions of the bolus in the pharynx may remain after the swallow **(pharyngeal residue)**, increasing a patient's risk for airway invasion.

Esophageal Component

As the bolus head enters the esophagus through the PES, it is propagated by sequential, involuntary contractions of the circular muscle in the esophageal body (i.e., primary peristalsis) (Castell, Diederrich, & Castell, 2000; Levine, 1989), typically with the assistance of gravity **(esophageal clearance in the upright position)** (Allen, Zamani, & Dimarino, 1997; Borgström & Ekberg, 1989; Ku et al., 1990; Paterson, 2006). Subsequent local distension continues movement of the bolus as secondary contractions of the esophagus (Paterson, 2006). Observations in the upright position (i.e., torso upright) afford impressions of the potential impact of incomplete or slowed esophageal clearance on oropharyngeal swallowing function, the potential for aspiration of residual esophageal contents, and the nutritional status of the patient.

Clinical Implications of the Penetration-Aspiration Scale

The Penetration-Aspiration (PA) Scale (Robbins et al., 1999; Rosenbek et al., 1996) was developed by clinical researchers at the Veterans Administration and University of Wisconsin Swallowing Laboratory. Although both "penetration" and "aspiration" were terms used for many years in research and in clinical applications prior to the introduction of the PA Scale, neither term was sufficiently described insofar as the level (or depth), or clearing of

material from the airway (Rosenbek et al., 1996). Although interest remains in both clinical practice and research to determine the amount and timing of airway invasion, the PA Scale does not address these measures. Instead, it has greatly improved sensitivity of penetration and aspiration, moving from two clinical signs (i.e., penetration, aspiration) to eight clinical signs through its validated and reliable 8-point ordinal scale (Robbins et al., 1999; Rosenbek et al., 1996). Moreover, the PA Scale has provided an invaluable, internationally accepted, and *standardized* descriptive scale with language for penetration and aspiration (Table 16–2). Although implicit in these research publications, it is important to emphasize that the development of the PA Scale was never meant to address swallowing physiology. Penetration and aspiration are, by definition, *results* of impaired swallowing physiology.

The PA Scale was developed and validated using 3ml thin liquid swallows presented by spoon to 15 patients with multiple strokes (Rosenbek et al., 1996). In a follow-up study, 15 patients with multiple strokes and 16 patients with head and neck cancer were used to further validate the PA Scale with 98 healthy adults, again using 3ml thin liquid boluses presented by spoon (Robbins et al., 1999). At first glance, a researcher or clinician might be critical of the PA Scale because of its limited number of subjects and limited scope of the types of boluses presented and presentation method of the boluses, however good content validity and good face validity appear to override these criticisms. Regardless of whether the PA Scale was tested on more subjects, the 8-point scale addresses all possibilities for bolus entry into the airway, depth of bolus flow, patient response, and success of clearing the airway of the material, leaving only the concern for reliability in scoring. This concern, too, may be set aside with its tested

Table 16–2. *Penetration-Aspiration Scale*

Category	Score	Description
No Penetration/Aspiration	1	Material does not enter airway
Penetration	2	Material enters airway, remains above vocal folds, ejected without residue
	3	Material enters airway, remains above vocal folds, not ejected from airway
	4	Material enters airway, contacts vocal folds, ejected without residue
	5	Material enters airway, contacts vocal folds, not ejected from airway
Aspiration	6	Material passes below vocal folds, ejected from airway
	7	Material passes below vocal folds, not ejected from airway despite response
	8	Material passes below vocal folds, no effort to eject material (silent aspiration)

Source: Robbins et al. (1999); Rosenbek et al. (1996)

high interjudge reliability (interjudge intraclass correlation coefficient = 0.96) (Rosenbek et al., 1996).

There is a lot of value in a tool that uses a prescriptive language to describe observations that is valid and reliable and can be understood by the masses. With all of these advantages to the PA Scale, clinicians might be tempted to compute scores (e.g., determine a mean or median score) from the patient's swallow attempts during the VFSS in an effort to show change in swallowing physiology. Computing a mean has no meaning with this ordinal scale, yet reporting *frequency* of each PA Scale score for each bolus type could provide some meaning across more than one VFSS of the same patient. It is worth a note of caution when using the PA Scale for these purposes, however. Although the PA Scale has defined normal from abnormal airway protection (Robbins et al., 1999), *no norms*

have been developed for any patient population. As noted, there is some appeal in reporting PA Scale scores, however there is far greater qualitative benefit in its use of language for clinical reporting.

To summarize, the PA Scale is neither sufficient to address swallowing physiology, nor is it considered best practice to be used numerically in a clinical report. *It reports the consequences of disordered physiology* with respect to the airway. Using the standardized language in the PA Scale serves to describe clinical observations objectively and clearly: two goals of clinical report writing.

An Offer of Guidelines, Format, and Language for VFSS Reporting

Adhering to a standard is not a creative process. Neither is clinical reporting. Having a standard language and formula for writing clinical reports will provide consistency, but will neither guarantee value nor accuracy. This final section of the chapter is devoted to offering a formula for writing logical, concise, clear, thorough, and interpretive clinical reports.

General Guidelines

The basic philosophy behind all clinical writing is reporting objective findings with conclusions that are supported by the data. Fowles et al. (2004) maintained that clinical reports should be approached with the assumption that what is written *will be viewed* by the patient and/or family members. Bearing this in mind *at all times*, a few general guidelines are suggested:

- Use of correct spelling, grammar, and punctuation is essential to ease of understanding and being respected as a professional.
- Handwritten reports should be legible. Readers will not spend time on a report that cannot be read. It will either be ignored or the clinician who wrote the report can look forward to being contacted for interpretation.
- Present clinical findings using professional terminology, succinct wording, and simple explanations; the more complex the report, the more opportunity for questions, concerns, and/or avoidance of the report (and your recommendations).
- Opinions may be offered but stated as such, *not* stated as fact.
- Proofread your writing. Written reports may offer some latitude (i.e., crossing out text), but there is little opportunity to delete an electronically submitted report. An electronic submission becomes a *permanent* record in the reporting database, as databases are designed never to lose information. Despite the fact that you may have deleted a report, an image of it remains in the database.

General Format and Language Offered as a Guide

Each institution will have its own reporting format. The de facto, or "practice" standard in all VFSS clinical reports is reporting on the oral, pharyngeal, and esophageal phases of swallowing physiology, then summarizing and interpreting the results in an "Assessment (or Impression)" section (see Figure 16–3). Using the vocabulary in Table 16–1, described earlier in this chapter, below is an example of a patient's VFSS findings:

Sample Patient Report (Objective and Assessment Sections)

OBJECTIVE

Oral Phase

- Lip Closure: No labial escape.
- Tongue Control During Bolus Hold: Cohesive bolus between the tongue to palatal seal.
- Bolus Preparation/Mastication: Timely and efficient chewing and mashing.
- Bolus Transport/Lingual Motion: Brisk tongue motion.
- Oral Residue: Residue collection on oral structures: palate, tongue.
- Initiation of the Pharyngeal Swallow (at first hyoid motion): Bolus head at the posterior angle of the ramus.

Pharyngeal Phase

- Soft Palate Elevation: Trace column of contrast or air between soft palate and pharyngeal wall.
- Laryngeal Elevation: Partial superior movement of thyroid cartilage/partial approximation of arytenoids to the base of the epiglottis.
- Anterior Hyoid Excursion: Complete anterior movement.

■ Epiglottic Movement: Full inversion.

■ Laryngeal Vestibular Closure: Incomplete; narrow column air/contrast in the laryngeal vestibule.

■ Pharyngeal Stripping Wave: Present — complete.

■ Pharyngeal Contraction: Complete.

■ Pharyngoesophageal Segment Opening: Complete distension and complete duration; no obstruction of flow.

■ Tongue Base Retraction: Trace column of contrast or air between tongue base and posterior pharyngeal wall.

■ Pharyngeal Residue: Trace residue within or on pharyngeal structures: tongue base, valleculae, pharyngeal wall, aryepiglottic folds, and pyriform sinuses.

Esophageal Phase

Esophageal Clearance in Upright Position: Esophageal retention with retrograde flow through the pharyngoesophageal segment (PES). **A barium esophagram was completed by the radiologist following the VFSS. The patient was placed in the right anterior oblique prone position. Aspiration from retrograde bolus flow through the PES was noted with thin liquids. Please see radiologist's report for details.**

Laryngeal Penetration/Aspiration

Laryngeal penetration was observed with thin and nectar-thick liquids, especially with larger volumes and drinking by cup. Material entered the laryngeal vestibule, remained above the vocal folds, and was ejected without residue with completion of the swallow. No throat clearing, coughing, or wet vocal quality was observed. No aspiration was observed during the VFSS at any time. Aspiration was noted with 5 mL thin liquid barium via retrograde flow through the PES during the barium swallow performed by the radiologist.

Compensatory Strategies

Oral residue and pharyngeal residue were easily cleared with a double swallow. No additional compensatory strategies were indicated.

Additional Comments

Patient presents with small cervical osteophytes at C_4, C_5, and C_6. These do not appear to have any functional consequence on the pharyngeal swallow.

ASSESSMENT

Patient presents with mild oropharyngeal dysphagia characterized by reduced lingual strength and reduced hyolaryngeal excursion, leading to an open laryngeal vestibule during the swallow that resulted in laryngeal penetration with larger volumes and consecutive swallows of liquids. Penetrated material was expelled with completion of the swallow. Esophageal retention with retrograde flow through the PES leads to increased risk for aspiration.

FORMULAS

Throughout the *Objective* section of the clinical report, note that *observations* (not conclusions) are made. Observations should be stated using anatomical and physiological terms in a logical, sequential order. Time and timing are often important concepts for describing swallowing physiology (e.g., x *occurred before* y; or *following* the x event, the y event *occurred*). Describe observations succinctly using professional language (not necessarily jargon) so readers (e.g., medical team, private health insurance providers, government sponsored health care, family/patients) of the medical chart are easily able to understand the report (e.g., avoid: "the esophageal anastomosis *extravasated* barium"; use: "the esophageal anastomosis *leaked* barium"). Be detailed enough in your report to create a clear understanding for other clinicians to treat the impaired mechanisms. The terms "within normal limits" or "within functional limits" do not offer observations or measurements. They are drawn *conclusions* and are not appropriate for use in the *Objective* section of the report. The best place for the use of these terms is the *Assessment* section (if at all).

The *Assessment* section of the clinical report offers *conclusions* based on the *objectively observed* "grocery list" of findings. To get to these conclusions logically, there needs to be a "story" that answers the questions of *why* and *how*. This story is effectively the clinician's subjective interpretation of the findings. In the context of a statement from the sample report, the following "formula" (Figure 16–4) is offered to get to logical conclusions that are anatomically and physiologically linked to the objective findings.

The notes in the sections *Laryngeal Penetration/Aspiration*, *Compensatory Strategies*, and *Additional Comments* flow with similar logic. The language in the *Laryngeal Penetration/Aspiration* section is borrowed from the PA Scale (Table 16–2). Note there are no numerical values in the report. Note also that there must always be a cause for something to "result in"/"lead to." Cause is the finding stated in the *Objective* section of the report. For every cause, there *must* be a result. For every result, there *must* be a response; and *no response* is *indeed* a response (e.g., silent aspiration). Most clinics and institutions "note by exception" (i.e., normal findings are omitted to concentrate on or highlight the non-normal findings, effectively abbreviating the clinical report). For *each* impairment listed in the *Objective* section, there should be a statement that follows the formula suggested above in the *Assessment* section of the clinical report.

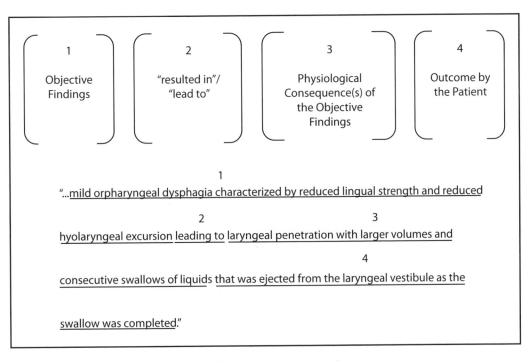

Figure 16–4. Schematic of physiological assessment interpretation.

SUMMARY

The preceding chapters have addressed the anatomy, physiology, and consequences of impairments. This chapter offers a "plug 'n' chug" method with standardized language for clinical report writing. The sample patient report and the formulas provided herein are starting points, ultimately leading to a long and successful career as a clinician for patients with swallowing disorders. It is important to emphasize that an explanation of findings goes a long way, more than any number, measurement, statistic, or simple observation. Following the *Assessment* section is arguably the most important section of the clinical report. This is the section that leads to patient recommendations, not only from the clinician assessing and treating the patient's dysphagia, but clinical decisions made by the patient's entire medical team.

REFERENCES

Allen, M. L., Zamani, S., & Dimarino, A. J., Jr. (1997). The effect of gravity on oesophageal peristalsis in humans. *Neurogastroenterology and Motility, 9*(2), 71–76.

Ardran, G. M., & Kemp, F. H. (1952). The protection of the laryngeal airway during swallowing. *British Journal of Radiology, 25*, 406–416.

American Speech-Language-Hearing Association. (2004). Knowledge and skills needed by speech-langage pathologists performing videofluoroscopic swallowing studies. *ASHA Supplement, 24*, 178–183.

Atkinson, M., Kramer, P., Wyman, S., & Ingelfinger, F. (1957). The dynamics of swallow. I. Normal pharyngeal mechanisms. *Journal of Clinical Investigation, 36*, 581–598.

Borgström, P. S., & Ekberg, O. (1989). Peristalsis in pharyngeal constrictor musculature in relation to positioning and gravity. *Acta Radiologica, 30*(2), 183–185.

Castell, D. O., Diederrich, L. L., & Castell, J. A. (2000). *Esophageal motility and pH testing* (3rd ed.). Highlands Ranch, CO: Sandhill Scientific.

Castell, J. A., Dalton, C. B., & Castell, D. O. (1990). Pharyngeal and upper esophageal sphincter manometry in humans. *American Journal of Physiology, 258*(2 Pt. 1), G173–G178.

Cook, I. J., Dodds, W. J., Dantas, R. O., Kern, M. K., Massey, B. T., Shaker, R., & Hogan, W. J. (1989). Timing of videofluoroscopic, manometric events, and bolus transit during the oral and pharyngeal phases of swallowing. *Dysphagia, 4*(1), 8–15.

Cook, I. J., Dodds, W. J., Dantas, R. O., Massey, B., Kern, M. K., Lang, I. M., . . . Hogan, W. J. (1989). Opening mechanisms of the human upper esophageal sphincter. *American Journal of Physiology, 257*(5 Pt. 1), G748–G759.

Dantas, R. O., Dodds, W. J., Massey, B. T., Shaker, R., & Cook, I. J. (1990). Manometric characteristics of glossopalatal sphincter. *Digestive Diseases and Sciences, 35*(2), 161–166.

Dodds, W. J., Logemann, J. A., & Stewart, E. T. (1990). Radiologic assessment of abnormal oral and pharyngeal phases of swallowing. *American Journal of Roentgenology, 154*(5), 965–974.

Dodds, W. J., Stewart, E. T., & Logemann, J. A. (1990). Physiology and radiology of the normal oral and pharyngeal phases of swallowing. *American Journal of Roentgenology, 154*(5), 953–963.

Doty, R. W. (1968). Neural organization of deglutition. In C. F. Code (Ed.), *Handbook of physiology* (Vol. 4). Washington DC: American Physiologic Society.

Dua, K., Shaker, R., Ren, J., Arndorfer, R., & Hofmann, C. (1995). Mechanism and timing of nasopharyngeal closure during swallowing and belching. *American Journal of Physiology, 268*(6 Pt. 1), G1037–G1042.

Ekberg, O., & Nylander, G. (1982). Cineradiography of the pharyngeal stage of deglutition in 150 individuals without dysphagia. *British Journal of Radiology, 55*(652), 253–257.

Ekberg, O., & Sigurjónsson, S. V. (1982). Movement of the epiglottis during deglutition. A cineradiographic study. *Gastrointestinal Radiology, 7*(2), 101–107.

Fowles, J. B., Kind, A. C., Craft, C., Kind, E. A., Mandel, J. L., & Adlis, S. (2004). Patients' interest in reading their medical record: Relation with clinical and sociodemographic characteristics and patients' approach to health care. *Archives of Internal Medicine, 164*(7), 793–800.

Hiiemae, K., Heath, M. R., Heath, G., Kazazoglu, E., Murray, J., Sapper, D., & Hamblett, K. (1996). Natural bites, food consistency and feeding behaviour in man. *Archives of Oral Biology, 41*(2), 175–189.

Hiiemae, K. M., & Palmer, J. B. (1999). Food transport and bolus formation during complete feeding sequences on foods of different initial consistency. *Dysphagia, 14*(1), 31–42.

Hiss, S. G., & Huckabee, M. L. (2005). Timing of pharyngeal and upper esophageal sphincter pressures as a function of normal and effortful swallowing in young healthy adults. *Dysphagia, 20*(2), 149–156.

Jacob, P., Kahrilas, P. J., Logemann, J. A., Shah, V., & Ha, T. (1989). Upper esophageal sphincter opening and modulation during swallowing. *Gastroenterology, 97*(6), 1469–1478.

Kahrilas, P. J., Dodds, W. J., Dent, J., Logemann, J. A., & Shaker, R. (1988). Upper esophageal sphincter function during deglutition. *Gastroenterology, 95*(1), 52–62.

Kahrilas, P. J., Logemann, J. A., Lin, S., & Ergun, G. A. (1992). Pharyngeal clearance during swallowing: A combined manometric and videofluoroscopic study. *Gastroenterology, 103*(1), 128–136.

Kibbee, P., & Lilly, G. (1988). Outcome-oriented documentation in a psychiatric facility. *Journal of Quality Assurance, 10*(5), 16–21.

Ku, D. N., Ma, P. P., McConnel, F. M., & Cerenko, D. (1990). A kinematic study of the oropharyngeal swallowing of a liquid. *Annals of Biomedical Engineering, 18*(6), 655–669.

Levine, M. S. (1989). *Radiology of the esophagus.* Philadelphia, PA: W. B. Saunders.

Logemann, J. (1983). *Evaluation and Treatment of Swallowing Disorders.* Austin, TX: Pro-Ed.

Logemann, J. A. (1998). *Evaluation and Treatment of Swallowing Disorders* (2nd ed.). Austin, TX: Pro-Ed.

Logemann, J. A., Kahrilas, P. J., Cheng, J., Pauloski, B. R., Gibbons, P. J., Rademaker, A. W., & Lin, S. (1992). Closure mechanisms of laryngeal vestibule during swallow. *American Journal of Physiology-Gastrointestinal and Liver Physiology, 262*(2), G338–G344.

Martin-Harris, B., Brodsky, M. B., Michel, Y., Castell, D. O., Schleicher, M., Sandidge, J., Blair, J. (2008). MBS measurement tool for swallow impairment—MBSImp: Establishing a standard. *Dysphagia, 23*(4), 392–405.

Martin-Harris, B., Brodsky, M. B., Michel, Y., Lee, F. S., & Walters, B. (2007). Delayed initiation of the pharyngeal swallow: normal variability in adult swallows. *Journal of Speech Language and Hearing Research, 50*(3), 585–594.

Matsuo, K., Hiiemae, K. M., & Palmer, J. B. (2005). Cyclic motion of the soft palate in feeding. *Journal of Dental Research, 84*(1), 39–42.

McConnel, F. M. (1988). Analysis of pressure generation and bolus transit during pharyngeal swallowing. *Laryngoscope, 98*(1), 71–78.

McConnel, F. M., Cerenko, D., & Mendelsohn, M. S. (1988). Manofluorographic analysis of swallowing. *Otolaryngologic Clinics of North America, 21*(4), 625–635.

Ohmae, Y., Logemann, J. A., Kaiser, P., Hanson, D. G., & Kahrilas, P. J. (1995). Timing of glottic closure during normal swallow. *Head and Neck, 17*(5), 394–402.

Palmer, J. B., Rudin, N. J., Lara, G., & Crompton, A. W. (1992). Coordination of mastication and swallowing. *Dysphagia, 7*(4), 187–200.

Paterson, W. G. (2006). Esophageal peristalsis. In R. K. Goyal & R. Shaker (Eds.), *GI Motility Online.* Retrieved from http://www.nature.com/ gimo/index.html

Perlman, A. L., Booth, B. M., & Grayhack, J. P. (1994). Videofluoroscopic predictors of aspiration in patients with oropharyngeal dysphagia. *Dysphagia, 9*(2), 90–95.

Royal College of Speech and Language Therapists. (2006). *Videofluoroscopic evaluation of oropharyngeal swallowing disorders (VFS) in adults: The role of speech and language therapists.* RCSLT Policy Statement.

Robbins, J., Coyle, J., Rosenbek, J., Roecker, E., & Wood, J. (1999). Differentiation of normal and abnormal airway protection during swallowing using the penetration-aspiration scale. *Dysphagia, 14*(4), 228–232.

Robbins, J., Hamilton, J. W., Lof, G. L., & Kempster, G. B. (1992). Oropharyngeal swallowing in normal adults of different ages. *Gastroenterology, 103*(3), 823–829.

Rosenbek, J. C., Robbins, J. A., Roecker, E. B., Coyle, J. L., & Wood, J. L. (1996). A penetration-aspiration scale. *Dysphagia, 11*(2), 93–98.

Shaker, R., Dodds, W. J., Dantas, R. O., Hogan, W. J., & Arndorfer, R. C. (1990). Coordination of deglutitive glottic closure with oropharyngeal swallowing. *Gastroenterology, 98*(6), 1478–1484.

Shaker, R., Ren, J., Kern, M., Dodds, W. J., Hogan, W. J., & Li, Q. (1992). Mechanisms of airway protection and upper esophageal sphincter opening during belching. *American Journal of Physiology, 262*(4 Pt. 1), G621–G628.

Sokol, E. M., Heitmann, P., Wolf, B. S., & Cohen, B. R. (1966). Simultaneous cineradiographic and manometric study of the pharynx, hypopharynx, and cervical esophagus. *Gastroenterology, 51*(6), 960–974.

Storey, A. T. (1976). Interactions of alimentary and upper respiratory tract reflexes. In B. Sessle & A. Hannam (Eds.), *Mastication and swallowing: Biological and clinical correlates* (pp. 22–36). Toronto, Canada: University of Toronto Press.

World Health Organization. (2006). *eHealth: Standardized terminiology*. (EB118/8). Geneva, Switzerland: World Health Organization.

GLOSSARY

Achalasia: A rare disorder of the esophagus, affecting its ability to propel food or fluid toward the stomach. A narrowing of the lower esophagus, potentially caused by neurological damage to the lower esophageal sphincter, cancer, or, very rarely, it may be inherited.

Action potential: A short-term change in the electrical potential associated with the passage of an impulse on the surface of a cell in response to stimulation.

ALARP (As Low as Reasonably Practicable): An important principle of health and safety in UK case law, where risks and harm are weighed against potential benefits. It must be possible to demonstrate that the cost, time and effort involved in reducing the risk further would be grossly disproportionate to the benefit gained. The ALARP principle is applied to radiation protection, and ensures that imaging staff reduce doses to well below dose limits. All medical exposures should be undertaken with a dose that is as low as reasonably practicable consistent with producing satisfactory image quality. The principle of ALARA is referred to in the USA (as low as reasonably achievable) which takes into account economic and social perspectives.

Anastomotic dehiscence

    Anastomosis: *(medical)* Surgical joining together of two vessels with eventual healing, usually after resection, e.g., removal of part of the gastrointestinal tract.

    Dehiscence: Splitting open of natural or surgical fusion.

Anastomotic dehiscence is therefore defined as the failure of the fusion, through either bursting open or the body's own rejection of the surgical joining. It is commonly seen in upper or lower gastrointestinal tract surgery, and increases the postoperative mortality rate due to peritonitis and septicemia.

Ankylosing spondylitis (AS): A chronic inflammatory spinal disease of unknown cause resulting in fibrosis of spinal ligaments.

Ansa cervicalis: A loop of cranial nerve fibers forming part of the cervical plexus.
Also known as: Ansa hypoglossi.

Apnea: Temporary absence or cessation of breathing, often found in the elderly or frail individual (usually with an underlying respiratory condition); or in the obese person whose breathing may become progressively difficult (particularly at night —known as *sleep apnea*).

Aspiration: The act of material entering the airway below the level of the true vocal folds.

Barium sulfate preparation: A radiopaque positive contrast agent used in videofluoroscopy, barium swallows, and barium enemas. Chemical element with atomic number 56 (Barium) and the formula $BaSO_4$ (Barium sulfate).

Barrett's esophagus: A condition in which normal stratified epithelial cells lining the esophagus are replaced with abnormal columnar cells (columnarization), that, in some people, develop into a type of cancer of the esophagus called adenocarcinoma. It is therefore classified as a potential premalignant condition. It is usually precipitated by gastroesophageal reflux disease whereby acid from the stomach flows back up into the esophagus due to weakness of the lower esophageal sphincter/gastroesophageal sphincter.

Bolting: Eating extremely quickly—a feature commonly seen in learning disabilities.

Brodmann's areas (BA): Schematic mapping of the brain created by German neurologist Korbinian Brodmann based on their histological characteristics. These areas denote *topographical* (detailed, precise description), and *functional* arrangements of cortical brain areas.

Bulbar: Medullary or brainstem involvement.

C-arm: Part of a modern fluoroscopy unit. The C-arm suspends the x-ray tube mechanism directly opposite the image receptor/image intensifier mechanism, but enables the operator to pivot the equipment around the fluoroscopy table and patient. This is an advantage for patients with limited mobility.

Candidiasis: A fungal or yeast infection commonly referred to as *thrush*. Often found in immunosuppressed individuals, and is usually localized to the skin or mucosal membranes, including the oral cavity, pharynx, esophagus, and gastrointestinal tract. Oropharyngeal and esophageal thrush is also a side effect of some antibiotic treatments, and causes varying degrees of discomfort and pain upon swallowing. Severe cases of candidiasis are often found in cancer patients.

Caudal: Inferior; toward to tail. (*Antonym:* Rostral).

Cervical osteophytes: Bony outgrowths of the bodies of the anterior cervical spine associated with vertebral degenerative disease.

Chaperone: An independent person who acts as a "witness" to protect both patient and staff. Particularly recommended in intimate examinations.

Collimation: The process of limiting an x-ray beam by actively closing the tube diaphragms. Collimation has the potential to reduce dose and increase image quality by reducing the amount of scattered radiation.

Compensatory strategies: Techniques often used in the acute onset of dysphagia whereby various adaptation strategies are used to swallow safely and effectively. However, for long-term disorders in both adults and children, such compensatory strategies may be used indefinitely.
These include:

Modification of posture to redirect bolus flow, e.g., head turn, chin tuck, head tilt, neck extension.

Consistency of food or fluid intake, e.g., softer foods, puréed meals, thickened liquids.

Swallowing techniques, e.g., Mendelssohn maneuver; effortful swallow; supraglottic swallow; super-supraglottic swallow.

Rate of food intake, e.g., "little and often" to avoid fatigue while eating/drinking, teaspoon feeding, smaller cups to promote slower drinking.

Surgery, e.g., cricopharyngeal myotomy, surgical prosthesis such as a forearm flap reconstruction following resection of the oropharynx after tumor excision.

Taste and temperature, e.g., sour/cold/fizzy bolus to stimulate the oropharyngeal neuroreceptors to trigger a stronger and more effective swallow.

Compensatory strategies could also include the route of feeding via alternative means, such as nasogastric/gastrostomy tube feeding, etc.

Confidentiality: A professional requirement to maintain privacy of patients and research participants. Personal information (including medical records) should only be passed on to those directly involved in the patient's care, or with their permission.

Congenital: Existing at, or dating from, birth. Usually relating to a medical condition.

Consent: The act of seeking permission from a patient to proceed with an examination or test—considered a process rather than a "one off" event. Consent should always be informed (full knowledge of what the procedure entails and the associated risks). It may be expressed or implied, verbal or written. Written consent is normally required where there are significant inherent risks of a procedure (including anesthesia).

Controlled area: Following a risk assessment, an employer will be required to designate a controlled area where it is necessary for a person who enters to follow special procedures designed to restrict exposure, or the exposure of any employee is likely to exceed three tenths of any relevant dose limit. Fluoroscopy rooms are controlled areas, and they must be clearly identified with radiation warning signs. Access is permissible only with observation of special radiation protection regulations.

Cramming: Forcing excessive amounts of food into the mouth at once—a feature commonly seen in learning disabilities.

Cricopharyngeus: The horizontal sphincter muscle located at the top of the esophagus. Also known as the upper esophageal sphincter (UES).

Cricopharyngeal: Pertaining to the cricopharyngeus.

Cricopharyngeal bar: A smooth, posterior bar or bandlike posterior protrusion at the junction of the hypopharynx and cervical esophagus at about the level of C5-C6.

Cricopharyngeal myotomy: Surgical sectioning of cricopharyngeal muscle to improve upper esophageal sphincter opening during swallowing.

Decussate: In neurology, *decussation* relates to the oblique crossing of nerve fibers from one lateral part of the spinal cord to the other at a level other than their origin.

Defecating proctography: A fluoroscopic examination of the lower gastrointestinal tract whereby barium paste is inserted into the rectum until there is sufficient distension. The patient is then transferred to a commode, situated next to a fluoroscopy unit which records the defecation/opening of the bowel.

Deglutition: The act or process of swallowing.

Density: The measure of the relative "heaviness" of objects with a constant volume. The quantity of something per unit measure. For example the density of barium sulfate preparations are calculated by a measurement of weight (mg) per volume (ml)—e.g., 100% w/v.

Diagnostic reference level (DRL): It is recommended by the International Commission of Radiological Protection (ICRP) that diagnostic reference levels (DRLs) should be used by regional, national and local authorized bodies. The DRL is a form of investigation level to identify unusually high levels, which calls for local review if consistently exceeded. Diagnostic reference levels are advisory and will be set at different levels in different localities, but can be used to identify outliers and educate imaging personnel.

Diffuse idiopathic skeletal hyperostosis (DISH): A skeletal disease characterized by ossification of the anterolateral side of the spine and various extraspinal ligaments. *Also known as:* Forestier's disease.

Diplopia: Double vision.

Diverticulum: An out-pouching of a hollow (or a fluid-filled) structure in the body, commonly seen in the pharynx and gastrointestinal tract. A "true" diverticulum extends through all layers of the gastrointestinal tract wall, whereas a "false" diverticulum extends through the mucosa and submucosal layers only.

Zenker's diverticulum: The most common form of out-pouching of the upper gastrointestinal tract, situated in the distal hypopharynx/proximal esophagus (see *Pharyngeal pouch*).

Dorsal: Pertaining to the rear or posterior aspect of any structure. (*Antonym:* Ventral).

Dose: Absorbed dose is a measure of the energy imparted by ionizing radiation into a tissue per unit mass. A dose equivalent adds a weighting factor dependent upon the type of radiation, giving a more realistic measure of the likely biological effects. Effective dose adds a weighting factor dependent on the relative sensitivity of the irradiated tissues.

Absorbed dose is reported in gray (Gy), with equivalent dose reported in sieverts (Sv). 1 Gy or 1 Sv is equal to 1 joule per kilogram. Non-SI units are still prevalent in the USA, where dose is often reported in rads and dose equivalent in rems. By definition, 1 Gy = 100 rad and 1 Sv = 100 rem.

Dosimetry: Radiation dosimetry is the measurement and calculation of the absorbed dose in matter and tissue resulting from the exposure to indirect and direct ionizing radiation. It is focused on the calculation of internal and external doses from ionizing radiation.

Dysarthria: Collective name for a group of neurological disorders frequently affecting speech intelligibility, usually resulting in a slurring of speech output.

Dysphagia: A disorder of swallowing food or fluid from the mouth to the stomach. Classified as high dysphagia (pertaining to the oropharynx) or low dysphagia (esophagus and stomach).

El Escorial criteria: Set of diagnostic criteria for amyotrophic lateral sclerosis (ALS)/motor neuron disease (MND) devised by the World Federation of Neurologists.

Emotional lability: Involuntary laughing or crying.

Esophageal manometry: Measurement of the strength of esophageal muscle contractions during swallowing via the passage of a pressure-sensitive tube through the nose, pharynx, and esophagus.

Exposure factors: The operating parameters available to a radiographer to manipulate the x-ray exposure. These factors include kVp (kilovoltage peak), mA (milliamperes), seconds, source image distance, source object distance, and focal spot.

Fasciculation: Involuntary wavelike muscle twitches, frequently seen as an initial presenting symptom of amyotrophic lateral sclerosis (ALS)/motor neuron disease (MND).

FEES: Fiberoptic Endoscopic Evaluation of Swallowing.

FEEST: Flexible Endoscopic Evaluation of Swallowing with Sensory Testing.

Flaccid: Low muscle tone due to lower motor neuron disorder.

Fluoroscopy: Real-time acquisition and display of x-ray images using an image intensification system.

Fluoroscopy time: The total amount of time that x-rays have been generated during a fluoroscopic procedure (also known as screening time). May be significantly reduced when using pulsed fluoroscopy rather than continuous fluoroscopy.

Fluoroscopy unit (C-arm/remote/over-couch): A specialized x-ray machine comprising of an x-ray tube and image intensifier system connected via a TV camera to a display monitor. The unit may be an undercouch configuration (x-ray tube under the fluoroscopy table), overcouch configuration (x-ray tube above the table, often operated remotely), or a C-arm configuration (see *C-arm*).

Functional magnetic resonance imaging (fMRI): A magnetic resonance neuroimaging technique enabling the identification of the various areas of the brain that are involved in a task, process, or emotion.

Gastrointestinal: Referring collectively to the esophagus, stomach, and small and large intestines.

Gastroesophageal: Pertaining to the stomach and the esophagus.

Gastrostomy: The surgical formation of an artificial opening through the abdominal wall and insertion of a tube into the stomach, usually used for alternative feeding.

Globus pharyngeus: The constant sensation of a lump in the throat.

Halitosis: The term used to describe bad breath. This is usually associated with dental disease and poor oral hygiene, and is frequently seen in patients who are unable to swallow. Also one of the symptoms of a *pharyngeal pouch* due to food residue remaining in the pouch for an extended period of time.

Hiatus hernia: A disorder where part of the stomach pushes up into the thoracic cavity through a defect in the diaphragm. It may be asymptomatic, but it increases the likelihood of acid reflux into the esophagus, causing heartburn and other symptoms.

Hypopharynx: The distal portion of the pharynx which lies inferior to the epiglottis and is continuous with the proximal esophagus.
Hypopharyngeal: Pertaining to the hypopharynx.
Also known as: Laryngopharynx.

Image intensifier: Part of a fluoroscopy unit. The image intensifier is designed to detect the x-rays emitted from the x-ray tube and convert them into light photons which greatly increases the quantity of photons (and therefore reduced the dose required to form an image). These are then converted into an electrical signal for display via a TV camera to a monitor. Modern fluoroscopy units may be fully digital, converting x-ray photons directly into a digital signal.

Innervation: The distribution, or supply of nerves to a particular part of the body.

Justification: Justification is one of the three main principles of the International Commission on Radiological Protection (ICRP 60) system of radiological protection, and has been adopted by the UK Ionising Radiations Medical Exposure Regulations (2000). Justification, together with Optimization and Limitation, are used as the basis of Radiation Protection internationally. Justification requires that no practice involving exposures to radiation should be adopted unless it produces sufficient benefit to the exposed individual or to society to offset the detriment it causes. The decision to undertake a clinical radiation procedure to determine or affect the clinical management of a patient, screening participant or research volunteer must take into account the benefit of the procedure and potential detriment including specific aspects such as age, gender, and pregnancy status.

Killian's dehiscence: A small triangular area on the posterior hypopharyngeal wall between the oblique fibers of the thyropharyngeus muscle and the transverse fibers of the cricopharyngeus muscle.
Also known as: Killian's triangle.

kVp: Kilovoltage peak (see *Exposure factors*).

Kyphosis: Exaggerated antero-posterior curvature of the thoracic spine, causing a "humped" appearance of the back. It can be caused by degenerative diseases associated with aging, developmental defects, and trauma.

Laryngopharynx: See *Hypopharynx.*
Laryngopharyngeal: Pertaining to the laryngopharynx.

Lead rubber protection: Ancillary radiographic equipment that contains a minimum quantity of lead equivalent material that is used to absorb scattered radiation (e.g. personnel aprons and thyroid shields). Higher lead equivalent materials may be used to absorb the primary beam (e.g., leaded gloves, gonad shields).

Lower motor neuron: A neuron (nerve cell) connecting the spinal cord to muscle fibers.

mA: Milliamperes (see *Exposure factors*).

Malignant/Malignancy: Literal meaning: tending to be severe and become progressively worse. With regard to cancer or tumors, malignancy relates to cells that are invasive and tend to metastasize (spread) to other parts of the body. Malignant tumor cells are characterized by uncontrolled growth and have the potential to cause death.

Maneuvers: Airway protection strategies designed to specifically assist the strength and safety of swallowing (see *Compensatory strategies*).

Manometry: See *Esophageal manometry*.

Micturating cystography: A radiographic examination of the bladder and urinary tract, whereby the bladder is filled with x-ray contrast, and the patient is asked to pass urine while being examined by fluoroscopic x-ray.

Mucosa: Also known as mucous membrane of the gastrointestinal tract. Made up of epithelial tissue, the mucosa is the innermost layer of the gastrointestinal tract wall and is involved in digestive absorption and secretion.

Nasal regurgitation: Incomplete/insufficient articulation of the soft palate and posterior pharyngeal wall during swallowing, causing escape of the bolus into the nasopharynx. Usually seen most with fluids.

Nasogastric tube (NGT): A plastic tube (of varying widths/bores) passed through the nose, pharynx, esophagus, and into the stomach. Used for short-term administration of nutrition, fluids and medication in a patient whose swallowing is deemed unsafe, or in individuals who are unable to maintain their nutritional balance via oral feeding alone.

An NGT may also be used to drain the contents of the stomach, either following gastrointestinal (GI) surgery where the lower GI tract may not be functioning, or in emergency situations where ingestion of toxic materials has occurred.

Passage of an NGT is contraindicated in some circumstances, including gastroesophageal reflux; upper gastrointestinal stricture; esophageal fistula; nasal injuries; and base of skull fractures.

Nasopharynx: The uppermost part of the pharynx extending from the base of the skull to the upper surface of the soft palate. *Nasopharyngeal:* Pertaining to the nasopharynx.

Nucleus ambiguus (NA): The nucleus of the origin of the motor fibers of the vagus (CN X), glossopharyngeal (CN IX), and accessory (CN XI) nerves in the medulla oblongata.

Nucleus tractus solitarius (NTS): The cell group in the brainstem lying on each side of the upper medulla that receives *viscerosensory* information (see *Visceral*).

Operator (radiation): Any person undertaking a practical task associated with a medical exposure does so as an operator (IRMER 2000 regulations). For example the operator may take an x-ray or authorize (approve) a referral. Operators are responsible for the radiation dose delivered to the patient and undertaking all tasks that affect that dose correctly and in adherence to the employer's procedures.

Oropharynx: The part of the pharynx between the soft palate and the epiglottis. *Oropharyngeal:* Pertaining to the oropharynx.

Osteophytes: Commonly referred to as bone spurs, protrusions of bone and cartilage are very common and develop in areas of a degenerating joint. They are associated with aging and the most common type of arthritis, osteoarthritis. Frequently seen on cervical vertebrae (see *Cervical osteophytes*).

Penetration: The act of material entering the airway and remaining above the level of the true vocal folds.

Percutaneous endoscopic gastrostomy (PEG): An endoscopic medical procedure in which a plastic tube of varying lengths (depending on the size and weight of the patient) is endoscopically inserted into the mouth and pulled through the esophagus, into the stomach cavity, and out through the abdominal wall via a small incision previously marked during the procedure. A PEG is used for long-term administration of nutrition, fluids, and medication in a patient whose swallowing is unsafe, or in individuals who are unable to maintain their nutritional balance via oral feeding alone. The patient will usually have had a period of nasogastric tube feeding prior to PEG insertion.

Pharyngeal pouch: A herniation of the posterior pharyngeal wall through *Killian's dehiscence* between the thyropharyngeus and cricopharyngeus muscles. The pouch fills with fluids and food during swallowing and may increase with size over a period of time. Usual clinical presentations are *globus pharyngeus*; regurgitation, aspiration, chronic cough, and weight loss. Another symptom may be *halitosis* due to food decaying in the pouch.

Pharynx: The part of the aerodigestive tract situated behind the nasal cavities, mouth, and larynx. Lined with mucous membrane, the pharynx can be subdivided into the naso-, oro-, and hypo-/laryngopharynx. *Pharyngeal:* Pertaining to the pharynx.

Positron emission tomography (PET): A nuclear medicine imaging technique that produces a detailed, three-dimensional image of functional processes in the body.

Postcricoid web: A thin, membranous tissue covered with squamous epithelium forming on the anterior surface of the esophagus immediately inferior to the cricopharyngeal sphincter.

Practitioner: Practitioners (IRMER 2000 legislation) are radiation-trained clinical specialists entitled to undertake IRMER duties as an oncologist, radiologist, nuclear medicine physician, cardiologist, or dentist. Practitioners are responsible for justifying medical radiation procedures and for all clinical aspects that influence the dose received by the person undergoing examination or treatment.

Presbyphagia: The age-related changes in the oropharyngeal and esophageal swallowing of healthy adults.

Primary beam: The collimated x-ray beam that is emitted from the x-ray tube.

Ptosis: Drooping of one or both eyelids.

Radiation dose: See *Dose.*

Radiation protection: The process of minimizing doses to patients and staff by following appropriate procedures.

Radiographer: A registered/licensed health professional trained in the use of ionizing and non-ionizing radiation to produce high quality diagnostic images while caring for the safety and well-being of the patient. Known as a radiological technologist in the USA. In some countries the radiographers' scope of practice may include performing complex procedures and reporting of imaging examinations.

Radiologic technologist: See *Radiographer.*

Radiologically inserted gastrostomy (RIG): A plastic tube of varying lengths (depending on the size and weight of the patient) passed directly into the stomach through an incision in the abdominal wall using fluoroscopy to ensure correct positioning. It is carried out under sedation by an interventional radiologist in the x-ray department following ingestion of barium to highlight the outline of the gastrointestinal tract. It varies from *percutaneous endoscopic gastrostomy* (PEG) insertion as the patient may not be suitable for an endoscopic procedure (e.g., due to pharyngeal cancers), or PEG may already have been attempted and failed.

Radiologist: A registered/licensed medical doctor who has specialized following postgraduate training in diagnostic radiology. The radiologist may then subspecialize (e.g., gastrointestinal radiology, neuroradiology).

Radiotherapy/Radiation therapy: The exposure of a focused area of malignant growth to high dosage radiation, usually delivered in fractionated (divided) doses, in an attempt to control cancerous cell growth while reducing effects on normal tissues. Radiation has a greater harmful effect on the DNA of rapidly dividing cells (e.g., cancer cells).

Referrer (imaging examinations): A referrer (according to IRMER, 2000 regulations) is a medical or dental practitioner, or other approved health professional, who is entitled to refer individuals for medical exposure to a practitioner. Referrals must give sufficient information to enable the appropriate procedure to be undertaken on the correct individual, taking account of any patient dependent factors, e.g., pregnancy, breastfeeding.

Reflux: The retrograde flow of fluid in the body. In terms of the gastrointestinal tract it is associated with reflux from the stomach into the esophagus, or duodenal contents into the stomach.

Rostral: Superior/toward the head. (*Antonym:* Caudal).

Sarcopenia: The specific age-related process that describes the degree of loss of skeletal muscle mass, organization, and strength.

Scattered radiation: The x-ray beam that has passed through tissue and is then deflected in varying directions. This adversely affects image quality and increased dose. Good collimation can reduce the scatter produced. A higher kVp reduces the scatter produce, but it is more energetic and therefore more likely to affect the image receptor.

Scintigraphy: A nuclear medicine test whereby a bolus labeled with a radionuclide marker is given to the patient to swallow which is then monitored by a gamma camera by imaging the radiation emitted from it.

Scoliosis: Abnormal lateral curvature of the spine, the cause of which is largely unknown, but can be attributed to birth defects, muscular dystrophy, and connective tissue disorders.

Screening time: See *Fluoroscopy time.*

Spasticity: High muscle tone due to upper motor neuron involvement.

Speech-language pathologist (SLP)/Speech and language therapist (SLT): The lead experts in communication and swallowing disorders, whose role will overlap with other members of the multidisciplinary team to assist in the differential diagnosis and treatment of patients with communication and/or swallowing disorders.

Tegmentum: Anterior aspect of the midbrain.

Tensilon test: Diagnostic test for myasthenia gravis whereby administration of short-acting anticholinesterase and provides transient relief of clinical symptoms.

> **Anticholinesterase:** A drug that causes the nerve transmitter *acetylcholine* to accumulate at the junctions of certain nerve fibers, allowing continuous stimulation throughout the central and peripheral nervous systems.

Thermoluminescent dosimeter: One type of dosimeter which can be used for personnel (staff) or patient monitoring.

Upper esophageal sphincter (UES): The involuntary sphincter muscle consisting of striated muscle at the superior section of the esophagus. Relaxation and subsequent opening of the UES is triggered by the swallow reflex (see *Cricopharyngeus*).

Upper motor neuron: A neuron originating in the cerebral cortex and terminating in the brainstem or spinal cord.

Ventral: Pertaining to the front or anterior aspect of any structure (*Antonym:* Dorsal).

Visceral: Pertaining to the internal organs.

> **Viscerosensory:** Relating to the sensory innervation of internal organs.

Xerostomia: Dry mouth, or the sensation of dry mouth.

X-linked recessive inherited disorder: Condition inherited through the X chromosome. X-linked diseases usually occur in males who have XY sex chromosomes, but can also occur in females if both XX sex chromosomes carry the same disorder.

X-ray tube: An evacuated glass tube containing a source of electrons (cathode and filament) and a target (anode). When a large potential difference is applied, electrons emitted by the filament are fired at high velocity to the anode target. The electrons interact with the target material and energy in the form of both heat (99%) and x-rays (1%) are produced. The x-ray tube is shielded with lead apart from the tube port through which the x-rays are able to pass.

INDEX

Note: Page numbers in **bold** reference non-text material.

A

Abduction, defined, 67
Acromegaly, cervical osteophytes and, 263
Adduction, defined, 67
Adults with Incapacity (Scotland) Act, 47
Aging
    dentition changes, 125–126
    respiration and, 130–131
    swallowing and, 123–132
        changes in physiology, 124
        cortical processing and, 131–132
        esophageal stage, 129–130
        transit time changes, 124–125
Agnosia, 227
Airway, aging/protection of, 128
Airway closure, 113
    biometrics of impaired, 115–117
Airway protection, changes with age, 128
ALS (Amyotrophic lateral sclerosis), 177–181
    clinical presentation, 179–180
    ethical dilemmas, 180–181
    findings/images, 181
    VFSS and, 180
ALS Severity Scale (ALSSS), 180
Alzheimer's disease, 228–229
    sense of smell and, 232
    swallowing and, 231
Amyotrophic lateral sclerosis (ALS), 177–181
    clinical presentation, 179–180
    ethical dilemmas, 180–181
    findings/images, 181
    VFSS and, 180
Ankylosing spondylitis (AS), cervical osteophytes
    and, 263–264
Anterior, defined, 67
Aphasia, 227
Apraxia, 227
AS (Ankylosing spondylitis), cervical osteophytes
    and, 263–264
Aspiration, 67
    prandial, 234

Aspiration pneumonia, dementia and, 230
Audit Commission, NHS (National Health
    Service), 40

B

Barium sulfate, videofluoroscopy and, 24
Barium swallow, options, 21
Barrett's esophagus, esophagoscopy and, 22
Best available evidence, evidence-based practice
    and, 48
Biomechanics
    impaired airway closure and, 115–117
    oropharyngeal, 108–112
    of pharyngeal onset delay versus oral
        containment impairment, 112–115
    of pharyngeal residue, 117–119
    purposes of, 107–108
    of swallowing, 108
Boyle's law, 109
Bullous pemphigoid, 270

C

Cancer
    clinical dilemmas, 256–257
    head/neck
        aspiration and, 254–255
        (chemo-)radiotherapy and, 240–241
        fistula, 252–253
        laryngeal conservation surgery, 255
        pseudodiverticulum, 252
        reduced propulsion in neopharynx,
            253–254
        reflux and, 255
        stricture, 253
        videofluoroscopy examination and, 6
    larynx, removal of, 243–252
    oral/oropharyngeal, surgery for, 241–243
    VFSS (Videofluoroscopic swallowing study)
        and, 256
    videofluoroscopy examination and, 6

Cardiac presentation, pediatric, 203
Celiac disease, 270
Cerebral palsy (CP), dysphagia and, 214–215
Cervical osteophytes, 21, 263–267
    clinical presentation, 265–266
    ethical dilemmas, 266–267
    pathophysiology, 264
Chemesthesis, aging and, 126
(Chemo-)radiotherapy, 240–241
Chewing, dementia and, 231
Chin lift, **9**
Chin tuck, **9**
Chronic obstructive pulmonary disease (COPD),
        impaired airway closure and, 115
Cine magnetic resonance imaging, 21
Clinical experience
    evidence-based practice and, 48
Clinical reporting
    defining components of
        esophageal components of, 289
        pharyngeal components, 288–289
        swallowing physiology, 286–288
    formulas, 292–293
    guidelines, format, language, 290–291
    need for standardization of, 281–286
    penetration-aspiration scale, 289–290
    sample report, 291–292
    VFSS clinical report proforma, 286
Clinical swallowing evaluation (CSE), 19
    guide to as evaluation tool, 20
    options, 20–28
        barium swallow, 21
        esophagoscopy, 21–22
    stroke and, 161–163
Cognitive impairment, vascular, 229
Communication, errors in, 39
Compliance, pediatric, 207
Confidentiality, patients, 43–44
Consent, 12–13
    adults without capacity, 47–48
    capacity to, 47
    importance of, 43–44
    pediatric, 207
    process, 45–46
    types of, 46
    voluntary, 44–45
Contrast, x-ray, 7
COPD (Chronic obstructive pulmonary disease),
        impaired airway closure and, 115

Cortical processing, aging and, 131–132
CP (Cerebral palsy), dysphagia and, 214–215
Cricopharyngeal myotomy, 267
Cricopharyngeal prominence, 272–273
Critical incident, defined, 39
CSE (Clinical swallowing evaluation), 19
    guide to as evaluation tool, 20
    options, 20–28
        barium swallow, 21
    stroke and, 161–163

D

DAP (Dose Area Product), 149
Dehydration, dementia and, 230
Delayed laryngeal closure, 112–113
Delirium, 227
Dementia
    Alzheimer's disease, 228–229
    clinical presentation, 230–232
    cognitive/behavioral aspects of, 229
    described, 227–228
    incidence of, 228
    multi-infarct, 229
    physiological aspects
        motor, 230
        sensory, 230
    semantic, 232
    swallowing difficulties and, 231
    vascular, 229
    vascular impairment and, 232
    videofluoroscopy examination and, 5–6
Dementia frontotemporal, 232
Dentition, aging and, 125–126
Depression, 227–228
Depressor, defined, 67
Dieticians, VFSS and, 11
Diffused idiopathic skeletal hyperostosis (DISH),
        cervical osteophytes and, 263–264
Discrepancies, defined, 39
DISH (Diffused idiopathic skeletal
        hyperostosis), cervical osteophytes and,
        263–264
DMD (Duchenne muscular dystrophy),
        186–191
    clinical presentation, 188
    ethical dilemmas, 191
    VFSS and, 188
Doppler images, 23

Dose Area Product (DAP), 149
Down's syndrome (DS), dysphagia and, 214–215
Dry mouth, 126
DS (Down's syndrome), dysphagia and, 214–215
DST (Duration of stage transition), 113–115
Duchenne muscular dystrophy (DMD),
        186–191
   clinical presentation, 188
   ethical dilemmas, 191
   VFSS and, 188
Duplex images, 23
Duration of stage transition (DST), 113–115
Dysphagia, 22, 159
   defined, 4
   dementia and, 228
   head/neck cancers, pretreatment, 239
   learning disabilities and, 214
   management of, 233–234
   NMC and, 177
   structural causes of high, 263–276
      cervical osteophytes, 263–267
      cricopharyngeal prominence, 272–273
      postcricoid web, 270–272
   VFSS (Videofluoroscopic swallowing study)
        and, 273–275
   videofluoroscopy examination and, structural
        causes, 6

E

Ear, Nose, and Throat (ENT)
   structural conditions, 202
   surgeons, VFSS and, 11
Effortful swallow, 9–10
El Escorial criteria, 179
Embryo, development of, 198–199
End of life considerations, pediatric, 208
ENT (Ear, Nose, and Throat), structural
        conditions, 202
ENT surgeons, VFSS and, 11
Epidermolysis bullosa, 270
Error, defined, 38–39
Esophageal, stage of swallowing, 67, 78–79
Esophageal sphincter
   lower, 130
   upper, 129–130
Esophagoscopy, 21–22
Evidence-based practice, elements of, 48
Executive functioning, reduction in, 227

F

False negatives, 39
False positives, over reporting, 39
Feeding, nonoral, 208
Feeding disorders, sensory-based, 204–205
FEES (Fiberoptic endoscopic evaluation of
        swallowing), 19, 25–27
FEEST (Fiberoptic endoscopic evaluation of
        swallowing with sensory testing), 26
   versus VFSS, 27–28
Fiberoptic endoscopic evaluation of swallowing
        (FEES), 19, 25–27
Fiberoptic endoscopic evaluation of swallowing
        with sensory testing (FEEST), 26
Fiberoptic nasendoscope, FEES and, 25
Fluoroscopy, principles of, 140–142
Fluorosis, cervical osteophytes and, 263
Frontotemporal dementis, 232

G

Gastroenterological presentation, pediatric,
        202–203
Gastroesophageal reflux disease, 22, 201, 270
General Medical Council, 37
*Gillick v. West Norfolk and Wisbech Area Health
        Authority*, 48
Globus pharyngeus, 271

H

Head cancer, 20
   aspiration and, 254–255
   (chemo-)radiotherapy and, 240–241
   clinical dilemmas, 256–257
   dysphagia and, pretreatment, 239
   fistula, 252–253
   laryngeal conservation surgery, 255
   pseudodiverticulum, 252
   reduced propulsion in neopharynx, 253–254
   reflux and, 255
   stricture, 253
   VFSS (Videofluoroscopic swallowing study)
        and, 256
   videofluoroscopy examination and, 6
Head turn, **9**
Health Professions Council, 37
High Resolution Manometry (HRM), 22

Hiroshima, radiation studies, 143
HLE (Hyolaryngeal excursion), 108–116, 118
HRM (High Resolution Manometry), 22
Huntington's disease, 229
Hyolaryngeal excursion (HLE), 108–116, 118
Hypoparathyroidism, cervical osteophytes and, 263

I

ICF (International Classification of Functioning), 19
ID (Intellectual disabilities). *See* Learning disabilities
IM (Inflammatory myopathies), 184–186
Inclusion body myositis, 180, 184–186
Infant, development of, 199
Inferior, defined, 67
Inflammatory myopathies (IM), 184–186
Informed consent, 45
   see also Consent
Intellectual disabilities (ID). *See* Learning disabilities
International Classification of Functioning (ICF), 19
Interpretation, errors in, 39

K

Kennedy's disease, 180
Killian's triangle/dehiscence, 267
Knowledge and Skills Needed by Speech-Language Pathologists Performing Videofluoroscopic Swallowing Studies, 286

L

Lacunar infarctions, 229
Laryngectomy, 243–252
   stoma, placement marker, 249
   swallowing after, 249
   voicing after, 246–249
Laryngopharyngeal reflux disease, 22
Larynx
   removal of, 243–252
      stoma placement marker, 249
      swallowing after, 249
      voicing after, 246–249
Lateral, defined, 67

LD (Learning disabilities). *See* Learning disabilities
Lead rubber gown, as shielding, 7
Lean/head tilt, **9**
Learning disabilities
   clinical presentation of, 216–218
   prevalence/pathophysiology of, 214–216
   VFSS (Videofluoroscopic swallowing study) and, 213–222
      dysphagia and, 218–220
      ethical dilemmas, 220–221
   videofluoroscopy examination and, 5
Levator, defined, 67
Lewy bodies, 230, 231
Lie down, **9**
Lou Gehrig's disease, 177–181
   clinical presentation, 179–180
   ethical dilemmas, 180
   findings/images, 181
   VFSS and, 180
Ludlow, Abraham, 267

M

Magnetic resonance imaging (MRI), 21
Malnutrition, dementia and, 230
Manometry, 22
Maxillofacial surgeons, VFSS and, 11
MBS (Modified barium swallow). *See* Videofluoroscopic swallowing study (VFSS)
Mendelsohn maneuver, 9
Mental Capacity (England) Act, 47
MG (Myasthenia gravis), 181–184
   clinical presentation, 181–183
   ethical dilemmas, 183
   findings/images, 184
   VFSS and, 183
MND (Motor neuron disease), 177–181
Modernisation Agency, National Health Service (NHS), 41
Modified barium swallow (MBS). *See* Videofluoroscopic swallowing study (VFSS)
Motor neuron disease (MND), 177–181
MRI (Magnetic resonance imaging), 21
Multi-infarct dementia, 229
Multiple sclerosis, 20
Muscles, involved in swallowing, **54–60**

Myasthenia gravis (MG), 181–184
   clinical presentation, 181–183
   ethical dilemmas, 183
   findings/images, 184
   VFSS and, 183

N

Nagasaki, radiation studies, 143
National Health Service (NHS)
   Audit Commission, 40
   complaints about, 37
   Modernisation Agency, 41
   VFSS and, 10
NBM (Nil by mouth), VFSS and, 7
Neck cancer, 20
   aspiration and, 254–255
   (chemo-)radiotherapy and, 240–241
   clinical dilemmas, 256–257
   dysphagia and, pretreatment, 239
   fistula, 252–253
   laryngeal conservation surgery, 255
   pseudodiverticulum, 252
   reduced propulsion in neopharynx, 253–254
   reflux and, 255
   stricture, 253
   VFSS (Videofluoroscopic swallowing study) and, 256
   videofluoroscopy examination and, 6
Neurological disorders/diseases, videofluoroscopy examination and, 5
Neuromuscular conditions (NMC), 177–192
   amyothrophic lateral sclerosis, 177–181
   clinical presentation, 179–180
   dysphagia and, 177
   ethical dilemmas, 180–181
   findings/images, 181
   motor neuron disease, 177–181
   myasthenia gravis, 181–184
   oropharyngeal dysphagia on videofluoroscopy across neuromuscular conditions, **189–191**
   overview of, **178**
   VFSS and, 180
NHS (National Health Service)
   Audit Commission, 40
   complaints about, 37
   Modernisation Agency, 41
   VFSS and, 10

Nil by mouth (NBM), VFSS and, 7
Nil per oris (NPO), VFSS and, 7
NMC (Neuromuscular conditions), 177–192
   amyotrophic lateral sclerosis, 177–181
   clinical presentation, 179–180
   dysphagia and, 177
   ethical dilemmas, 180–181
   findings/images, 181
   motor neuron disease, 177–181
   oropharyngeal dysphagia on videofluoroscopy across neuromuscular conditions, **189–191**
   overview of, **178**
   VFSS and, 180
Non-nutritive sucking, 199
Non-oral feeding, 208
NPO (Nil per oris), VFSS and, 7
Nurses/staff, VFSS and, 11
Nutritive sucking, 199

O

OA (Osteoarthritis), cervical osteophytes and, 263
Obesity, VFSS and, 7
Ochronosis, cervical osteophytes and, 263
OPSE (Oropharyngeal Swallowing Efficiency), 23–24
Oral, stage of swallowing, 67–68, 73
Oral cancer, surgery for, 241–243
Oral containment impairment, 112–113, 115
Oral dryness, aging and, 126
Oral preparatory, stage of swallowing, 67–68
Oropharyngeal biomechanics, 108–112
Oropharyngeal scintigraphy, 22–23
Oropharyngeal swallowing disorder. *See* Dysphagia
Oropharyngeal Swallowing Efficiency (OPSE), 24
Oropharyngeal tumors, surgery for, 241–243
Osteoarthritis (OA), cervical osteophytes and, 263

P

PACS (Picture Archiving and Communications System), 43–44, 142
Parkinson's disease, 20, 229–230
   metabolic aspects of, 230
   motor functions and, 231

Pathophysiology, stroke, 160–161
Patient positioning
    modifications, 8–10
    VFSS (Videofluoroscopic swallowing study)
        and, 8
Patient preference, evidence-based practice and,
        48
Patients
    advocacy, 49
    children/young people, 48–49
    confidentiality, 43–44
    experience of, 36–37
        consequence of poor, 37
    information, 40
    quality of care for, 36
    radiation safety for, 144–145
Pediatrics
    cardiac presentation, 203
    degenerative conditions, 204
    end of life considerations, 208
    feeding disorders, sensory-based, 204–205
    gastroenterological presentation, 202–203
    swallowing difficulties, 201
        signs of, **201–202**
    VFSS and, 197–211
        clinical presentation, 201–205
        data/scoring, 210
        pathophysiology, 198–201
        technique modification, 209–210
    videofluoroscopy examination and, 5
Penetration-Aspiration (PA) Scale, 24, 289–290
Perception errors, 39
Peristalsis, 130
Pernicious anemia, 270
Personal Protective Equipment (PPE), 148
Personnel monitoring, radiation, 148–149
Pharyngeal manometry, 22
Pharyngeal onset delay, 112–113
Pharyngeal residue, biomechanics of, 117–119
Pharyngeal, stage of swallowing, 67, 73–78
Physiology, change with age, 124
Physiotherapists, VFSS and, 11
Pick's disease, 229
Picture Archiving and Communications System
        (PACS), 43–44, 142
Plastic surgeons, VFSS and, 11
Plummer-Vinson/Paterson-Kelly syndrome, 270
Pneumonia, aspiration, 230

Postcricoid web, 21, 270–272
Posterior, defined, 67
Posterior oral containment, impaired, 112–113,
        115
PPE (Personal Protective Equipment), 148
Prandial aspiration, 234
Pregnancy, VFSS and, 7
Premature spillage, 112
Primary peristalsis, 130
Protocols
    key elements of, **42–43**
    role of, 40–43
    steps in developing, **41**

Q

Quality of care, 36

R

Radiation
    distance/staff location and, 146–148
    dose reduction strategies, **146**
    dosimetry, 149–150
    Personal Protective Equipment (PPE), 148
    personnel monitoring, 148–149
    risk of, 142–144
        pediatrics and, 207–208
    safety
        for patients, 144–145
        for personnel, 145–149
Radiation Protection Advisor (RPA), 145
Radiation Protection Supervisors (RPS), 145
Radiation Safety Officers (RPO), 145
Radiation science, introduction to, 138–142
Radiobiology, risk of radiation and, 142–144
Radiography, emergence of, 138
Radiology professions
    emergence of, 138
Reporting
    clinical
        defining components of, 286–289
        formulas, 292–293
        guidelines, format, language, 290–291
        need for standardization of, 281–286
        penetration-aspiration scale, 289–290
        sample report, 291–292
        VFSS clinical report proforma, 286

Respiration
   pediatric, 201
   swallowing and, 130–131
Rheumatoid arthritis, 270
Riluzole, 179
Roentgen, Wilhelm, 138
Rooting, defined, 199
Royal College of Radiologists, 43–44
Royal College of Speech and Language Therapists
   (RCSLT), VFSS defined by, 4
RPA (Radiation Protection Advisor), 145
RPO (Radiation Safety Officers), 145
RPS (Radiation Protection Supervisors), 145

S

Scintigraphy, 22–23
Secondary peristalsis, 130
Semantic dementia, 232
*Sidaway v. Board of Governors of the Bethlem Royal
   and the Maudsley Hospital*, 45
Smell
   aging and, 126
   sense of, Alzheimer's disease, 232
Solid state manometry, 22
Spondylosis deformans, cervical osteophytes and,
   263
Stroke
   clinical presentation, 161–163
   ethical dilemmas, 170–171
   incidence of, 159–160
   pathophysiology, 160–161
   VFSS (Videofluoroscopic swallowing study)
      and, 163–165, 170
      images, 172–173
   videofluoroscopy examination and, 5
Sucking, 199
Superior, defined, 67
Super-supraglottic swallow, 8–9
Supraglottic swallow, 8
Swallowing
   aging and, 123–132
      changes in physiology, 124
      cortical processing and, 131–132
      esophageal stage, 129–130
      pharyngeal stage, 126–128
      respiration and, 130–131
      transit time changes, 124–125

anatomy/physiology of, 68–79
   esophageal stage, 78–79
   oral preparatory stage, 68
   oral stage, 68, 73
   pharyngeal stage, 73–78
biomechanical analysis of, 108
dementia and, 231
difficulties
   pediatric, 201
   signs of, **201–202**
esophageal parameters of, 101–103
infant, 199
muscles involved in, **54–60**
oral parameters of, 88–95
   central motor preparation/planning, 91, 93
   central sensory processing/perception, 89–90
   peripheral motor output, 93–95
   peripheral sensory reception, 88–89
oropharyngeal biomechanics, 108–112
pharyngeal parameters of, 95–101
   central motor preparation/planning, 97–98
   central sensory processing/perception, 95,
      97
   peripheral motor output, 98, 100–101
   peripheral sensory reception, 95
pre-oral parameters of, 83–88
   central mechanisms of motor contribution,
      86
   central sensory processing/perception, 84,
      86
   peripheral motor output, 86, 88
   peripheral sensory reception, 83–84
reasons for, 67
stages of, 67
structures involved in, **61–67**

T

Taste, aging and, 126
Thymus gland, myasthenia gravis and, 181–184
Thyroiditis, 270
TNE (Transnasal esophagoscopy), office-based,
   22
Tracheostomy, pediatric, 203
Transnasal esophagoscopy (TNE), office-based,
   22
Trauma, cervical osteophytes and, 263
Tune-Motion ultrasound images, 23

U

UES (Upper esophageal sphincter)
   anterior hyoid movement and, 98
   cricopharyngeal bar and, 130
   oropharyngeal biomechanics and, 108
   pharyngeal plexus and, 100
   supraglottic structures closure and, 128
Ultrasound, 23–24
United Kingdom, National Health Service
         (NHS), VFSS and, 10
Upper esophageal sphincter (UES)
   anterior hyoid movement and, 98
   cricopharyngeal bar and, 130
   oropharyngeal biomechanics and, 108
   pharyngeal plexus and, 100
   supraglottic structures closure and, 128

V

Vascular cognitive impairment, 229
Vascular dementia, 229
   swallowing and, 232
Vascular impairment, dementia and, 232
VFSS (Videofluoroscopic swallowing study), 3
   obesity and, 7
   cancer and, 256
   chair, 150, 153
   contraindications to, 6
   defined, 4
   dementia and, 233–234
   dysphagia and, 273–275
   evolution of, 10–11
   feeding apparatus, 153
   versus FEEST, 27–28
   functional versus structural interpretation,
         4–5
   images, stroke, 172–173
   image storage, 142
   learning disabilities and, 213–222
   legal/ethical considerations, 12–15
   neuromuscular conditions and, **192**
   patient positioning and, 8
   patients experience and, 38–39
   pediatric, 197–211
      clinical presentation, 201–205
      data/scoring, 210
      ethical dilemmas, 207–208

   incidence of, 197–198
   pathophysiology, 198–201
   technique modification, 209–210
   procedure, 38
   professionals involved in following, 12
   purpose of, 6
   radiographer role in, **151–153**
   reporting procedure, 38–39
   stroke and, 163–165, 170
   study score sheet example, **166–170**
   suction apparatus, 153
Videofluoroscopy, 24–25
   deterministic/nondeterministic effects, 25
   uses of, 4
Videofluoroscopy examination, indicators for,
         5–6
Videofluoroscopic swallowing study (VFSS),
         6–10
   cancer and, 256
   chair, 150, 153
   defined, 4
   dementia and, 233–234
   dysphagia and, 273–275
   evolution of, 10–11
   feeding apparatus, 153
   versus FEEST, 27–28
   functional versus structural interpretation,
         4–5
   images, stroke, 172–173
   image storage, 142
   lack of standards, 3
   learning disabilities and, 213–222
   legal/ethical considerations, 12–15
   neuromuscular conditions and, **192**
   patients experience and, 38–39
   pediatric, 197–211
      clinical presentation, 201–205
      data/scoring, 210
      pathophysiology, 198–201
      technique modification, 209–210
   procedure, 38
   professionals involved in following, 12
   purpose of, 6
   radiographer role in, **151–153**
   reporting procedure, 38–39
   stroke and, 163–165, 170
   study score sheet example, **166–170**
   suction apparatus, 153

W

Water-soluble nonionic isotonic agents, videofluoroscopy and, 24
Weight loss, dementia and, 230
Wet voice, 20
World Alzheimer's Report, 228

X

Xerostomia, 126

X-ray
  production of
    beams, 138–139
    image, 139
X-ray contrast, 7

Z

Zenker, Friedrich Albert von, 267
Zenker's diverticulum, 21, 267–270